Handbook of
Systemic Autoimmune Diseases

Volume 1

The Heart in Systemic Autoimmune Diseases

Handbook of
Systemic Autoimmune Diseases

Series Editor: Ronald A. Asherson

Volume 1 The Heart in Systemic Autoimmune Diseases
Edited by: Andrea Doria and Paolo Pauletto

Handbook of
Systemic Autoimmune Diseases

Volume 1

The Heart in Systemic Autoimmune Diseases

Edited by:

Andrea Doria and Paolo Pauletto
University of Padova, Padova, Italy

Series Editor

Ronald A. Asherson

2004

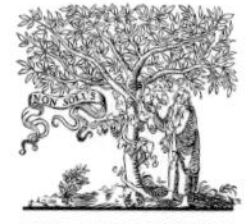

ELSEVIER

Amsterdam – Boston – Heidelberg – London – New York – Oxford
Paris – San Diego – San Francisco – Singapore – Sydney – Tokyo

ELSEVIER B.V.
Sara Burgerhartstraat 25
P.O. Box 211, 1000 AE Amsterdam, The Netherlands

First edition 2004

Library of Congress Cataloging in Publication Data
A catalog record from the Library of Congress has been applied for.

British Library Cataloguing in Publication Data
A catalogue record from the British Library has been applied for.

ISBN: 0-444-51398-1
ISSN: 1571-5078 (Series)

⊗ The paper used in this publication meets the requirements of ANSI/NISO Z39.48-1992 (Permanence of Paper).
Printed in The Netherlands.

Preface

Systemic autoimmune diseases comprise a family of conditions which share common pathogenetic mechanisms as well as a multi-organ involvement including the heart. Moreover, a growing body of evidence supports the view that autoimmune mechanisms are involved in the pathogenesis of cardiovascular disease.

By looking at the recent literature, we realized that a comprehensive, systematic overview of recent progress in this field was lacking. Therefore, we enthusiastically accepted the invitation of Ronald Asherson to be the editors of the series volume dealing with the heart in the setting of the "Handbook of Systemic Autoimmune Diseases". This prompted us to propose leading scientists and physician-scientists in this field to produce this book.

This volume is subdivided into three parts. In the first part, the immune mechanisms involved in cardiac damage are considered. The role of proinflammatory and regulatory cytokines in driving an autoimmune response to cardiac self-tissues as well as the prevalence, the clinical meaning and the hypothetical pathogenicity of a broad spectrum of anti-heart antibodies are discussed in detail. It is worthy to note that two chapters of this part are devoted to the possible pathogenetic implications of some non-organ specific antibodies including not only the anti-Ro/SSA and antiphospholipid antibodies, on which attention had largely been focused, but also other autoantibodies whose role as mediators of cardiac damage has not been systematically explored until now.

In the second part of the volume, the role of the immune system in promoting the development of atherosclerotic plaque is extensively reviewed. The role of cellular, humoral and innate immunity as well as that of the inflammatory process potentially exerted by them are discussed, along with the newly discovered anti-inflammatory property of statins.

These two parts of the volume deal with the most exciting aspects of this topic, suggesting a very close connection between cardiology and immunology which may generate a new field in medicine, namely, cardio-immunology.

Finally, in the third part, the cardiac manifestations observed in the major systemic autoimmune conditions are comprehensively reviewed.

We would like to thank all our distinguished contributors who have accepted our invitation giving concrete support in the realization of this project.

It is our feeling that the awareness of the role of autoimmune mechanisms in heart disease as well as the knowledge of the spectrum of cardiac manifestations in autoimmune systemic disease would stimulate a specific search for and, ultimately, produce a better diagnostic capacity. In turn, this would disclose the use of specific immune therapy, hence opening a new horizon for treating cardiovascular disease.

Andrea Doria
Paolo Pauletto

Padova, January 2004

Volume Editors

Andrea Doria

Andrea Doria graduated in Medicine at University of Padova in 1982. He trained at the Division of Rheumatology at the same University, and in 1986 became Specialist in Rheumatology. From 1986 to 1990 he was research fellow in Rheumatology at the University of Padova, and in 1990 he was appointed Assistant Professor of Rheumatology. In 1991 he became Lecturer at the Postgraduate School of Rheumatology. Since 1995 he has collaborated in teaching Rheumatology at Padova University School of Medicine.

He is a member of Italian Society of Rheumatology (SIR) and American College of Rheumatology (ACR). Since 1999 he has been a Council member of Italian College of Rheumatology (CRO).

He has a long-standing experience in clinical management of connective tissue disease patients. The Unit in which he works is a 3rd referral rheumatological Centre, of prominence within Italy, for the diagnosis and management of patients affected with systemic connective diseases. In addition, he has expertise in the management and follow-up of pregnant patients with systemic rheumatic diseases.

His research group is primarily involved in the clinical as well as immunological aspects of autoimmune diseases and he is author of many publications in this field. Recently he has focused his interest on the prevalence of atherosclerosis in systemic lupus erythematosus and on the traditional and non traditional risk factors which influence its development. For this research project he has begun to collaborate with Prof. Paolo Pauletto, the co-editor of this volume.

Paolo Pauletto

Paolo Pauletto graduated in Medicine at the University of Padua in 1972. His career and clinical activity started as a Research Fellow in the Department of Clinical Medicine at the University of Padua, where he has spent almost all his working life. In 1992 he was appointed as Associate Professor of Internal Medicine. Starting from 1996 he has been responsible for the section of Vascular Medicine which included both ultrasound facilities and a laboratory of vascular biology. This enabled him to carry out not only clinical practice but also substantial basic and applied research in the field of vascular disease. In 2002 he was appointed as Head of Internal Medicine at the Hospital of Treviso (Italy). His teaching activity to students of medicine at the University of Padua consists of seminars and lessons of Clinical Pathophysiology and of Medical Therapy. He is a lecturer in the Postgraduate Schools of Cardiology, Internal Medicine, and Vascular Surgery. Among his institutional duties, he has acted as a member of the Scientific Committee of the University of Padua and of the Committee for the Development of the University of Padua. He is a member of the following scientific Institutions: Council of the European Vascular Biology Association, European Council for Blood Pressure and Cardiovascular Research, Working Group on Dyslipidemias and Atherosclerosis of the Italian Society of Cardiology, Working Group "Pathogenesis of Atherosclerosis" of the European Society of Cardiology. He is on the Editorial Board of Arteriosclerosis, Thrombosis and Vascular Biology. His research activities deal with basic and applied vascular medicine, and in particular the pathophysiological mechanisms of vascular disease.

Volume Editors

Series Editor

Ronald A. Asherson

Ronald A. Asherson, MD. FACP, MD (Hon) (London), FCP (SA), FACR, is Honorary Consultant Physician at the Rheumatic Disease Unit, Department of Medicine, University of Cape Town Health Sciences Centre in Cape Town, as well as being Consultant Rheumatologist at the Rosebank Clinic in Johannesburg, South Africa. He is also Visiting Professor at the Systemic Autoimmune Diseases Unit at the Hospital Clinic, Barcelona, Spain where he regularly visits and co-ordinates research projects.

Dr Asherson qualified in Medicine at the University of Cape Town in 1957 and, after completing his internship, became H/P to Prof. Sir Christopher Booth at the Hammersmith Hospital, London, in 1960. In 1961 he accepted a Fellowship at the Columbia Presbyterian Hospital in New York, returning in 1962 to become Registrar and then Senior Registrar at Groote Schuur Hospital in Cape Town to 1964. After 10 years as a Clinical Tutor in the Department of Medicine, he returned to the United States and was appointed as Assistant Clinical Professor of Medicine at the New York Hospital - Cornell Medical Centre under the late Professor Henry Heineman. From 1981 to 1986 he was associated with the Rheumatology Department at the Royal Postgraduate Medical School of London. It was at that time that he developed his interest in Connective Tissue Diseases and Antiphospholipid Antibodies.

In 1986 he moved to the Rayne Institute and St. Thomas' Hospital in London, where he was appointed Honorary Consultant Physician and Senior Research Fellow. In 1991 he took a sabbatical at St Luke's Roosevelt Hospital Centre in New York, working with Prof. Robert Lahita. In 1992 he returned to South Africa to private practice in Johannesburg.

In 1998 he was elected as Fellow of the American College of Physicians (FACP) as well as a Founding Fellow of the American College of Rheumatology (FACR). From 1988 to 1991 he was on the Council of the Royal Society of Medicine in London. In 1992 he was co-winner of the European League Against Rheumatism (EULAR) Prize and in 1993 was the co-recipient of the International League Against Rheumatism (ILAR) Prize, both for his research on antiphospholipid antibodies. In 1994 he was elected as a Fellow of the Royal College of Physicians (FRCP) of London. In 2002 he was awarded an Honorary Doctorate in Medicine from the University of Pleven, the second largest University in Bulgaria.

Dr Asherson has been an invited speaker at many universities and International conferences both in the USA and in Europe. He is the author of more than 280 papers on connective tissue diseases and has contributed to more than 30 textbooks of medicine, rheumatology and surgery as well as having co-edited two editions of the "*Phospholipid Binding Antibodies*". He is currently engaged in research on connective tissue diseases, particularly on the antiphospholipid syndrome and is involved in clinical practice in South Africa. In 1999, he was the co-recipient of the Juan Vivancos Prize in Spain and in 2003 was the co-recipient of the Abbott Prize, awarded at the European League Against Rheumatism (EULAR) International Meeting held in Lisbon, Portugal.

His original description of the "Catastrophic Antiphospholipid Syndrome" and the publishing of more than 40 papers on this new disease was rewarded by the attachment of the eponym "Asherson's Syndrome" to this condition at the November 2002 International Phospholipid Conference held in Sicily.

He is currently editing a series of 12 volumes entitled "The Handbook of Systemic Autoimmune Diseases" (Elsevier, The Netherlands) and in September 2003 was Co-Chairman of the First Latin American Congress on Autoimmunity, held in the Galapagos Islands, Ecuador. He will also co-chair a Session at the forthcoming Conference to be held in Milan in February 2004 on the "Heart, Rheumatism, and Autoimmunity" as well as contributing to another session.

He has been appointed to the International Advisory Board of the International Conference on Systemic Lupus Erythematosus to be held in New York in May 2004.

Series Editor

List of Contributors

Marina Afanasyeva
Department of Pathology
Johns Hopkins Medical Institutions
720 Rutland Avenue
Baltimore, MD 21205, USA

Luigi Boiardi
Division of Rheumatology
Department of Internal Medicine
Arcispedale S. Maria Nuova
V.le Umberto 1° N 50
42100 Reggio Emilia, Italy

Antonio Brucato
Divisione Medica Brera and Rheumatology
Ospedale Niguarda
Milan, Italy
For correspondence: Antonio Brucato
Via Del Bollo 4
20123 Milano, Italy
brucato.guareschi@libero.it

Jill Buyon
Department of Rheumatology
Hospital for Joint Diseases
New York University School of Medicine
301 E 17th Street
New York, NY 10003, USA
jill.buyon@med.nyu.edu

Alida Caforio
Division of Cardiology
Department of Clinical and Experimental Medicine
University of Padua
Policlinico Universitario
Centro 'V. Gallucci'
via N. Giustiniani 2
35128 Padova, Italy
alida.caforio@unipd.it

Ricard Cervera
Institut Clinic d'Infeccions i Immunologia (ICII)
Hospital Clinic
Institut d'Investigacions Biomediques
August Pi i Sunyer (IDIBAPS)
Barcelona, Catalonia, Spain
rcervera@clinic.ub.es

Robert Clancy
Hospital for Joint Diseases
NYU School of Medicine
Research Associate Professor
Department of Rheumatology
301 E 17th Street
New York, NY 10003, USA
Bobdclancy@aol.com

Gerry Coghlan
Royal Free Hospital
London, UK

Chris Denton
Center for Rheumatology
Royal Free Campus
University College London
Rowland Hill Street
Hampstead, NW3 2PF, UK
c.denton@rfc.ucl.ac.uk

Andrea Doria
Division of Rheumatology
Department of Medical and
Surgical Sciences
University of Padova
Via Giustiniani 2
35128 Padova, Italy
adoria@unipd.it

Doruk Erkan
Hospital for Special Surgery
535 East 70th Street
New York, NY 10021, USA
derkan@pol.net

DeLisa Fairweather
Department of Pathology
Johns Hopkins Medical Institutions
720 Rutland Avenue
Baltimore, MD 21205, USA

Maria Gerosa
Allergy, Clinical Immunology and
Rheumatology Unit
Department of Internal Medicine
University of Milan
Via L. Ariosto, 13
20145 Milan, Italy

Nicola Goodson
Arthritis Research Campaign
Epidemiology Unit
Stopford Building University of Manchester
Oxford Road
Manchester M13 9PT, UK
nicola.goodson@man.ac.uk

Loïc Guillevin
Department of Internal Medicine
Hôpital Cochin, 27, rue du Faubourg Saint-Jacques
Paris, F-75014, France
loic.guillevin@cch.ap-hop-paris.fr

Victor Gurevich
Mechnicov's State Medical Academy
The Center of Atherosclerosis
and Lipid Disorders, Chair of Cardiology
194291 pr. Kultury 4
CMSD-122 Saint-Petersburg, Russia
Gur@cards.lanck.net

Michael Lockshin
Barbara Volcker Center
Hospital for Special Surgery
Joan and Sanford I. Weill Medical College
Cornell University
New York, USA
lockshinm@hss.edu

Ingrid Lundberg
Rheumatology Unit
Department of Medicine
Karolinska Institutet
and Rheumatology Clinic
Karolinska Hospital
Stockholm, Sweden
Ingrid.Lundberg@medks.ki.se

William McKenna
Cardiological Sciences
St. George's Hospital Medical School
Cranmer Terrace, Tooting
London SW 17 0RE, UK
wmckenna@sghms.ac.uk

Pier Luigi Meroni
Allergy, Clinical Immunology &
Rheumatology Unit
IRCCS Istituto Auxologico Italiano
Via L. Arioso, 13
20145 Milan, Italy
pierluigi.meroni@unimi.it

Christian Pagnoux
Department of Internal Medicine
Hôpital Cochin
27, rue du Faubourg Saint-Jacques
Paris, F-75014, France

Paolo Pauletto
Dipartimento di Medicina
Clinica e Sperimentale
Università di Padova and
Medicina Interna I^-Ospedale Ca'Foncello
Piazza Ospedale, 1-31100 Treviso, Italy
ppauletto@ulss.tv.it

Michelle Petri
Johns Hopkins, University School of Medicine
Baltimore, Maryland, USA
mpetri@welch.jhu.edu

Marcello Rattazzi
Dipartimento di Medicina Clinica e Sperimentale
Università di Padova and Medicina Interna
1^- Ospedale Ca'Foncello
Via Ospedale, 1
31100 Treviso, Italy

Piersandro Riboldi
Allergy, Clinical Immunology and
Rheumatology Unit
Department of Internal Medicine
University of Milan
Via L. Ariosto, 13
20145 Milan, Italy

Mary Roman
Division of Cardiology
Weill Medical College of Cornell University
New York, NY 10021, USA

Noel Rose
Department of Pathology
Johns Hopkins Medical Institutions
720 Rutland Avenue
Baltimore, MD 21205, USA
nrrose@jhsph.edu

Carlo Salvarani
Division of Rheumatology
Department of Internal Medicine
Arcispedale S. Maria Nuova
V.le Umberto 1° N 50
42100 Reggio Emilia, Italy
salvarani.carlo@asmn.re.it

Piercarlo Sarzi-Puttini
Rheumatology Unit
University Hospital L
Sacco
Milan, Italy
sarzi@tiscalinet.it

Yaniv Sherer
Department of Medicine 'B'
Center of Autoimmune Diseases
Sheba Medical Center, Tel-Hashomer
Sackler Faculty of Medicine
Tel-Aviv University
Tel-Aviv, Israel

Yehuda Shoenfeld
Department of Medicine 'B'
Sheba Medical Center
Tel-Hashomer, 52621, Israel
Shoenfel@post.tau.ac.il
shoenfel@sheba.helath.gov.il

Felicia Tenedios
Department of Rheumatology
Hospital for Special Surgery
Weill Medical College of Cornell University
535 East 70th Street
New York, NY 10021, USA

Angela Tincani
Rheumatology Unit, Spedali Civili
Pizza Spedali Civili, 1
25100 Brescia, Italy
ati.gba@tin.it

Francesco Tona
Division of Cardiology
Department of Experimental and Clinical Medicine
Centro 'V. Gallucci'
University of Padova-Policlinico
Via Giustiniani, 2
35128 Padova, Italy

Maurizio Turiel
Istituto Ortopedico Galeazzi
Cardiology Unit
University of Milan
Via Galeazzi 4
20161 Milan, Italy
Maurizio.turiel@unimi.it

Contents

Preface v
Volume Editors vii
Series Editor ix
List of Contributors xi

I Immune and Autoimmune Mechanisms Involved in Cardiac Damage
Cellular Immunity: A Role for Cytokines 3
DeLisa Fairweather, Marina Afanasyeva, Noel R. Rose
Organ-Specific Autoimmunity Involvement in Cardiovascular Disease 19
Alida L.P. Caforio, Francesco Tona, William J. McKenna.
Non-organ Specific Autoimmunity Involvement in Cardiovascular Disease 41
Piersandro Riboldi, Maria Gerosa, Angela Tincani, Pier Luigi Meroni
Pathogenesis of Anti-SSA/Ro-SSB/La Associated Congenital Heart Block 53
Robert M. Clancy, Jill P. Buyon

II Immune Mechanisms Involved in Atherosclerosis
Innate Immunity, Inflammation, and Atherogenesis 75
Marcello Rattazzi, Yehuda Shoenfeld, Paolo Pauletto
Atherosclerosis and Autoimmunity 89
Yaniv Sherer, Paolo Pauletto, Yehuda Shoenfeld
Statins and Autoimmunity 97
Victor S. Gurevich

III Cardiac Involvement in Autoimmune Connective Tissue Diseases
Cardiac Imaging Techniques in Systemic Autoimmune Diseases 109
Maurizio Turiel, Piercarlo Sarzi-Puttini, Ricard Cervera
Cardiac Involvement in Rheumatoid Arthritis 121
Nicola J. Goodson
Cardiac Involvement in Systemic Lupus Erythematosus 145
Andrea Doria, Michelle Petri
Neonatal Lupus Syndromes: Clinical Features 163
Antonio Brucato, Jill P. Buyon
Cardiac Involvement in Scleroderma 189
J. Gerry Coghlan, Christopher P. Denton
Cardiac Involvement in Autoimmune Myositis and Overlap Syndromes 197
Ingrid E. Lundberg
Cardiac Involvement in the Antiphospholipid Syndrome 213
Doruk Erkan, Mary J. Roman, Felicia Tenedios, Michael D. Lockshin
Cardiac Involvement in Systemic Vasculitis 227
Christian Pagnoux, Luigi Boiardi, Carlo Salvarani, Loïc Guillevin

Index 255

PART I

Immune and Autoimmune Mechanisms Involved in Cardiac Damage

Handbook of Systemic Autoimmune Diseases, Volume 1
The Heart in Systemic Autoimmune Diseases
A. Doria and P. Pauletto, editors

CHAPTER 1

Cellular Immunity: A Role for Cytokines

DeLisa Fairweather[a], Marina Afanasyeva[a], Noel R. Rose[*,a,b]

[a]*Department of Pathology, and*
[b]*Department of Molecular Microbiology and Immunology, Johns Hopkins Medical Institutions, 720 Rutland Avenue, Baltimore, MD 21205, USA*

1. Introduction

The heart is a remarkably durable and efficient pump that provides all cells of the body with nutrients and removes waste products. If cardiac dysfunction occurs for any reason, it can have devastating results. Consequently, heart disease accounts for the majority of illness and death in Western populations (Schoen, 1999). Myocarditis or inflammation of the heart muscle is a significant contributor to heart disease, especially in infants, children, and young adults, and its treatment remains problematic (Drory et al., 1991; Rose and Afanasyeva, 2003). Importantly, myocarditis often precedes the development of dilated cardiomyopathy (DC), which can lead to heart failure and the need for cardiac transplantation.

Myocardial inflammation is a major diagnostic characteristic of myocarditis. According to the current histologic definition based on the Dallas criteria, myocarditis is a "process characterized by an inflammatory infiltrate of the myocardium with necrosis and/or degeneration of adjacent myocytes not typical of the ischemic damage associated with coronary artery disease" (Aretz, 1987). Although inflammation can also occur as a result of ischemic injury, in myocarditis the inflammatory infiltrate plays a primary role in causing the myocardial damage.

The true incidence of myocarditis in the human population is unknown, but up to 10% of routine post-mortem examinations show histological evidence of myocardial inflammation (Gore and Saphir, 1947; Gravanis and Sternby, 1991). Because myocarditis is often difficult to diagnose with standard cardiologic tests, a definitive diagnosis depends on an endomyocardial biopsy, a relatively insensitive procedure due to the focal nature of the inflammation. Histologically defined disease has been confirmed in only approximately 30% of the patients with clinically suspected myocarditis, and in 30–60% of patients with DC (Marboe and Fenoglio, 1988; Peters and Poole-Wilson, 1991). The wide range in the rate of detection of myocarditis in biopsy specimens probably reflects local differences in diagnostic criteria and patient selection as well as the insensitivity of biopsy in general.

To further complicate diagnosis, myocarditis can be induced from many different agents including infections, immune-mediated reactions or drugs (Table 1). Viral infections, such as Coxsackievirus B3 (CB3) and cytomegalovirus (CMV), are widespread in the population, and most individuals in Western populations will be infected with one or both of these two viruses at some point, although acute viral myocarditis may occur frequently without clinical detection (Forbes, 1989; Grist and Reid, 1993). Advances in molecular techniques, such as genomic hybridization and the polymerase chain reaction (PCR), have confirmed the presence of

* Corresponding author.
E-mail address: nrrose@jhsph.edu (N.R. Rose).

DOI: 10.1016/S1571-5078(03)01001-8

Table 1
Major causes of clinical myocarditis

Infections
Viruses (e.g. Coxsackievirus, CMV, influenza)
Bacteria (e.g. streptococci, *Borrelia burgdorgferi* (Lyme disease), chlamydia)
Protozoa (e.g. *Trypanosoma cruzi* (Chagas' disease))
Immune-mediated reactions
Postviral
Poststreptococcal (rheumatic fever)
Systemic lupus erythematosus
Drug hypersensitivity (e.g. sulfonamides)
Transplant rejection
Chemical
Drugs (e.g. adriamycin, cocaine, lead)
Physical
Radiation
Hyperpyrexia
Exercise stress
Unknown
Sarcoidosis

Modified from Huber (1997) and Schoen (1999).

infectious agents like CB3 in the hearts of some myocarditis and DC patients, but the high prevalence of these infections in the population makes it difficult to relate infection with disease. Because these viruses are so common, diagnostic tests based on detection of viral antibody tend to be overly sensitive and the viral infection has usually cleared from the blood stream by the time heart disease occurs. Hence, a better understanding of the pathogenesis of disease is needed in order to find measures that both confirm diagnosis and determine whether the disease is at an early viral or later immune-mediated stage. When viruses directly damage myocytes or initiate immune-mediated damage is often unclear (Huber, 1997; Fairweather et al., 2001).

A number of infectious agents other than viruses are associated with myocarditis. Parasites such as *Trypanasoma cruzi* (the causative agent of Chagas' disease) are the primary cause of myocarditis in Latin American populations where parasites are estimated to infect 16 to 18 million people (Table 1) (Cunha-Neto et al., 1996). Chagas' disease can afflict nearly 50% of endemic populations with 80% of infected individuals developing myocarditis (Schoen, 1999). Likewise, bacterial infection with *Streptococcus pyogenes* may result in rheumatic heart disease, which remains a major cause of heart disease in many developing countries. Myocarditis has also been associated with systemic autoimmune diseases such as systemic lupus erythematosus and polymyositis.

2. Autoimmunity in myocarditis

Soon after autoimmune diseases were first recognized more than a century ago, researchers began to associate them with infectious organisms. The basic task of the immune system is to recognize the myriad of foreign molecules that enter the body from the environment and to avoid harming self (Rose, 2002). Despite such protective mechanisms, autoimmune diseases are common in industrialized societies. Although autoimmune diseases present differently in different organs, they share many common mechanisms.

In order to better understand the relationship between infection and autoimmune disease, we established a mouse model of myocarditis induced by CB3 (Fairweather et al., 2001). Coxsackievirus is believed to account for the majority of cases of myocarditis in North America and Europe (Fujioka et al., 1996; Friman and Fohlman, 1997), and the same virus is capable of inducing myocarditis in humans and mice. Following CB3 infection, BALB/c mice develop an acute, focal inflammatory myocarditis with a mixed cellular infiltrate peaking around day 12 after infection (Fig. 1). Infectious virus can be detected in the heart during this time, but viral levels do not correlate with the severity of inflammation (Fairweather et al., 2001, 2003). Inflammation subsides by day 21 after infection, when heart sections look relatively normal under the microscope. A similar course also occurs following murine CMV (MCMV) infection of BALB/c mice (Fairweather et al., 2001). We surmise that a parallel sequence of events occurs in humans infected with diverse types of viruses such as CB3 (a small, non-enveloped RNA virus) or CMV (a large, enveloped DNA virus). That is, individuals typically develop acute but self-limiting viral myocarditis that heals without residual lesions. In some individuals, as in susceptible

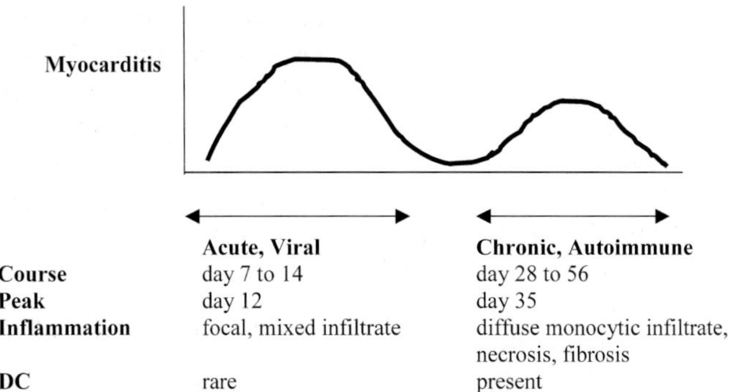

Figure 1. Progression to autoimmune myocarditis following CB3 infection of BALB/c mice. Infection of BALB/c mice with CB3 results in the development of acute, viral myocarditis. During this time, infectious virus can be detected in the heart, but does not correlate with the level of inflammation. The acute inflammatory infiltrate in CB3 infection is comprised predominantly of macrophages, $CD4^+$ T cells, $CD8^+$ T cells, and B cells. The inflammation subsides by day 21 after infection. In BALB/c mice, the chronic, autoimmune stage of the disease emerges around day 28 after infection. Acute myocarditis is characterized by a mixed cellular infiltrate but very little necrosis or fibrosis, in contrast to the autoimmune chronic phase where the lymphocytic infiltrate is associated with large regions of fibrosis and necrosis that may be followed by the development of DC.

mouse strains, the disease develops a chronic phase associated with inflammation and fibrosis accompanied by an autoimmune response to cardiac myosin and other cardiac antigens. The pathogenic process sometimes progresses to DC.

We propose that certain cytokines released in response to viral infection are key in driving the progression to chronic, autoimmune heart disease in mice. We have studied the influence of the immune response to the virus on the subsequent development of myocarditis using mice deficient in immune cells or cytokines due to antibody treatment or genetic manipulation. This chapter will focus on the role of these cells and cytokines in the pathogenesis of myocarditis in mice.

3. Pathogenesis: the role of cells and cytokines

Although a number of animal species (such as primate, pig, dog, rabbit, guinea pig, and rat) have been used in myocarditis research, most animal investigations utilize mice (Huber, 1997). A number of experimental mouse models of myocarditis and DC have been developed, which closely reflect the course of human disease. These include immunization of animals with antigens, such as cardiac myosin, or the use of infectious agents such as viruses. The viruses most often studied in animal models include reovirus, encephalomyocarditis virus, MCMV, and CB3.

Animal models have provided valuable information on factors important for susceptibility to viral infection, such as age, sex, nutritional status, pregnancy, and genetic background (Khatib et al., 1980; Huber et al., 1981; Wolfgram et al., 1986; Fairweather et al., 2001). Infants are more susceptible to Coxsackievirus infections than are young children or adults (Kaplan, 1988), and similarly, susceptibility in mice decreases with increasing age (Khatib et al., 1980). Furthermore, individuals in the human population respond differently to the same infectious agent, with similar observations reported with different mouse strains. Studies to determine the genetic predisposition for myocarditis involved infecting many types of inbred mouse strains with CB3 (Wolfgram et al., 1986). Susceptibility to autoimmune myocarditis, whether inoculating with CB3, MCMV, or cardiac myosin plus adjuvant, is under strict genetic control (Rose et al., 1988; Lawson et al., 1990; Fairweather et al., 2001; Rose and Afanasyeva, 2003). For example, A/J mice are highly susceptible, BALB/c mice are intermediate, and C57BL/6 mice are resistant to the development of the chronic, autoimmune phase of myocarditis (Fig. 1). Surprisingly, this susceptibility is due primarily to genes that are not part of the major histocompatibility complex (MHC) (Rose and Afanasyeva, 2003).

Key in our understanding of the control of susceptibility to autoimmune disease was the finding that inoculation with bacterial lipopolysaccharide (LPS), interleukin (IL)-1β, or tumor necrosis factor (TNF)-α after viral infection resulted in the development of the chronic, autoimmune phase of disease in resistant strains of mice (Lane et al., 1991, 1992; Lenzo et al., 2002). Moreover, when genetically susceptible A/J mice are treated with agents that block IL-1 or TNF, they fail to develop myocarditis induced by cardiac myosin (Neumann et al., 1993). From this series of experiments, we conclude that inflammatory mediators are critical for the development of a pathogenic autoimmune response following viral infection. The production of key cytokines following infection may vary depending on the virus, the mouse strain, the conditions surrounding the infectious process, or the interplay of these and other genetic and environmental factors.

3.1. Viral mouse model

Infection of BALB/c mice with CB3 results in the development of acute myocarditis from day 7 to 14 after infection (Fig. 1). During this time, infectious virus can be detected in the heart, but does not correlate with the level of inflammation (Fairweather et al., 2003). The inflammatory infiltrate in CB3 infection is comprised predominantly of macrophages, natural killer (NK) cells, $CD8^+$ T cells, and $CD4^+$ T cells, B cells and neutrophils (Godeny and Gauntt, 1986, 1987a,b; Henke et al., 1995; Fairweather et al., 2001). The inflammation in the heart subsides by day 21 after infection, when heart sections look relatively normal under the microscope. In BALB/c mice, the chronic, autoimmune stage of the disease emerges around day 28 after infection and can be detected at least until day 56 (Fairweather et al., 2001). Acute myocarditis following viral infection is characterized by a focal, mixed cellular infiltrate but very little necrosis or fibrosis, in contrast to the autoimmune chronic phase where a diffuse lymphocytic infiltrate is associated with large regions of fibrosis and necrosis that may be followed by the development of DC (Fig. 1).

It is important to note that many of the studies of virally induced myocarditis used high doses of virus that resulted in death during the acute phase of myocarditis (Huber, 1997; Horwitz et al., 2000; Fong, 2003). In these models, necrosis of myocytes and fibrosis can be observed during acute myocarditis with few animals surviving to the chronic phase. In contrast, a low dose of virus results in virtually no deaths, allowing 100% of mice to survive to develop chronic myocarditis and DC (Fairweather et al., 2001). Since young adults rarely die from acute Coxsackievirus infections (Schoen, 1999), we feel that the low-dose model more closely resembles the disease as it occurs in human populations. Interestingly, inoculation of higher doses of CB3 actually results in lower levels of inflammation in the heart than inoculation of low doses (D. Fairweather, unpublished observations).

3.2. Cardiac myosin mouse model

Cardiac myosin is the major target of the autoimmune response in many cases of myocarditis in humans and mice (Neu et al., 1987; Caforio et al., 1996; Wang et al., 1999; Lauer et al., 2000). Evidence that persistent viral infection is not required for the development of myocarditis comes from the demonstration that inoculation of BALB/c mice with cardiac myosin, emulsified in complete Freund's adjuvant, induces an experimental autoimmune myocarditis (EAM) that closely resembles the myocarditis associated with CB3 infection (Fig. 1) (Neu et al., 1987; Lawson et al., 1992; Rose, 1996). Twenty-one days after immunization, the disease is characterized by a predominantly mononuclear infiltration of the myocardium and some cardiomyocyte death and replacement fibrosis (Fig. 1). The myocardial infiltrate contains many macrophages, $CD4^+$ T cell and some $CD8^+$ T cells, and $B220^+$ B cells (Pummerer et al., 1991; Wang et al., 1999). Among the infiltrating cells are eosinophils and occasional giant cells, both of which are more prominent in severe myocarditis as often occurs in highly susceptible A/J mice (Afanasyeva et al., 2001a). At later time points, inflammation recedes and myocardial fibrosis becomes the hallmark of disease, similar to the late chronic phase of myocarditis after viral infection (Fig. 1). Extensive myocardial damage eventually leads to the development of DC and congestive heart failure (Afanasyeva and Rose, 2002).

3.3. Role of cells

Both cellular and humoral autoimmunity are involved in the pathogenesis of CB3-induced myocarditis in susceptible mice, but distinct pathogenic mechanisms may function in different strains of mice. For example, CB3 infection of DBA/2 mice has an exclusively humoral pathogenesis, whereas BALB/c mice develop a primarily cell-mediated disease, and the pathogenesis of disease in A/J mice involves both autoimmune T cells and autoantibodies (Huber and Lodge, 1986; Lodge et al., 1987).

The involvement of autoimmune T cells in the pathogenesis of CB3-induced myocarditis was first inferred from the observation that T cell depleted mice have less severe disease than normal mice (Woodruff and Woodruff, 1974). In both CB3- and MCMV-induced myocarditis models, T cells have been shown to play a decisive role in disease pathogenesis (Lawson et al., 1989; Schwimmbeck et al., 1997). Athymic nude mice also develop less severe disease to either CB3 or MCMV infection (Hashimoto and Komatsu, 1978; Lawson et al., 1989). Furthermore, myocarditis can be transferred by inoculation of autoimmune $CD4^+$ T cells from virally infected mice to uninfected recipients (Guthrie et al., 1984; Huber, 1997). Infection of mice depleted of T cell subsets or mice genetically altered to be deficient in subsets of T cells results in reduced myocarditis (Henke et al., 1995; Schwimmbeck et al., 1997; Fairweather et al., 2001). Table 2 indicates the important role T cells, particularly $CD8^+$ T cells, play in the development of acute MCMV-induced myocarditis in BALB/c mice (Fairweather et al., 2001). Although depletion of $CD4^+$ T cells from MCMV-infected BALB/c mice reduces myocardial inflammation, the reduction is far more dramatic if $CD8^+$ alone or both $CD4^+$ and $CD8^+$ T cells are removed. Furthermore, acute myocarditis is more severe in CD4 C57BL/6 knockout (KO) mice ($CD4^+$ T cells are absent due to gene deletion) following CB3 infection (Henke et al., 1995). These studies confirm that the development of myocarditis, although requiring virus to initiate the process, also needs components of adaptive immunity for disease progression.

Autoreactive T cells and autoantibodies are also present in myosin-induced EAM (Neu and Ploier, 1991; Pummerer et al., 1995). T cells are necessary for the development of disease in this model, with myosin-stimulated T cells capable of transferring myocarditis into immunodeficient SCID mice (Smith

Table 2
Role of immune cells in MCMV-induced myocarditis

Genetic background[a]	Depletion[b]	Myocarditis[c]	p[d]
BALB/c (no NK1.1)	Control	24 ± 2	
	Anti-NK1.1	15 ± 4	<0.05
	Anti-CD4	14 ± 4	<0.05
	Anti-CD8	7 ± 2	<0.01
	Anti-CD4/8	5 ± 1	<0.01
BALB.B6 congenic (BALB/c + NK1.1)	Control	5 ± 1	
	Anti-NK1.1	23 ± 5	<0.01
C57BL/6 (NK1.1)	Control	5 ± 1	
	Anti-NK1.1	19 ± 2	<0.01

Modified from Fairweather et al. (2001).

[a] BALB/c (do not have $NK1.1^+$ cells), BALB.B6-*Cmv1*^{r} (BALB.B6 congenic) (have $NK1.1^+$ cells on a BALB/c genetic background), or C57BL/6 (have $NK1.1^+$ cells on a C57BL/6 genetic background) mice were infected with MCMV intraperitoneally.

[b] Mice were also treated with antibodies that deplete $NK1.1^+$ cells, $CD4^+$ T cells, $CD8^+$ T cells, both $CD4^+$ and $CD8^+$ T cells, or saline control. Successful cell depletions were confirmed by FACS analysis (data not shown).

[c] Myocarditis (number of foci per heart section) was examined at day 9 after MCMV infection and scored as the standard error of the mean number of foci.

[d] Values significantly different (p) from the control group by Student's t-test are shown.

and Allen, 1991, 1993; Pummerer et al., 1995). Depletion of $CD4^+$ or $CD8^+$ T cells from myosin-immunized susceptible mice diminishes myocarditis, suggesting that both cell types are important in the pathogenesis of EAM, as in virally induced models (Pummerer et al., 1991; Smith and Allen, 1991, 1993; Penninger et al., 1993). However, while CD4 KO mice have reduced inflammation, myocarditis is exacerbated in CD8 KO mice following immunization (Penninger et al., 1993; Pummerer et al., 1995). Thus, $CD8^+$ T cells may sometimes suppress the disease in this model. $CD4^+$ T cells are involved in the pathogenesis of EAM through recognition of antigen presented by MHC class II (Smith and Allen, 1992a; Donermeyer et al., 1995), which may be important regulatory molecules for the induction of autoimmunity (Todd et al., 1988; Nepom, 1993). An understanding of the cellular mechanisms driving the autoimmune response in EAM may help to distinguish the role of the cellular response to viral infection from the response directed against cardiac myosin.

NK cells are an important first line of defense against viral infections where they efficiently limit replication of both CB3 and MCMV (Godeny and Gauntt, 1987a; Bancroft, 1993; Tay et al., 1998). When antigen-presenting cells detect viral infection of host tissues, they release cytokines and chemokines, which attract NK cells to the site of infection. The ability of NK cells to rapidly produce interferon (IFN)-γ after infiltrating infected tissues, before clonal expansion of T cells, is critical for an effective innate immune response (Fairweather and Rose, 2002). Depletion of NK cells with anti-asialo GM_1 (a pan-NK marker) resulted in increased myocarditis in outbred CD-1 mice following CB3 infection (Godeny and Gauntt, 1986), suggesting that NK cells primarily protect against myocarditis by inhibiting viral replication. In order to examine the role of NK cells in the development of MCMV-induced acute myocarditis, $NK1.1^+$ cells were depleted from normal C57BL/6 or BALB.B6-*Cmv1^r^* congenic mice using antibodies against NK1.1 (Table 2) (Fairweather et al., 2001). BALB.B6-$Cmv1^r$ is a congenic mouse strain that carries the NK cell gene complex found in B10 mice (e.g. NK1.1) on a BALB/c genetic background (Scalzo et al., 1995). Since BALB/c mice do not have NK1.1 cells, they primarily clear MCMV infection through the cytolytic activity of $CD8^+$ T cells (Lathbury et al., 1996). Depletion of $NK1.1^+$ cells from C57BL/6 or BALB.B6-$Cmv1^r$ congenic mice significantly increased myocarditis to levels found in BALB/c control mice (Table 2). The role for NK cells in $NK1.1^-$ BALB/c mice is not yet clear. These results indicate that the protection mediated by NK cells during acute myocarditis is more important in reducing myocarditis than other traits in the BALB/c genetic background, since the only difference between congenic and regular BALB/c mice is the NK cell gene complex.

The innate immune response to pathogens has become a topic of great interest in recent years. In the past, innate immunity was considered only to provide rapid, but incomplete antimicrobial host defense until the slower, more definitive acquired immune response developed (Fearon and Lockley, 1996; Parish and O'Neill, 1997; Hoffmann et al., 1999). However, recent research indicates that innate immunity critically impacts the subsequent development of the adaptive immune response and autoimmunity (Carroll and Prodeus, 1998; Seder and Gazzinelli, 1999; Kadowski et al., 2000; Kaya et al., 2001). How innate immunity controls the initiation of an adaptive response and the development of autoimmune disease is not well understood, but is likely to involve innate immune cell release of proinflammatory cytokines.

3.4. Role of cytokines

Many of the mediators associated with the innate immune response, particularly cytokines, can act in a long-range endocrine manner so that antigen-presenting cells far removed from the site of infection are activated to present either viral or autoantigens to T and B cells (Parish and O'Neill, 1997; Carnaud et al., 1999; Kadowski et al., 2000). Moreover, recent evidence suggests that a bidirectional relationship exists between innate and adaptive immunity (Kos and Engelman, 1996).

IFN-α production following viral infection stimulates an effective NK cell response. The type 1 IFNs belong to a multigene family that include multiple IFN-α subtypes and IFN-β (Bellardelli, 1995). IFNs also provide an important link between the innate and adaptive immune responses (Kadowski et al., 2000).

Previous studies have shown that administration of IFN-α subtypes or IFN-β to MCMV-infected BALB/c mice not only reduces viral replication but also decreases acute and chronic myocarditis (Table 3) (Lawson et al., 1997; Yeow et al., 1998; Fairweather et al., 2001). These results emphasize the role of innate cytokines in modulating the adaptive immune response and autoimmune disease.

As pointed out previously, cytokines can determine whether mice develop autoimmune myocarditis. For example, administration of IL-1 or IL-2 augments disease in CB3-infected susceptible mice (Table 3) (Huber et al., 1994), while blocking these receptors inhibits the development of myocarditis (Neumann et al., 1993). On the other hand, C57BL/6 mice, which are resistant to the development of chronic myocarditis following CB3 or MCMV infection, can be induced to develop chronic myocarditis by administration of LPS (a generator of several proinflammatory cytokines), IL-1β, or TNF-α with the virus (Table 3) (Lane et al., 1991, 1992; Lenzo et al., 2001). Cytokines may play a number of different roles. They may provide second signals after viral infection that stimulate an effective protective immune response or a deleterious response in individuals susceptible to autoimmune disease (Fairweather et al., 2001). Thus, certain cytokines can influence whether chronic autoimmune disease develops in response to viral infection, bridging the gap between the innate and adaptive immune response.

LPS and TNF-α are also important in the development of cardiac myosin-induced myocarditis. Neutralization of TNF-α effectively inhibits the initiation of EAM, although neutralization is not

Table 3
Role of cytokines and cytokine signaling in virus-induced myocarditis

Cytokine	Method studied[a]	Effect on myocarditis	References
Promotes myocarditis			
LPS	CB3 + LPS (using BL/6 mice)	Develop chronic myocarditis by increasing IL-1 and TNF	Lane et al. (1991), Lenzo et al. (2001)
TLR4	TLR4 KO	Reduces myocarditis, IL-1, and IL-18	Fairweather et al. (2003)
TNF-α	CB3 + TNF-α (using BL/6 mice)	Develop chronic myocarditis	Lane et al. (1992), Lenzo et al. (2001)
IL-1β	CB3	IL-1 levels correlate with increased myocarditis	Fairweather et al. (2003)
	IL-1 administration	Increases myocarditis	Huber et al. (1994)
	CB3 + IL-1β (using BL/6 mice)	Develop chronic myocarditis	Lane et al. (1992)
IL-12Rβ1	IL-12Rβ1 KO (signaling for IL-12p70 and IL-23)	Decreases myocarditis, IL-1, and IL-18	Fairweather et al. (2003)
IL-18	CB3	IL-18 levels correlate with increased myocarditis	Fairweather et al. (2003)
Reduces myocarditis			
IFN-α	IFN-α administration	Decreases viral replication	Fairweather et al. (2001)
IL-12p35	IL-12p35 KO (effect of IL-12p70)	Decreases viral replication, no effect on acute myocarditis	Unpublished
IL-12p40	IL-12p40 KO (effect of IL-12p70, $p40_2$, IL-23)	Increases acute myocarditis, IL-1, and IL-18	Unpublished
STAT4	STAT4 KO	Decreases viral replication, no effect on myocarditis	Unpublished
IFN-γ	IFN-γ KO	Decreases viral replication, increases chronic myocarditis, fibrosis, and DC	Unpublished
IL-4	IL-4 KO	Increases myocarditis	Unpublished
STAT6	STAT6 KO	Increases myocarditis	Unpublished

C57BL/6, BL/6; Coxsackievirus B3, CB3; dilated cardiomyopathy; DC, interferon-α/γ, IFN-α/γ; interleukin, IL; knockout, KO; lipopolysaccharide, LPS; receptor, R; p40 homodimer, $p40_2$; signal transducer and activator of transcription, STAT; toll-like receptor 4, TLR4; tumor necrosis factor, TNF.

[a] BALB/c mice are used unless otherwise stated.

beneficial in suppressing ongoing disease (Table 4) (Smith and Allen, 1992b). TNF-α is believed to be necessary for upregulating MHC class II binding of self-reactive peptides on antigen-presenting cells in EAM, since upregulation of MHC and accessory molecules fails to occur in TNF deficient mice (Smith and Allen, 1992a). Furthermore, myocarditis can be transferred by injection of cardiac myosin-specific T cells into mice pretreated with LPS or TNF-α (Penninger et al., 1997). Thus, the primary role of virus or adjuvant, in the EAM model, may be to provide an optimal cytokine environment (i.e. increased IL-1β and TNF-α) in the context of self-antigen thereby allowing an autoimmune response to occur.

According to the current dogma, inflammatory autoimmune diseases are primarily attributable to Th1 responses, of which IFN-γ is the prototypic cytokine, while Th2 responses, where IL-4 predominates, should reduce autoimmunity (Cunningham, 2001). Th1-mediated immune responses have been implicated in the pathogenesis of a number of autoimmune diseases including inflammatory bowel disease, type I diabetes, multiple sclerosis, and rheumatoid arthritis (O'Garra, 1998). IFN-γ stimulates Th1 cell development, activates macrophages, induces MHC class I and II expression, promotes delayed-type hypersensitivity reactions, induces certain immunoglobulin class switching, recruits Th1 cells to the site of inflammation, and is important for clearing intracellular bacteria, parasites, and viral infections (Boehm et al., 1997). IL-4, on the other hand, stimulates Th2 cell development, activates B cells, induces MHC class II expression on B cells, promotes allergic reactions, induces immunoglobulin class switching to IgG1 and IgE, recruits eosinophils and Th2 cells to the site of inflammation, and is important for clearing parasites (Nelms et al., 1999). Thus, determining whether a predominantly Th1 or Th2 immune response occurs to virus or cardiac myosin immunization may promote understanding the pathogenesis of autoimmune heart disease.

IL-12 is produced by phagocytic and antigen-presenting cells. Produced during the early phase of an infection, IL-12 promotes the differentiation of T cells to a Th1 phenotype with IFN-γ production,

Table 4
Role of cytokines and cytokine signaling in cardiac myosin-induced myocarditis

Cytokine	Method studied[a]	Effect on myocarditis	References
Promotes myocarditis			
TNF-α	Blocking Ab	Prevents EAM	Smith and Allen (1992a,b)
TNFRp55	TNFRp55 KO	Reduces EAM	Bachmaier et al. (1997)
IL-12p40	IL-12p40 KO (effect of IL-12p70, $p40_2$, IL-23)	Reduces EAM	Eriksson et al. (2001a,b)
IL-12p70	IL-12p70 administration	Exacerbates EAM	Afanasyeva et al. (2001b)
IL-12Rβ1	IL-12Rβ1 KO (signaling for IL-12p70 and IL-23)	Prevents EAM	Afanasyeva et al. (2001b)
STAT4	STAT4 KO	Reduces EAM	Afanasyeva et al. (2001b)
IL-4	Blocking Ab	Reduces EAM	Afanasyeva et al. (2001a)
Reduces myocarditis			
IFN-γ	Blocking Ab	Increases EAM and DC	Afanasyeva et al. (2001a,b)
	IFN-γ KO	Increases EAM and DC	Afanasyeva et al. (2001b), Eriksson et al. (2001a), Kurrer et al. (2002)
IFN-γ R	IFN-γ R KO	Increases EAM and DC	Eriksson et al. (2001b)
IL-10	Blocking Ab	Increases EAM	Kaya et al. (2002)

Antibody, Ab; interferon-α/γ, BL/6, C57BL/6, IFN-α/γ; experimental autoimmune myocarditis, EAM; interleukin, IL; knockout, KO; p40 homodimer, $p40_2$; receptor, R; signal transducer and activator of transcription, STAT; tumor necrosis factor, TNF.

[a] Using A/J or BALB/c mouse strains.

which in turn supports cell-mediated immunity, cytotoxic T cell generation, activation of phagocytic cells, and eventual eradication of intracellular pathogens (Ma and Trinchieri, 2001). IL-12 is a heterodimer composed of IL-12p35 and IL-12p40 subunits bound via disulfide bonds and secreted as a biologically active IL-12p70 molecule. IL-12 receptors (R) are primarily expressed on activated NK and T cells, and signaling requires coexpression of the IL-12Rβ1 and IL-12Rβ2 chains for the generation of high affinity IL-12p70 binding and maximal IFN-γ production. In the mouse, IL-12R signaling activates the signal transducer and activator of transcription (STAT)1, STAT3, and STAT4, with STAT4 being responsible for most of the biological activities of IL-12 through the production of IFN-γ (O'Garra, 1998; Moser and Murphy, 2000). IL-12p40 is also produced as a monomer and homodimer ($p40_2$) in great excess over IL-12p70. The IL-12p40 homodimer has been found to antagonize IL-12p70 activity by competitively binding the IL-12R (Mattner et al., 1993).

IL-18 has emerged as an important cytokine along with IL-12 for increasing IFN-γ production from immune cells. The synergistic effect is mediated through the induction of IL-18Rα by IL-12 and the upregulation of IL-12Rβ2 by IL-18 on naïve T cells (Yoshimoto et al., 1998). In contrast, NK cells constitutively express IL-18R and IL-12Rβ2 and are able to immediately respond to these cytokines (Nakanishi et al., 2001). The IL-18R has been identified as a member of the IL-1R/toll-like receptor (TLR) superfamily and shares a common signal transduction pathway with IL-1R (O'Neill and Dinarello, 2000). Importantly, IL-18 can also stimulate IFN-γ production through STAT-independent pathways (O'Neill and Dinarello, 2000; Nakanishi et al., 2001). IL-18 is produced by a wide range of immune and non-immune cells as a biologically inactive precursor that is activated in the same manner as IL-1 by cleavage with caspase-1. Likewise, caspase-1 undergoes proteolytic cleavage to produce its active form after stimulation through TLR4 (Akira et al., 2001). Respiratory syncytial virus was discovered to be a ligand for TLR4, along with LPS, suggesting that activation of TLR may be involved in protecting the host from viral infections (Kurt-Jones et al., 2000).

Recently, we examined the role of IL-12-induced IFN-γ on the development of CB3-induced myocarditis using mice deficient in IL-12p35 (lacking IL-12p70), IL-12p40 (lacking IL-12p70, IL-23, and $p40_2$), IL-12Rβ1 (lacking signaling induced by IL-12p70 and IL-23), STAT4, IFN-γ, or TLR4 (Fairweather et al., 2003). We found that decreased levels of IL-1β and IL-18 in the heart following CB3 infection of IL-12Rβ1 or TLR4 deficient mice was directly associated with decreased myocardial inflammation (Table 3). Unexpectedly, deficiency of either of these two receptors also decreased viral replication in the heart. These results suggest that IL-12Rβ1 and TLR4 share common downstream pathways that directly influence IL-1β and IL-18 production and viral replication. Examination of IL-12p35 (IL-12p70), IFN-γ, or STAT4 deficient mice confirmed that IFN-γ protects against viral replication in the heart but did not affect acute myocardial inflammation, indicating that the role of the IL-12R in exacerbating acute myocarditis is not via IFN-γ production (Table 3) (D. Fairweather, unpublished results). Furthermore, we found evidence that IL-12p40 (probably the p40 homodimer) protects against acute CB3 myocarditis by reducing the level of IL-1β and IL-18 in the heart. In contrast, IL-12p70 facilitates viral clearance by increasing IFN-γ levels.

A good candidate to explain the increased production of IL-1β and IL-18, and the myocardial inflammation observed in wild type BALB/c mice following CB3 infection is IL-23, which has been shown to be released following viral infection (Oppmann et al., 2000; Pirhonen et al., 2002). IL-23 is a heterodimer composed of IL-12p40 and a p19 subunit. The IL-12p40 subunit binds to IL-12Rβ1 and the p19 subunit binds to a recently identified IL-23R (Parham et al., 2002). Although IL-23 can activate STAT4, STAT3 is believed to be the primary transcription factor activated following IL-23R ligation (Parham et al., 2002; Lankford and Frucht, 2003). Interestingly, transgenic mice that ubiquitously express the p19 subunit of IL-23 develop severe multiorgan inflammation and elevated levels of TNF-α and IL-1 (Wiekowski et al., 2001). Recently, IL-23, rather than IL-12p70, was discovered to be primarily responsible for exacerbating EAE (Cua et al., 2003; Zhang et al., 2003); IL-12p70 has been considered the key cytokine mediating EAE and many other autoimmune diseases (Caspi, 1998; Watford and O'Shea, 2003). Our findings corroborate and extend the studies by Cua et al. and Zhang et al. demonstrating that IL-12p70 is not responsible for increasing IL-1β/IL-18 levels or inflammation in the heart. However, IL-23 does not account for the increased inflammation and IL-1β/IL-18 levels in IL-12p40 deficient hearts since this cytokine is absent. In this case, signaling via TLR4, perhaps exacerbated by other molecules such as Epstein-Barr virus-induced gene 3 (EBI3)/IL-12p35, can lead to increased IL-1β/IL-18 levels and myocarditis (Fairweather et al., 2003).

In the EAM model, IL-12Rβ1 deficient mice do not develop myocarditis, suggesting a role for this receptor in increasing inflammation (Table 4) (Afanasyeva et al., 2001b). In the absence of IL-12Rβ1, IL-1β production from splenocyte cultures was also significantly reduced (Afanasyeva et al., 2001b), further suggesting an important role for this cytokine in the development of autoimmune heart disease. While STAT4 deficiency has no affect on inflammation in CB3-induced myocarditis (Table 3), inflammation is reduced in STAT4 deficient mice in the EAM model (Table 4). IL-23 is also a likely candidate for the increased disease that is mediated via IL-12Rβ1 and STAT4 in the EAM model. In contrast to CB3-induced myocarditis, IL-12p40 deficient mice do not develop EAM (Eriksson et al., 2001a,b). It may be that IL-1β levels are regulated by different mechanisms in the EAM model.

In contrast to the role for IL-12Rβ1 and STAT4 in exacerbating EAM, IFN-γ plays a protective role in both EAM and CB3-induced myocarditis. Mice genetically deficient in either IFN-γ or IFN-γ R or mice treated with IFN-γ neutralizing antibody develop severe EAM with large, dilated hearts and some mice even developed congestive heart failure (Table 4) (Afanasyeva et al., 2001a,b; Eriksson et al., 2001b; Rose and Afanasyeva, 2003). The role for IFN-γ in mediating Th1-mediated autoimmune responses has been attributed to its ability to expand autoreactive $CD4^+$ T cells. However, the simplistic distinction between Th1 and Th2 responses and autoimmune disease requires re-evaluation in light of these findings (Gor et al., 2003; Rose and Afanasyeva, 2003). The mechanisms whereby IFN-γ protects against EAM and the chronic phase of CB3 myocarditis remain to be understood.

Conflicting data exist regarding the role of IL-4 and a Th2-mediated immune response in autoimmune myocarditis. Blocking IL-4 with neutralizing antibody reduces the severity of EAM (Table 4) and produces a shift from a Th2 to a Th1-like response indicated by increased IFN-γ and decreased IL-4, IL-5, and IL-13 production from splenocyte cultures (Afanasyeva et al., 2001a). However, IL-4 and IL-4 receptor KO mice are not protected from the development of EAM (Table 4) (Eriksson et al., 2001a; Kurrer et al., 2002). These contrasting findings may be due to the differential effect of antibody administration versus complete lack of the molecule and other factors such as the dose of cytokine, timing of administration, or difference in the strain of mice (A/J mice used in antibody blocking experiments versus genetically deficient BALB/c mice). Eosinophils and multinucleated giant cells are prominent in EAM (Afanasyeva et al., 2001a). Eosinophils are known to be associated with Th2 type cytokines such as IL-4, IL-5, IL-10, and IgE antibodies (Cunningham, 2001). Although IL-4 can also lead to the formation of multinucleated giant cells, these cells have long been associated with the granulomatous lesions formed in response to intracellular bacterial infections such as *Mycobacterium tuberculosis*, which is a component of the adjuvant used in the EAM model (Cunningham, 2001). Thus it appears that components of both Th1 and Th2 responses contribute to severe autoimmune myocarditis. In CB3-induced myocarditis, however, infection of IL-4 and STAT6 KO mice (STAT6 mediates signaling through the IL-4 receptor) results in increased acute and chronic myocarditis indicating a protective role for IL-4 in virally induced autoimmune myocarditis (Table 3) (D. Fairweather, unpublished results). These findings suggest that a delicate balance of key cytokines determines whether an autoimmune response occurs following viral infection or cardiac myosin and adjuvant inoculation (Fairweather et al., 2001; Rose and Afanasyeva, 2003). A better understanding of the individual cytokines involved in mediating the immune response, particularly the early innate response that determines the profile of key cytokines, will be necessary in order to develop therapies for human autoimmune heart disease.

3.5. Summary of pathogenic mechanisms

The development of autoimmune heart disease following viral infection involves the production of key cytokines by immune cells such as macrophages and NK cells. Activation of TLRs by virus (Fig. 2a) or the bacterial component of complete Freund's adjuvant (Fig. 2b) leads to the production of IL-1β and TNF-α. Overproduction of these proinflammatory cytokines increases the inflammatory infiltrate in the heart. Regulatory cytokines such as IL-10, and possibly the IL-12p40 homodimer, decrease the severity of inflammation in the heart. However, if environmental or genetic factors allow overproduction of proinflammatory cytokines, then progression to chronic autoimmune myocarditis may follow.

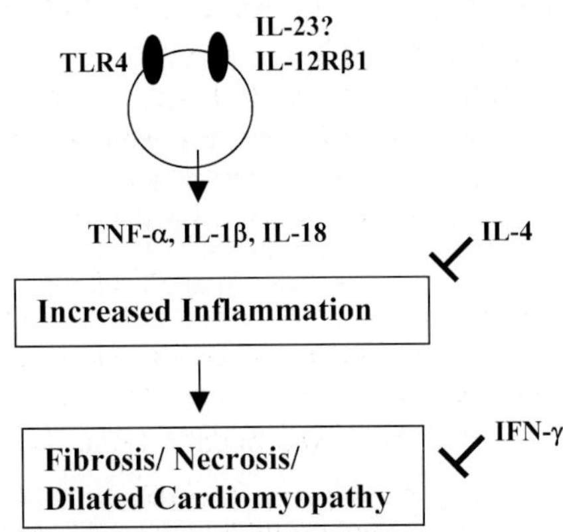

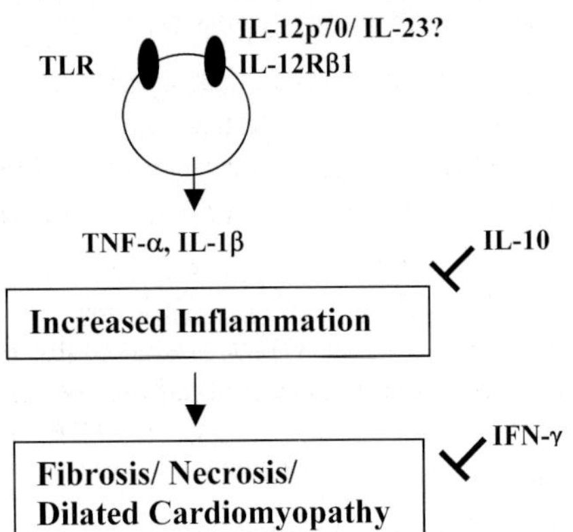

Figure 2. Proposed model for the development of autoimmune heart disease. The development of autoimmune heart disease following (a) viral infection or (b) cardiac myosin injection involves production of key cytokines by immune cells such as macrophages or NK cells after release of cardiac myosin by viral infection of myocytes or by inoculation. Activation of TLRs by CB3 or the bacterial component of complete Freund's adjuvant leads to the production of proinflammatory cytokines such as IL-1β, TNF-α, and possibly IL-4. Overproduction of these cytokines increases the inflammatory infiltrate in the heart. Cytokines such as IL-10, and possibly the IL-12p40 homodimer, reduce inflammation in the heart. However, if environmental or genetic factors allow overproduction of proinflammatory cytokines, then progression to chronic autoimmune myocarditis and DC may follow.

Key points

- Proinflammatory cytokines (e.g. IL-1β and TNF-α) released after viral infection or adjuvant stimulation are capable of driving an autoimmune response to cardiac self-tissues resulting in chronic autoimmune myocarditis.
- Key proinflammatory cytokines involved in this process do not adhere to a strict Th1–Th2 dichotomy.
- IL-12Rβ1 and TLR4 signaling stimulate IL-1β production in the heart that relates to increased acute inflammation.
- The IL-12p70–STAT4–IFN-γ pathway does not significantly influence the severity of acute myocardial inflammation but protects against viral replication in the heart, whereas IFN-γ reduces chronic inflammation, fibrosis, and the development of DC.
- The regulatory cytokines IL-10 and the IL-12p40 homodimer reduce inflammation in the heart.

References

Afanasyeva, M., Rose, N.R. 2002. Immune mediators in inflammatory heart disease: insights from a mouse model. Eur. Heart J. Suppl. 4 (Suppl. I), I31.

Afanasyeva, M., Wang, Y., Kaya, Z., Park, S., Zilliox, M.J., Schofield, B.H., Hill, S.L., Rose, N.R. 2001a. Experimental autoimmune myocarditis in A/J mice is an interleukin-4-dependent disease with a Th2 phenotype. Am. J. Pathol. 159, 193.

Afanasyeva, M., Wang, Y., Kaya, Z., et al. 2001b. Interleukin-12 receptor/STAT4 signaling is required for the development of autoimmune myocarditis in mice by an interferon-γ-independent pathway. Circulation 104, 3145.

Akira, S.A., Takeda, K., Kaisho, T. 2001. Toll-like receptors: critical proteins linking innate and acquired immunity. Nat. Immunol. 2, 675.

Aretz, H.T. 1987. Myocarditis: the Dallas criteria. Hum. Pathol. 18, 619.

Bachmaier, K., Pummerer, C., Kozieradzki, I., et al. 1997. Low-molecular-weight tumor necrosis factor receptor p55 controls induction of autoimmune heart disease. Circ. 95, 655.

Bancroft, G.J. 1993. The role of natural killer cells in innate resistance to infection. Curr. Opin. Immunol. 5, 503.

Bellardelli, F. 1995. Role of interferons and other cytokines in the regulation of the immune response. APMIS 103, 161.

Boehm, U., Klamp, T., Groot, M., et al. 1997. Cellular responses to interferon-γ. Annu. Rev. Immunol. 15, 749.

Caforio, A.L., Goldman, J.H., Haven, A.J., et al. 1996. Evidence for autoimmunity to myosin and other heart-specific autoantigens in patients with dilated cardiomyopathy and their relatives. Int. J. Cardiol. 54, 157.

Carnaud, C., Lee, D., Donnars, O., et al. 1999. Cutting edge: cross-talk between cells of the innate immune system: NKT cells rapidly activate NK cells. J. Immunol. 163, 4647.

Carroll, M.C., Prodeus, A.P. 1998. Linkages of innate and adaptive immunity. Curr. Opin. Immunol. 10, 36.

Caspi, R.R. 1998. IL-12 in autoimmunity. Clin. Immunol. Immunopathol. 88, 4.

Cua, D.J., Sherlock, J., Chen, Y., et al. 2003. Interleukin-23 rather than interleukin-12 is the critical cytokine for autoimmune inflammation of the brain. Nature 421, 744.
This report shows that IL-23 is predominantly responsible for increasing autoimmune disease in the brain, rather than IL-12p70. Similar findings have been found in CB3-induced myocarditis.

Cunha-Neto, E., Coelho, V., Guilherme, L., et al. 1996. Autoimmunity in Chagas' disease: identification of cardiac myosin-B13 *Trypanosoma cruzi* protein crossreactive T cell clones in heart lesions of a chronic Chagas' cardiomyopathy patient. J. Clin. Invest. 98, 1709.

Cunningham, M.W. 2001. Cardiac myosin and the Th1/Th2 paradigm in autoimmune myocarditis. Am. J. Pathol. 159, 5.
An excellent review of myocarditis with an emphasis on the role of molecular mimicry and Th1 versus Th2 cytokines on the pathogenesis of disease.

Donermeyer, D.L., Beisel, K.W., Allen, P.M., et al. 1995. Myocarditis-inducing epitope of myosin binds constitutively and stably to I-A^k on antigen presenting cells in the heart. J. Exp. Med. 182, 1291.

Drory, Y., Turetz, Y., Hiss, Y., et al. 1991. Sudden unexpected death in persons less than 40 years of age. Am. J. Cardiol. 68, 1388.

Eriksson, U., Kurrer, M.O., Sebald, W., et al. 2001a. Dual role of the IL-12/IFN-γ axis in the development of autoimmune myocarditis: induction by IL-12 and protection by IFN-γ. J. Immunol. 167, 5464.

Eriksson, U., Kurrer, M.O., Bissinger, R., et al. 2001b. Lethal autoimmune myocarditis in interferon-γ receptor-deficient mice: enhanced disease severity by impaired inducible nitric oxide synthase function. Circulation 103, 18.

Fairweather, D., Kaya, Z., Shellam, G.R., et al. 2001. From infection to autoimmunity. J. Autoimmun. 16, 175.

Fairweather, D., Rose, N.R. 2002. Type I diabetes: virus infection or autoimmune disease? Nat. Immunol. 3, 338.

Fairweather, D., Yusung, S., Frisancho, S., et al. 2003. IL-12Rβ1 and TLR4 increase IL-1β and IL-18-associated myocarditis and Coxsackievirus replication. J. Immunol. 170, 4731.
Results reveal a mechanism where LPS, TNF-α and IL-1β can lead to increased myocarditis following CB3 infection. Here IL-12p70 and a Th1 response are primarily important in producing IFN-γ to protect against viral infection, but are not directly responsible for inflammation of the heart.

Fearon, D.T., Lockley, R.M. 1996. The instructive role of innate immunity in the acquired immune response. Science 272, 50.

Fong, I.W. 2003. New insights and updates for established entities. In: I.W. Fong (Ed.), Infections and the Cardiovascular System: New Perspectives. Kluwer Academic/Plenum Publishers, New York, p. 20.

Forbes, B.A. 1989. Acquisition of cytomegalovirus infection: an update. Clin. Micro. Rev. 2, 204.

Friman, G., Fohlman, J. 1997. Infectious myocarditis and dilated cardiomyopathy. Cur. Opin. Infect. Dis. 10, 202.

Fujioka, S., Koide, H., Kitaura, Y., et al. 1996. Molecular detection and differentiation of enteroviruses in endomyocardial biopsies and pericardial effusions form dilated cardiomyopathy and myocarditis. Am. Heart J. 131, 760.

Godeny, E.K., Gauntt, C.J. 1986. Involvement of natural killer cells in Coxsackievirus B3-induced murine myocarditis. J. Immunol. 137, 1695.

Godeny, E.K., Gauntt, C.J. 1987a. Murine natural killer cells limit Coxsackievirus B3 replication. J. Immunol. 139, 913.

Godeny, E.K., Gauntt, C.J. 1987b. In situ immune autoradiographic identification of cells in heart tissues of mice with Coxsackievirus B3-induced myocarditis. Am. J. Pathol. 129, 267.

Gor, D.O., Rose, N.R., Greenspan, N.S. 2003. Th1–Th2: a procrustean paradigm. Nat. Immunol. 4, 503.
A commentary on recent findings in experimental models of autoimmunity that indicate that many diseases are a mix of Th1 and Th2 responses.

Gore, I., Saphir, O. 1947. Myocarditis: a classification of 1402 cases. Am. Heart J. 34, 827.

Gravanis, M.G., Sternby, N.H. 1991. Incidence of myocarditis. Arch. Pathol. Lab. Med. 15, 309.

Grist, N.R., Reid, D. 1993. Epidemiology of viral infections of the heart. In: J.E. Banatvala (Ed.), Viral Infections of the Heart. Edward Arnold, London, p. 23.

Guthrie, M., Lodge, P.A., Huber, S.A. 1984. Cardiac injury in myocarditis induced by Coxsackievirus group B, type 3 in BALB/c mice is mediated by $Lyt2^+$ cytolytic lymphocytes. Cell. Immunol. 88, 558.

Hashimoto, I., Komatsu, T. 1978. Myocardial changes after infection with Coxsackievirus B3 in nude mice. Br. J. Exp. Pathol. 59, 13.

Henke, A., Huber, S.A., Stelzner, A., et al. 1995. The role of $CD8^+$ T lymphocytes in Coxsackievirus B3-induced myocarditis. J. Virol. 69, 6720.

Hoffmann, J.A., Kafatos, F.C., Janeway, C.A. Jr., et al. 1999. Phylogenetic perspectives in innate immunity. Science 284, 1313.

Horwitz, M.S., La Cava, A., Fine, C., et al. 2000. Pancreatic expression of interferon-γ protects mice from lethal Coxsackievirus B3 infection and subsequent myocarditis. Nat. Med. 6, 693.

An important paper illustrating that cytokines can directly influence the development of myocarditis.

Huber, S.A. 1997. Autoimmunity in myocarditis: relevance of animal models. Clin. Immunol. Immunopathol. 83, 93.

Huber, S.A., Lodge, P.A. 1986. Coxsackievirus B3 myocarditis in mice: evidence for an autoimmune disease. Am. J. Pathol. 122, 284.

Huber, S.A., Job, L.P., Auld, K.R., et al. 1981. Sex-related differences in the rapid production of cytotoxic spleen cells active against infected myofibers during Coxsackievirus B3 infection. J. Immunol. 126, 1336.

Huber, S.A., Polgar, J., Schultheiss, H.-P., et al. 1994. Augmentation of pathogenesis of Coxsackievirus infections in mice by exogenous administration of interleukin-1 and interleukin-2. J. Virol. 68, 195.

Kadowski, N., Antonenko, S., Lau, J.Y.-N., et al. 2000. Natural interferon α/β-producing cells link innate and adaptive immunity. J. Exp. Med. 192, 219.

A study showing that early cytokines produced by cells of the innate immune response following viral infection can directly modulate the adaptive immune response, which has important implications for the development of autoimmune disease.

Kaplan, M.H. 1988. Coxsackievirus infection in children under 3 months of age. In: M. Bendinelli, H. Friedman (Eds.), Coxsackievirus: A General Update. Plenum Press, New York, p. 241.

Kaya, Z., Afanasyeva, M., Wang, Y., et al. 2001. Contribution of the innate immune system to autoimmune myocarditis: a role for complement. Nat. Immunol. 2, 739.

Kaya, Z., Dohmen, K.M., Wang, Y., et al. 2002. Cutting edge: a critical role for IL-10 in induction of nasal tolerance in experimental autoimmune myocarditis. J. Immunol. 168, 1552.

Khatib, R., Chason, J.L., Silberberg, B.K., et al. 1980. Age-dependent pathogenecity of group B Coxsackieviruses in Swiss-Webster mice: infectivity for myocardium and pancreas. J. Infect. Dis. 141, 394.

Kos, F.J., Engelman, E.G. 1996. Immune regulation: a critical link between NK cells and CTLs. Immunol. Today 17, 174.

Kurrer, M.O., Kopf, M., Penninger, J.M., et al. 2002. Cytokines that regulate autoimmune myocarditis. Swiss Med. Wkly, 132, 408.

Kurt-Jones, E.A., Popova, L., Kwinn, L., et al. 2000. Pattern recognition receptors TLR4 and CD14 mediate response to respiratory syncytial virus. Nat. Immunol. 1, 398.

A study revealing that RSV can stimulate TLR4 in addition to LPS. Similar findings have been found for CB3 infection, resulting in modulation of inflammation in the heart.

Lane, J.R., Neumann, D.A., LaFond-Walker, A., et al. 1991. LPS promotes CB3-induced myocarditis in resistant B10.A mice. Cell. Immunol. 136, 219.

The initial study showing that LPS can induce the autoimmune phase of CB3-induced myocarditis in mice that are resistant to the development of chronic heart disease. These findings demonstrate that TLR4 stimulation early after infection, during the innate immune response, can influence the development of autoimmune disease.

Lane, J.R., Neumann, D.A., LaFond-Walker, A., et al. 1992. Interleukin 1 or tumor necrosis factor can promote Coxsackievirus B3-induced myocarditis in resistant B10.A mice. J. Exp. Med. 175, 1123.

These studies demonstrate that TNF-α or IL-1β induced by LPS/TLR4 stimulation following CB3 infection is capable of inducing autoimmune heart disease in resistant mice.

Lankford, C.S.R., Frucht, D.M. 2003. A unique role for IL-23 in promoting cellular immunity. J. Leukoc. Biol. 73, 49.

Lathbury, L.J., Allan, J.E., Shellam, G.R., et al. 1996. Effect of host genotype in determining the relative roles of natural killer cells and T cells in mediating protection against murine cytomegalovirus infection. J. Gen. Virol. 77, 2605.

Lauer, B., Schannwell, M., Kuhl, U., et al. 2000. Antimyosin autoantibodies are associated with deterioration of systolic and diastolic left ventricular function in patients with chronic myocarditis. J. Am. Coll. Cardiol. 35, 11.

Lawson, C.M., O'Donoghue, H., Reed, W.D. 1989. The role of T cells in mouse cytomegalovirus-induced myocarditis. Immunology 67, 132.

Lawson, C.M., O'Donoghue, H., Bartholomaeus, W.M., et al. 1990. Genetic control of mouse cytomegalovirus-induced myocarditis. Immunology 69, 20.

Lawson, C.M., O'Donoghue, H.L., Reed, W.D. 1992. Mouse cytomegalovirus infection induces antibodies that cross-react with virus and cardiac myosin: a model for the study of molecular mimicry in the pathogenesis of viral myocarditis. Immunology 75, 513.

Lawson, C.M., Yeow, W.-S., Lee, C.M., et al. 1997. *In vivo* expression of an interferon-α gene by intramuscular injection of naked DNA. J. Int. Cytokine Res. 17, 255.

Lenzo, J.C., Fairweather, D., Shellam, G.R., et al. 2001. Immunomodulation of murine cytomegalovirus-induced myocarditis in mice treated with lipopolysaccharide and tumor necrosis factor. Cell. Immunol. 213, 52.

This study illustrates that exacerbation of autoimmune heart disease by LPS/TLR4 or TNF-α is a common feature of viral infection, since two completely different viruses (MCMV or CB3) induce similar responses.

Lenzo, J.C., Fairweather, D., Cull, V., et al. 2002. Characterisation of murine cytomegalovirus myocarditis: cellular infiltration of the heart and virus persistence. J. Mol. Cell. Cardiol. 34, 629.

Lodge, P.A., Herzum, M., Olszewski, J., et al. 1987. Coxsackievirus B3 myocarditis: acute and chronic forms of the disease caused by different immunopathogenic mechanisms. Am. J. Pathol. 128, 455.

Ma, X., Trinchieri, G. 2001. Regulation of interleukin-12 production by antigen-presenting cells. Adv. Immunol. 79, 55.

Marboe, C.C., Fenoglio, J.J. 1988. Biopsy diagnosis of myocarditis. In: B.F. Waller (Ed.), Contemporary Issues in Cardiovascular Pathology. F.A. Davis Co., Philadelphia, p. 137.

Mattner, F., Fischer, S., Guckes, S., et al. 1993. The interleukin-12 subunit p40 specifically inhibits effects of the interleukin-12 heterodimer. Eur. J. Immunol. 23, 2202.

Moser, M., Murphy, K.M. 2000. Dendritic cell regulation of Th1–Th2 development. Nat. Immunol. 1, 199.

Nakanishi, K., Yoshimoto, T., Tsutsui, H., et al. 2001. Interleukin-18 regulates both Th1 and Th2 responses. Annu. Rev. Immunol. 19, 423.

Nelms, K., Keegan, A.D., Zamorano, J., et al. 1999. The IL-4 receptor: signaling mechanisms and biologic functions. Annu. Rev. Immunol. 17, 701.

Nepom, B.S. 1993. The role of the major histocompatibility complex in autoimmunity. Clin. Immunol. Immunopathol. 67, S50.

Neu, N., Ploier, B. 1991. Experimentally induced autoimmune myocarditis: production of heart myosin-specific autoantibodies within the inflammatory infiltrate. Autoimmunity 8, 317.

Neu, N., Rose, N.R., Beisel, K.W., et al. 1987. Cardiac myosin induces myocarditis in genetically predisposed mice. J. Immunol. 139, 3630.

An initial study showing that cardiac myosin with adjuvant could induce myocarditis in susceptible strains of mice, similar to viral infection.

Neumann, D.A., Lane, J.R., Allen, G.S., et al. 1993. Viral myocarditis leading to cardiomyopathy: do cytokines contribute to pathogenesis? Clin. Immunol. Immunopathol. 68, 181.

O'Garra, A. 1998. Cytokines induce the development of functionally heterogeneous T helper cell subsets. Immunity 8, 275.

O'Neill, L.A.J., Dinarello, C.A. 2000. The IL-1 receptor/toll-like receptor superfamily: crucial receptors for inflammation and host defense. Immunol. Today 21, 206.

Oppmann, B., Lesley, R., Blom, B., et al. 2000. Novel p19 protein engages IL-12p40 to form a cytokine, IL-23, with biological activities similar as well as distinct from IL-12. Immunity 13, 715.

Parham, C., Chirica, M., Timans, J., et al. 2002. A receptor for the heterodimeric cytokine IL-23 is composed of IL-12Rβ1 and a novel cytokine receptor subunit, IL-23R. J. Immunol. 168, 5699.

Parish, C.R., O'Neill, E.R. 1997. Dependence of the adaptive immune response on innate immunity: some questions answered but new paradoxes emerge. Immunol. Cell Biol. 75, 523.

Penninger, J.M., Neu, N., Timms, E., et al. 1993. The induction of experimental autoimmune myocarditis in mice lacking CD4 or CD8 molecules. J. Exp. Med. 178, 1837.

Penninger, J.M., Pummerer, C., Liu, P., et al. 1997. Cellular and molecular mechanisms of murine autoimmune myocarditis. APMIS 105, 1.

Peters, N.S., Poole-Wilson, P.A. 1991. Myocarditis—a controversial disease. J. R. Soc. Med. 84, 1.

Pirhonen, J., Matikainen, S., Julkunen, I. 2002. Regulation of virus-induced IL-12 and IL-23 expression in human macrophages. J. Immunol. 169, 5673.

Pummerer, C., Berger, P., Fruhwirth, M., et al. 1991. Cellular infiltrate, major histocompatibility antigen expression and immunopathogenic mechanisms in cardiac myosin-induced myocarditis. Lab. Invest. 65, 538.

Pummerer, C., Grassl, G., Neu, N. 1995. Cellular immune mechanisms in myosin-induced myocarditis. Eur. Heart J. 16 (Suppl. O), 71.

Rose, N.R. 1996. Myocarditis—from infection to autoimmunity. Immunologist 4, 67.

Rose, N.R. 2002. Mechanisms of autoimmunity. Semin. Liver Dis. 22, 387.

Rose, N.R., Afanasyeva, M. 2003. From infection to autoimmunity: the adjuvant effect. ASM News 69, 132.

Rose, N.R., Neumann, D.A., Herskowitz, A. 1988. Genetics of susceptibility to viral myocarditis in mice. Pathol. Immunopathol. Res. 7, 266.

Scalzo, A.A., Lyons, P.A., Fitzgerald, N.A., et al. 1995. The BALB.B6-*Cmv1*^{r} mouse: a strain congenic for *Cmv1* and the NK gene complex. Immunogenetics 41, 148.

Schoen, F.J. 1999. The heart. In: R.S. Cotran, V. Kumar, T. Collins (Eds.), Robbins Pathologic Basis of Disease. W.B. Saunders Co., Philadelphia, p. 544.

Schwimmbeck, P.L., Huber, S.A., Schultheiss, H.-P. 1997. The role of T cells in Coxsackie B-induced disease. In: S. Tracy, N.M. Chapman, B.W.J. Mahy (Eds.), The Coxsackie B Viruses. Springer, Berlin, p. 283.

Seder, R.A., Gazzinelli, R.T. 1999. Cytokines are critical in linking the innate and adaptive immune responses to bacteria, fungal, and parasitic infection. Adv. Intern. Med. 44, 353.

Smith, S.C., Allen, P.M. 1991. Myosin-induced acute myocarditis is a T cell mediated disease. J. Immunol. 147, 2141.

Smith, S.C., Allen, P.M. 1992a. Expression of myosin-class II major histocompatibility complexes in the normal myocardium occurs before induction of autoimmune myocarditis. Proc. Natl Acad. Sci. USA 89, 9131.

Smith, S.C., Allen, P.M. 1992b. Neutralization of endogenous tumor necrosis factor ameliorates the severity of myosin-induced myocarditis. Circ. Res. 70, 856.

This study shows that TNF-α is also critical for the development of myocarditis in the cardiac myosin-induced model, similar to its role in virally induced disease.

Smith, S.C., Allen, P.M. 1993. The role of T cells in myosin-induced autoimmune myocarditis. Clin. Immunol. Immunopathol. 68, 100.

Tay, C.H., Szomolanyi-tsuda, E., Welsh, R.M. 1998. Control of infections by NK cells. In: K. Karre, M. Colonna (Eds.), Current Topics in Microbiology and Immunology: Specificity, Function and Development of NK Cells. Springer, Berlin, p. 193.

Todd, J.A., Acha-Orbea, H., Bell, J.I., et al. 1988. A molecular basis for MHC class II-associated autoimmunity. Science 240, 124.

Wang, Y., Afanasyeva, M., Hill, S.L., et al. 1999. Characterization of murine autoimmune myocarditis induced by self and foreign cardiac myosin. Autoimmunity 31, 151.

Watford, W.T., O'Shea, J.J. 2003. A case of mistaken identity. Nature 421, 706.

Wiekowski, M.T., Leach, M.W., Evans, E.W., et al. 2001. Ubiquitous transgenic expression of the IL-23 subunit p19 induces multiorgan inflammation, runting, infertility, and premature death. J. Immunol. 166, 7563.

Wolfgram, L.J., Beisel, K.W., Herskowitz, A., Rose, N.R. 1986. Variations in the susceptibility to Coxsactievirus B3-induced myocarditis among different strains of mice. J. Immunol. 136, 1846.

Woodruff, J.F., Woodruff, J.J. 1974. Involvement of T lymphocytes in the pathogenesis of Coxsackievirus B3 heart disease. J. Immunol. 113, 1726.

One of the earliest studies showing that CB3-induced myocarditis is driven by a cellular immune response to infection.

Yeow, W.-S., Lawson, C.M., Beilharz, M.W. 1998. Antiviral activities of individual murine IFN-α subtypes in vivo: intramuscular injection of IFN expression contructs reduces cytomegalovirus replication. J. Immunol. 160, 2932.

Yoshimoto, T., Takeda, K., Tanaka, T., et al. 1998. IL-12 up-regulates IL-18 receptor expression on T cells, Th1 cells and B cells: synergism with IL-18 for IFN-γ production. J. Immunol. 161, 3400.

Zhang, G.-X., Gran, B., Yu, S., et al. 2003. Induction of experimental autoimmune encephalomyelitis in IL-12 receptor-β2-deficient mice: IL-12 responsiveness is not required in the pathogenesis of inflammatory demyelination in the central nervous system. J. Immunol. 170, 2153.

Handbook of Systemic Autoimmune Diseases, Volume 1
The Heart in Systemic Autoimmune Diseases
A. Doria and P. Pauletto, editors

CHAPTER 2

Organ-Specific Autoimmunity Involvement in Cardiovascular Disease

Alida L.P. Caforio*[,a], Francesco Tona[a], William J. McKenna[b]

[a]*Division of Cardiology, Department of Experimental and Clinical Medicine, Centro 'V. Gallucci', University of Padova-Policlinico, Via Giustiniani, 2, 35128 Padova, Italy*

[b]*The Heart Hospital, London, UK*

1. Introduction

Autoimmune disease occurs as a result of the loss of tolerance to self-antigens, which under physiological conditions is maintained. To be classified as autoimmune in nature a disease must fulfill at least two of the major criteria first proposed by Witebsky and later modified by Rose (Witebsky et al., 1957; Rose and Bona, 1993). There are also minor criteria, some of which are common to all autoimmune conditions, and others that are found in just a few of them. These criteria are summarized in Table 1.

Autoimmune disease is characterized by the presence of circulating autoantibodies, which are not always pathogenic but represent markers of ongoing tissue damage. In nonorgan-specific autoimmune disease, the autoantibodies are against ubiquitous autoantigens (e.g. nuclear antigens in systemic lupus erythematosus) and tissue damage is generalized. In organ-specific autoimmune disease, immunopathology is restricted to one organ or apparatus within the body, and the autoimmune process, antibody and/or cell-mediated, is directed against autoantigens, which are unique to the affected organ (e.g. thyroid peroxidase in Hashimoto's thyroiditis). The histological hallmark of organ-specific autoimmunity is an early mononuclear cell infiltrate in the affected organ, e.g. insulitis in type 1 insulin-dependent diabetes mellitus (IDDM), with inappropriate expression of HLA class II and adhesion molecules. At a later stage, inflammatory cells tend to disappear and the tissue undergoes profound fibrotic changes with ultimate atrophy and organ dysfunction (such as in Hashimoto's thyroiditis). However, in other instances organ-specific autoimmunity may lead to enhanced target organ function (e.g. Basedow's disease).

Organ-specific autoimmune diseases occur as a result of genetic predisposition and environmental influences. The genetic predisposition accounts for the fact that different autoimmune conditions may be associated in patients or their family members, as well as for the well-known feature that single autoimmune diseases often run in families. The inheritance of susceptibility is usually polygenic. Organ-specific autoimmune diseases are commonly associated with specific HLA class II antigens, but the precise mechanisms by which HLA may operate in determining disease predisposition are still undefined. The majority of organ-specific autoimmune diseases are chronic and apparently 'idiopathic'. Organ- and disease-specific antibodies are found in the affected patients. These antibodies are also detected in family members even years before the development of disease, and thus identify asymptomatic relatives at risk (Bottazzo et al., 1986). Involvement

* Corresponding author.
E-mail address: alida.caforio@unipd.it (A.L.P. Caforio).

DOI: 10.1016/S1571-5078(03)01002-X

Table 1
Criteria of autoimmune disease

Major
Mononuclear cell infiltration and abnormal HLA expression in the target organ (organ-specific disease) or in various organs (nonorgan-specific disease)
Circulating autoantibodies and/or autoreactive lymphocytes in patients and unaffected family members
Detection of autoantibody and/or autoreactive lymphocytes in situ within the affected tissue
Identification and isolation of autoantigen(s) involved
Disease induced in animal models following immunization with relevant autoantigen and/or passive transfer of serum, purified autoantibody and/or lymphocytes
Efficacy of immunosuppressive therapy
Minor
Common to all autoimmune disorders
Middle-aged women most frequently affected
Familial aggregation
HLA association
Hypergammaglobulinemia
Clinical course characterized by exacerbations and remissions
Autoimmune diseases associated in the same patient or family members
Peculiar of organ-specific autoimmune disorders
Presence of autoantigens at low concentration
Autoantibodies directly against organ-specific autoantigens
Immunopathology mediated by type II, IV, V, VI reactions

of organ-specific autoimmunity has been suspected in the following cardiovascular diseases: the post-pericardiotomy and post-myocardial infarction (Dressler) syndromes, rheumatic carditis, idiopathic forms of inflammatory cardiomyopathy and of brady or tachyarrhythmias, systemic arterial hypertension.

2. Post-myocardial infarction (Dressler's) syndrome

Post-myocardial infarction (Dressler) pericarditis may occur in 1–4% of patients at 2–4 weeks following an acute myocardial infarction (Dressler, 1956, 1959; Van der Geld, 1964). Clinical features include: (1) fever; (2) chest pain, that is often localized to retrosternal and left precordial regions with radiation to the trapezius ridge and neck, or the left arm, sharp or dull in quality, increased by deep inspiration, coughing and recumbence, relieved by sitting up and leaning forward, lasting few days to several weeks; (3) dyspnea of variable extent (mild or severe in the presence of tamponade) and nonproductive cough; (4) pericardial friction rub, of variable intensity in relation to patient posture and pressure of the stethoscope, best heard during inspiration and full expiration with the patient sitting up and leaning forward; and (5) leukocytosis and increased erythrocyte sedimentation rate. Pericardial effusion may be present, and is associated with pleural effusion in 70% of the cases of Dressler's syndrome. Less than one-third of patients with Dressler's syndrome develop pneumonitis, usually at the lung basis. The disease is often self-limiting, but can relapse in the following 28 months.

2.1. Anti-heart autoantibodies

Back in 1960, it was demonstrated that in the first 2 weeks following experimentally induced myocardial infarction, rabbits developed circulating anti-heart autoantibodies (Kleinsorge et al., 1960). Subsequently, anti-heart autoantibodies were found using complement fixation test (CFT) or standard indirect immunofluorescence (s-I IFL) in 43–56% of post-myocardial infarction patients with Dressler's syndrome and in 10% of those with uncomplicated disease course (Van der Geld, 1964). Antibody titers were reported to reach their highest peak at 4 weeks post-myocardial infarction, with subsequent slow reduction (Itoh et al., 1969). These antibodies were also detected in patients with coronary artery disease without recent myocardial infarction episodes, with variable frequencies, depending upon patient selection criteria and the technique used (Kaplan et al., 1961; Hess et al., 1964; Heine et al., 1966; Bauer et al., 1972; Nicholson et al., 1977; Caforio et al., 1990a). Anti-heart autoantibody frequencies in cardiovascular disease, including ischemic heart disease, are summarized in Tables 2 and 3.

Two studies emphasized that comparative evaluation of the anti-heart antibody results in various cardiac diseases, particularly in relation to the autoantibody patterns observed by s-I IFL, is difficult (Nicholson et al., 1977; Caforio et al., 1990a). In fact, different substrates (e.g. human adult, human neonatal or rat myocardium) were used and there is no

Table 2
Anti-heart autoantibody specificities in miscellaneous cardiac and noncardiac conditions

Autoantibody (Ab)	Disease: Ab positive %	Technique	Autoantigen (s)
Anti-heart (AHA), skeletal muscle cross-reactive or not tested	Dressler's syndrome: 43–56%	s-I IFL, CFT	Sarcolemma, sarcoplasm, myofibrils
	PPS: 73–100%	s-I IFL	Sarcolemma, sarcoplasm, myofibrils
	Rheumatic fever: inactive 12–21%; active 25–87%; carditis 47%	s-I IFL	Sarcolemma, sarcoplasm, myofibrils
Organ-specific AHA	APE: 17% DCM relatives: 30%	s-I IFL + absor, s-I IFL, ELISA	Sarcoplasm, α and β MHC
Anti-cardiac conducting tissue (CCTA)	Idiopathic CD: 9–34% Nonidiopathic CD: 4–30% RBBB + RA: 76%; RA: 20% Collagenopathy + CD: 14–21%; N: 4–11%	s-I IFL on ox heart false tendon	Purkinje fibers
Anti-β_1 adrenoceptor, stimulating	CD: 28.5%; VA: 47.6% AA: 13.6%; N: 19%	ELISA	β_1 adrenoceptor
Anti-β_2 adrenoceptor, stimulating	CD: 14.3%; VA: 23.8% AA: 4.5%; N: 14.7%	ELISA	β_2 adrenoceptor
Anti-α_1 adrenoceptor, stimulating	I mHTN: 20%; II mHTN: 64%; N: 12% I HTN: 44%, N:12%	ELISA Bioassay	α_1 adrenoceptor
Anti-angiotensin (AT1) receptor, stimulating	I mHTN: 14%; II mHTN: 33%; N: 14% II HTN: 18%	ELISA Bioassay	AT1 receptor

absor, absorption; AA, primary atrial arrhythmias; CD, conduction disturbances; CFT, complement fixation test; N, normal subjects; APE, autoimmune polyendocrinopathy; PPS, post-cardiotomy syndrome; VA, ventricular arrhythmias; I mHTN, primary malignant hypertension; II mHTN, secondary malignant hypertension; I HTN, primary HTN; other abbreviations as in text.

Table 3
Frequency of heart autoantibodies in acute myocarditis and DCM

Antibody type	Method	% Antibody positive				Reference
		AM	DCM	OCD	Normals	
Muscle-specific						
ASA	s-I IFL	47*	10	NT	25	Maisch et al. (1983a,b)
AMLA	AMC	41*	9	NT	12	Maisch et al. (1983a,b)
AFA	s-I IFL	28*	24*	NT	6	Maisch et al. (1983a,b)
IFA	s-I IFL	32*	41*	NT	3	Maisch et al. (1983a,b)
Heart-reactive	s-I IFL	59*	20*	NT	0	Neumann et al. (1990)
	s-I IFL	NT	12–28	21–33	4	Fletcher and Wenger (1968), Camp et al. (1969), Kirsner et al. (1973)
Anti-SNa/K-ATPase	ELISA + Western blot	NT	26*	NT	2	Baba et al. (2002)
Organ-specific cardiac	s-I IFL + abs	34*,**	26*,**	1	3	Caforio et al. (1990a, 1997a,b)
Anti-mitochondrial						
M7	ELISA	13*	31*	10	0	Klein et al. (1984)
ANT	SPRIA	91*,**	57*,**	0	0	Schultheiss and Bolte (1985), Schultheiss et al. (1990)
BCKD-E2	ELISA	100*,**	60*,**	4	0	Ansari et al. (1994)
Anti-laminin	ELISA	73	78	25–35	6	Wolff et al. (1989)
Anti-β1 receptor						
Inhibiting	LBI	NT	30–75*,**	37	18	Limas et al. (1989), Limas and Limas (1991)
Inhibiting	ELISA	NT	31*,**	0	12	Magnusson et al. (1990, 1994)
Stimulating	Bioassay	96*,**	95*,**	8	0	Wallukat et al. (1991)
	ELISA	NT	38**	6	19	Chiale et al. (1995)
	ELISA	NT	26*,**	10	1	Jahns et al. (1999)
Anti-M2 receptor	ELISA	NT	39*	NT	7.5	Fu et al. (1993)
Anti-α and β MHC	Western blot	NT	46*,**	8	0	Caforio et al. (1992)
Anti-MLC 1v	Western blot	NT	35	25	15	Caforio et al. (1992)
Nonmyofibrillar	Western blot	NT	46*,**	17	0	Caforio et al. (1992)
Anti-MHC	Western blot	NT	67**	42	NT	Latif et al. (1993)
Anti-MLC 1	Western blot	NT	17**	0	NT	Latif et al. (1993)
Anti-tropomyosin	Western blot	NT	55**	21	NT	Latif et al. (1993)
Anti-actin	Western blot	NT	71**	21	NT	Latif et al. (1993)
Anti-HSP-60	Western blot	NT	85**	42	NT	Latif et al. (1993)
Anti-HSP-60, 70	Western blot	NT	10–14**	1–2	3	Portig et al. (1997)
Anti-β MHC	ELISA	37*,**	44*,**	16	2.5	Lauer et al. (1994)
Anti-α MHC	ELISA	17*,**	20*,**	4	2	Goldman et al. (1995), Caforio et al. (1997a,b)

*$p < 0.05$ vs. normals; **$p < 0.05$ vs. OCD. +abs, +absorption; AFA, anti-fibrillary antibody; AM, acute myocarditis; AMC, antibody-mediated cytotoxicity; AMLA, anti-myolemmal antibody; ASA, anti-sarcolemmal antibody; IFA, anti-interfibrillary; NT, not tested; OCD, other cardiac disease; LBI, ligand binding inhibition; other abbreviations as in Table 2 and text.

standardized nomenclature for the anti-heart antibody patterns. In addition, some but not all workers tested sera on both skeletal muscle and myocardium; therefore, several studies did not differentiate between organ-specific cardiac and muscle-specific (e.g. cardiac and skeletal muscle reactive) antibody. Taking into account these limitations, the anti-heart antibody patterns seen in ischemic heart disease, with or without Dressler's syndrome, were described as

(1) more pronounced peripheral sarcoplasmic stain on human or rat heart, with progressive increase of the IFL from the center to the periphery of myofibers, but without clear-cut linear sarcolemmal stain (pattern defined as 'sarcolemmal', 'subsarcolemmal-sarcoplasmic', 'sarcolemmal-subsarcolemmal' or 'peripheral');
(2) diffuse sarcoplasmic stain, without a tendency to peripheral enhancement (pattern defined as 'diffuse-sarcoplasmic' or 'diffuse';
(3) longitudinal intermyofibrillar sarcoplasmic stain, perpendicular to myofibrillar striations (pattern defined as 'intermyofibrillar');
(4) patterns defined as combinations of those detailed above, or with superimposed striated IFL (pattern defined as 'striated' or 'anti-fibrillary');
(5) stain of the intercalated disks, isolated or in association with sarcolemmal and/or sarcoplasmic IFL (pattern defined as 'anti-intercalated disks').

3. Post-pericardiotomy syndrome

Post-pericardiotomy syndrome and pericarditis may occur at 2–4 weeks following heart surgery operations that require opening of the pericardium. In the 1950s–1970s, it could be observed in up to 40% of the patients, but nowadays it is rare. It is characterized by fever, pericardial or pleuropericardial effusion, chest pain and pericardial rub; it may relapse (Van der Geld, 1964; Engle et al., 1974). An identical clinical syndrome has been described after cardiac perforation following pacemaker implantation, blunt chest trauma, percutaneous diagnostic left ventricular puncture and coronary perforation due to balloon angioplasty (Peters et al., 1980; Escaned et al., 1992).

3.1. Anti-heart autoantibodies

Anti-heart autoantibodies, giving staining patterns similar to those described in Dressler's syndrome and cross-reacting with skeletal muscle, were found in 73–100% of patients with post-pericardiotomy syndrome (Table 2). There was significant correlation between autoantibody titer and severity of symptoms; in addition, the antibodies were undetectable in quiescent intervals between attacks and were again detected during symptomatic recurrent episodes, suggesting a potential pathogenic role (Van der Geld, 1964; Zabriskie et al., 1970; Engle et al., 1974). In a later study, the antibodies were detected in 95% of patients with full clinical criteria, in 72% of those with only some typical clinical features and in 29% of control subjects who had undergone cardiac surgery without developing symptoms of post-pericardiotomy syndrome (Maisch et al., 1979).

4. Rheumatic carditis

Rheumatic fever is an inflammatory multisystem disease, occurring few weeks to 6 months following group A streptococcal (GAS) infection of the tonsillopharynx. Its diagnosis is based upon Jones' criteria (Jones, 1944), which were recently updated (Dajani et al., 1992).

Major criteria include

(1) carditis;
(2) polyarthritis;
(3) chorea;
(4) erythema marginatum;
(5) subcutaneous nodules.

Minor criteria are represented by

(1) fever;
(2) arthralgia;
(3) elevated erythrocyte sedimentation rate or C-reactive protein;

(4) prolonged P-R interval on standard 12-lead surface electrocardiogram (ECG).

If supported by evidence of GAS, e.g. positive throat culture or rapid streptococcal antigen test, elevated or rising streptococcal antibody titer, the presence of two major criteria (or one major and two minor) indicates a high probability of acute rheumatic fever.

The diagnosis of cardiac involvement during acute rheumatic fever is based upon unequivocal fulfillment of any of the following criteria:

(1) new onset of nonfunctional cardiac murmurs;
(2) cardiac enlargement;
(3) sign and symptoms of heart failure;
(4) pericardial friction rubs or accumulation of pericardial fluid.

4.1. Immune pathogenesis of rheumatic carditis

Rheumatic carditis is thought to represent an autoimmune disorder triggered by streptococcal infection via molecular mimicry. Indeed streptococci and heart tissue have several antigenic components for which molecular mimicry has been documented (Robinson and Kehoe, 1992). During rheumatic fever, patients produce both anti-streptococcal antibodies and anti-heart autoantibodies, since rheumatogenic streptococci and heart tissue have shared antigens.

4.1.1. Anti-streptococcus antibodies

The external parietal layer of GAS contains distinct M protein types in different strains. More than 80 M protein types are known. M proteins of rheumatogenic streptococci share a long terminal antigen domain (Bessen et al., 1989) and contain epitopes that are shared with human heart tissue, particularly sarcolemmal membrane proteins, cardiac myosin and tropomyosin, as well as with skeletal muscle and smooth muscle, renal glomerular basement membrane (Krisher and Cunningham, 1985; Dale and Beachey, 1986). In addition, shared epitopes have been reported between *N*-acetyl-glucosamine of the mid parietal streptococcus cell layer and glycoproteins of mammalian cardiac valve tissue, and another cross-reaction has been found between streptococcal hyaluronate and protein polysaccharide of mammalian cartilage (Robinson and Kehoe, 1992). In addition, anti-streptococcal antibodies, cross-reactive with heart antigens and thalamus and subthalamus components, have been found in some patients with carditis and chorea (reviewed by Kaplan and Frengley, 1969). The heart cross-reactive anti-streptococcal antibodies, identified by a combination of immunofluorescent and precipitin-absorption techniques, were present in 55 and 58% of patients with active and inactive rheumatic heart disease, respectively, or with acute glomerulonephritis in 24% of patients with recent streptococcal infection and only rarely (2%) in disease controls without rheumatic heart disease or previous streptococcal infection, but the pathogenetic significance of these antibodies remained to be evaluated (Kaplan and Svec, 1964).

4.1.2. Anti-heart autoantibodies

Several methods were used, in the earliest studies, for detection of circulating anti-heart autoantibodies in rheumatic fever. These (reviewed by Kaplan and Frengley, 1969) were later abandoned and included: agglutination tests with collodion particles coated with saline extracts of the heart and other organs, CFT with saline extracts of the heart, liver and spleen, tanned red cell hemagglutination test and antiglobulin consumption with heart homogenate. Subsequently, s-I IFL on cryostat-cut sections became the method of choice; however, tissue substrates were various and included: human or rat myocardium (Van der Geld, 1964), normal human myocardium obtained at autopsy or surgery in subjects with congenital heart defects (Zabriskie et al., 1970; Engle et al., 1974), normal human myocardium of O blood group, obtained at surgery in subjects with congenital heart defects (Maisch et al., 1979). Cryostat-cut sections were fixed in acetone (Zabriskie et al., 1970) or unfixed (Engle et al., 1974; Van der Geld, 1964) and then incubated with serum diluted at 1:5 (Zabriskie et al., 1970; Engle et al., 1974) or undiluted (Van der Geld, 1964); sections were washed in PBS and then the autoantibody binding was revealed with fluoresceinated serum anti-human IgG. In a more recent study, patient serum, at 1:10 dilution, was incubated on unfixed cryostat-cut sections and after washing the section was stained with fluoresceinated serum anti-human IgG, -IgA or -IgM (Maisch et al., 1979). Clearly, the lack of a standard s-I IFL protocol makes it difficult to compare results from different studies, particularly in terms of anti-heart antibody frequency.

Taking into account such limitations, circulating anti-heart autoantibodies have been found, using s-I IFL, in sera from 25–87% of patients with active rheumatic fever, 12–21% of those with inactive rheumatic disease and 0–4% of normal subjects (Kaplan et al., 1961; Kaplan and Dallenbach, 1961; Hess et al., 1964; Zitnan and Bosmanski, 1966) (Table 2). In another study, these have been detected in 81% of patients with streptococcal infection, 80% of those with post-streptococcal nephritis, 87% with acute rheumatic fever, 47% with rheumatic carditis, 100% with post-cardiotomy syndrome and in none of the control subjects (Zabriskie et al., 1970) (Table 2). The autoantibody patterns observed in rheumatic disease were similar to those described in Dressler's and post-pericardiotomy syndromes, but the 'sarcolemmal-sarcoplasmic' or 'peripheral' pattern was found more frequently than the 'diffuse' stain (Nicholson et al., 1977). In rheumatic carditis, anti-conductive tissue antibodies were also reported (see Section 6.1) (Ledford and Espinoza, 1987). The anti-heart autoantibodies from rheumatic sera could be absorbed out by streptococcal membranes as well as myocardial extracts; conversely, those found in post-pericardiotomy sera reacted exclusively with myocardial extracts, suggesting that the antigenic determinants were different in the two cardiac conditions (Zabriskie et al., 1970). In terms of relations of anti-heart autoantibodies to clinical activity of rheumatic disease, as pointed out by the first investigators in this field (Kaplan and Frengley, 1969), overall the frequency of anti-heart antibodies was higher in clinically active than in clinically inactive disease, in patients with carditis than without and in those with a higher number of previous attacks of rheumatic fever (Hess et al., 1964; Zitnan and Bosmanski, 1966). The titer of autoantibodies in some patients correlated with clinical severity or grade of rheumatic activity, and was occasionally reported to be a useful tool in differential diagnosis from other infections or inflammatory conditions (Felsh, 1966). As far as the time course of antibody production is concerned, using s-I IFL or anti-globulin consumption tests, it was shown that anti-heart antibody was detected in some patients before and, in other patients, after the onset of clinical symptoms of rheumatic fever (Hess et al., 1964; Zabriskie, 1967). In the majority of cases, antibody was first detected within the first week of symptom onset, thereafter it rose to maximal titer. Subsequently, antibody titer declined, in some cases rapidly, possibly in relation to steroid treatment; in other cases, a more variable or slower pattern of decay was documented with persistence of low titer antibody up to 2–3 years after an attack of rheumatic fever (Zabriskie, 1967). On the other hand, autoantibodies not detected using s-I IFL or anti-globulin consumption, and directed against aqueous and alcoholic heart tissue extracts, seemed unrelated to clinical findings, suggesting that some but not all antibody specificities produced in rheumatic heart disease may be relevant to pathogenesis (Kaplan and Frengley, 1969). Bound immunoglobulin G and complement were also identified within the myocardial as well as pericardial and valvular tissues in post-mortem rheumatic hearts and surgical specimens of auricular appendages from patients with rheumatic heart disease (Kaplan and Dallenbach, 1961; Kaplan et al., 1964).

5. Dilated cardiomyopathy and myocarditis

Dilated cardiomyopathy (DCM) is a relevant cause of heart failure and a common indication for heart transplantation. According to the current WHO classification of cardiomyopathies, DCM is characterized by dilatation and impaired contraction of the left or both ventricles; it may be idiopathic, familial/genetic, viral and/or immune (Richardson et al., 1996). Clinical onset is generally with symptoms/signs of congestive heart failure, brady/tachyarrhythmia or thromboembolism. In most cases, the duration of the asymptomatic phase is uncertain. Occasionally, DCM may be diagnosed following the detection of an apical systolic murmur of mitral insufficiency, pathologic ECG or enlarged cardiac chambers with systolic dysfunction on echocardiography. DCM is familial in 20–30% of cases, has severe prognosis with 40–50% mortality, because of heart failure or sudden death in 2 years following diagnosis. The diagnosis of DCM requires exclusion of known, specific causes of heart failure, including coronary artery disease. Thus in DCM, coronary angiography is normal; on endomyocardial biopsy there is myocyte loss, compensatory hypertrophy, fibrous tissue and immunohistochemical findings consistent with chronic inflammation (myocarditis) in 30–40% of cases.

Myocarditis is an inflammatory disease of the myocardium, and is diagnosed by endomyocardial biopsy using established histological, immunological and immunohistochemical criteria; it may be idiopathic, infectious or autoimmune and may heal or lead to DCM (Aretz et al., 1985; Richardson et al., 1996; Caforio and McKenna, 1996). The clinical features of myocarditis are quite diverse. Cardiac manifestations may or may not be preceded (1–2 weeks) by a systemic flu-like illness. Myocarditis may be subclinical, causing minor symptoms (palpitation, atypical chest pain), electrocardiographic abnormalities (atrioventricular (AV) conduction disturbance (CD), bundle branch block, ST and T-wave changes) or arrhythmias (paroxysmal atrial fibrillation or ventricular arrhythmias (VAs)) in the absence of demonstrable change in global or regional left or right ventricular function. Pericarditis with or without chest pain, a pericardial effusion or rub commonly coexist with myocarditis. Other presentations of myocarditis include syncope, sudden death, acute right or left ventricular failure, cardiogenic shock or DCM. A syndrome mimicking acute myocardial infarction, but with normal coronary arteries, may also occur.

Prognosis of myocarditis is thought to be good, with complete recovery at least in the majority of patients. However, in neonates and young children, the elderly and the debilitated, the disease is often severe, causing fulminant and fatal heart failure. Relapses may occur, and a proportion of patients will develop residual mild left ventricular dysfunction or DCM. Thus, in a patient subset, myocarditis and DCM are thought to represent the acute and chronic stages of an inflammatory disease of the myocardium, which can be viral, post-infectious immune or primarily organ-specific autoimmune (Caforio, 1994; Richardson et al., 1996; Caforio and McKenna, 1996).

5.1. Immune pathogenesis of myocarditis and dilated cardiomyopathy

Autoimmune features in human myocarditis/DCM include familial aggregation (Baig et al., 1998), a weak association with HLA-DR4 (Anderson et al., 1984), lymph mononuclear cell infiltrate, abnormal expression of HLA class II and adhesion molecules on cardiac endothelium, on endomyocardial biopsy, in the affected patients and family members (Caforio et al., 1990b; Caforio and McKenna, 1996; Mahon et al., 2002), increased levels of circulating cytokines and cardiac autoantibodies in patients and family members (reviewed by Caforio et al., 2002), experimental models of both antibody-mediated and cell-mediated autoimmune myocarditis/DCM following immunization with relevant autoantigen(s), the best characterized of which is cardiac myosin (Rose, 2000; Kuan et al., 2000). Here we mainly focus on the circulating cardiac autoantibodies.

5.2. Anti-heart autoantibodies by s-I IFL

Several groups have found antibodies to various cardiac antigens in myocarditis and DCM, but the organ- and disease-specificity of these antibody types have not been always evaluated (reviewed by Caforio et al., 2002). Using s-I IFL, earlier studies identified antibodies to sarcolemmal and myofibrillar antigens, but these were either cross-reactive or untested on skeletal muscle. In addition, it remained unclear whether these antibodies were disease-specific for myocarditis/DCM because controls with other cardiac disease were not always included.

These autoantibodies were found in 12–75% of DCM/myocarditis patients and 4–34% of normal control subjects (Fletcher and Wenger, 1968; Camp et al., 1969; Kirsner et al., 1973; Maisch et al., 1983a, b) (Table 3). The observed antibody patterns were identical to those described in rheumatic heart disease, Dressler and post-pericardiotomy syndromes, the 'diffuse' being more frequent than the 'sarcolemmal-sarcoplasmic' staining pattern. A more recent study on rat heart tissue sections showed high titer ($\geq$1:20) antibodies of IgG class in 59% of patients with myocarditis, 20% of those with DCM and in no normal control subjects; interestingly these authors suggested that the three main antibody patterns ('diffuse', 'peripheral' or 'sarcolemmal' and 'fibrillary' or 'striated') could coexist (Neumann et al., 1990).

Using indirect s-I IFL on 4 μm thick unfixed fresh frozen cryostat sections of blood group O normal human atrium, ventricle and skeletal muscle, and absorption with human heart and skeletal muscle and rat liver, organ-specific antibodies of IgG class were found in about one-third of myocarditis/DCM patients and their symptom-free family members, 1% of patients with other cardiac disease, 3% of normal subjects and 17% of patients without cardiac disease, but with autoimmune polyendocrinopathy (Caforio et al., 1990a, 1991, 1994, 1997a) (Tables 2 and 3). Cardiac antibodies of the cross-reactive 1 type, which exhibited partial organ-specificity for heart antigens by absorption, were also more frequently detected in DCM/myocarditis patients or in patients with autoimmune polyendocrinopathy than in controls. Conversely, cardiac antibodies of the cross-reactive 2 type, which were entirely skeletal muscle cross-reactive by absorption, were found in similar proportions among groups. No patients with Dressler or post-pericardiotomy syndromes or active rheumatic heart disease were included in these studies.

Sera were tested at 1/10 dilution; cardiac antibody titers in all sera classified as positive were determined by doubling dilutions of sera in phosphate-buffered saline solution. Immunoglobulin classes of the antibodies in the positive sera were also assessed using fluorescein isothiocyanate-labeled sheep anti-human IgG, IgM and IgA class-specific anti-sera (Caforio et al., 1990a, 1991, 1997a). The s-I IFL patterns (figures in Caforio et al., 1990a; Betterle et al., 1997) were as follows:

(1) *Organ-specific*. Sera were observed which gave diffuse cytoplasmic staining of both atrial and ventricular myocytes. The staining was stronger in atrial than in ventricular myocytes. These sera were negative on skeletal muscle. The titer range of these antibodies was 1/10 to 1/80 on atrial tissue and 1/10 to 1/20 on ventricular tissue. All positive sera contained antibodies of IgG class and 10% of IgM class. Organ-specific cardiac antibodies' titers fell after absorption with heart homogenate, but were not affected by incubation with skeletal muscle or rat liver.

(2) *Cross-reactive 1* or 'partially organ-specific'. Antibodies which gave a fine striational staining pattern on atrium and to a lesser extent on ventricle, but were negative or only weakly stained skeletal muscle sections were classified as 'cross-reactive 1' or 'partially organ-specific'. Their titers ranged from 1/20 to 1/80 on the atrial substrate and from 1/10 to 1/40 on ventricular tissue. All positive sera contained antibodies of IgG class and a few also contained IgM antibodies. Antibody titers in the sera classified as 'cross-reactive 1' or 'partially organ-specific' were reduced to the same extent after absorption with heart and skeletal muscle, and were not affected by absorption with rat liver.

(3) *Cross-reactive 2*. Antibodies which gave a broad striational pattern on longitudinal sections of heart and skeletal muscle were classified as 'cross-reactive 2'. This pattern had been previously found in 30–40% of sera from myasthenia gravis patients without thymoma and in all myasthenic patients with thymoma (Zweiman and Arnason, 1987). These striational antibodies have been shown to react with the A band of the myofibrils of striated muscle and cross-react with thymus myoepithelial cells. Cardiac antibodies in the sera classified as 'cross-reactive 2' were absorbed by human skeletal muscle and to a lesser extent by heart tissue and not by rat liver.

5.3. Anti-heart autoantibodies by s-I IFL: technical considerations and proposed nomenclature

(1) It is preferable to employ O blood group human heart and skeletal muscle to avoid false positive reactions due to heterophile or anti-ABO antibodies. Testing sera on skeletal muscle is necessary to differentiate heart-specific (organ-specific) from cross-reactive patterns (positive on heart and skeletal muscle), and on rat liver and kidney to detect nonorgan-specific mitochondrial or smooth muscle antibodies, which give false positive 'muscle reactive' IFL (Nicholson et al., 1977; Caforio et al., 1990a; Betterle et al., 1997).

The pattern defined as 'intermyofibrillary') is rather rare and might represent anti-mitochondrial antibodies (Nicholson et al., 1977). A pseudo-sarcolemmal or 'endomysial' interstitial pattern can be observed on some tissue substrates (heart and muscle). It lacks species and tissue-specificity, gives a 'brush border' staining on proximal tubules of rat kidney and represents a false positive reaction (Nicholson et al., 1977; Betterle et al., 1997).

(2) More recent studies suggest that there is no pure 'sarcolemmal' or 'peripheral' pattern; these authors observed that sera giving 'striated' patterns seem to react more intensely with the periphery of the myofiber, if the section does not include longitudinally cut fibers (Nicholson et al., 1977; Neumann et al., 1990; Caforio et al., 1990a; Betterle et al., 1997). It is important that the section includes longitudinally cut fibers, in order to identify 'striated' patterns, not visible on transverse sections.

(3) It is important to use standard positive and negative control sera titrated up to end-dilution in every assay, to minimize inter-assay variability (Caforio et al., 1990a; Betterle et al., 1997).

(4) New potentially organ-specific patterns (positive on heart, negative or weak positive on muscle) should be confirmed as heart-specific by absorption (Caforio et al., 1990a; Betterle et al., 1997).

(5) If absorption is not performed, patterns of anti-heart autoantibodies by s-I IFL should be classified according to those already described and characterized (Nicholson et al., 1977; Caforio et al., 1990a; Betterle et al., 1997), as follows:
   (a) 'diffuse' (also defined 'diffuse-sarcoplasmic' or 'organ-specific);
   (b) 'striated, nonmyasthenic' (also defined 'cross-reactive type 1' or 'partially organ-specific' or 'anti-fibrillary');
   (c) 'striated, myasthenic' (also defined ' cross-reactive type 2');
   (d) 'diffuse/striated, nonmyasthenic', if a 'striated, nonmyasthenic' pattern is superimposed on a diffuse sarcoplasmic stain resulting in a combination of patterns (a) and (b);
   (e) 'anti-intercalated disks', isolated or in combination with diffuse or striated stain;

5.4. Autoantibodies to myosin heavy chain and other autoantigens by immunoblotting techniques

Two of the autoantigens recognized by the cardiac autoantibodies detected by IFL were identified as α and β myosin heavy chain (MHC) isoforms, as well as ventricular light chain type 1 (MLC-1v), by Western blotting; several bands due to yet unknown antigens were also detected in DCM-positive sera (Caforio et al., 1992). These unknown antigens had apparent molecular weight of 30–35 kDa in 50% of positive sera, 55–60 kDa in 21%, 100 kDa in 14% and 130–150 kDa in 14% (Caforio et al., 1992). The β MHC is expressed in slow skeletal and ventricular myosin and is therefore only partially cardiac-specific. The α isoform is expressed solely within the atrial myocardium. Antibodies to this molecule represent truly organ-specific cardiac autoantibodies. The identification of α and β MHC as relevant autoantigens in DCM patients parallels what is seen in the experimental model of autoimmune myocarditis/DCM (Neu et al., 1987; Smith and Allen, 1991) and in human myocarditis (Caforio et al., 1997a,b; Neumann et al., 1990; Lauer et al., 2000). The finding of anti-MHC and MLC-1v antibodies of IgG class in DCM patients has been independently confirmed using Western blotting (Latif et al., 1993) or enzyme-linked immunosorbent assay (ELISA) (Limas et al., 1995; Goldman et al., 1995; Michels et al., 1994); a recent study has suggested that the disease-specific anti-myosin antibodies in DCM sera are mainly of IgG3 subclass (Warraich et al., 1999). By Western blot, antibodies to heat shock protein-60 (HSP-60), tropomyosin and actin have also been found more frequently in DCM sera than in ischemic heart disease controls, but normal sera were not tested (Latif et al., 1993) (Table 3). Portig et al. found antibodies to HSP-60 and -70 at higher frequency in DCM sera than in ischemic or normal control subjects (Table 3). Latif et al. (1994) later developed a microcytotoxicity assay and showed complement-mediated cytotoxic activity of DCM sera containing anti-heart antibodies by Western blot. DCM, ischemic and normal control sera were screened used W1, a transformed human fetal cardiac cell line, and also EA.hy 926, an endothelial and IRB3, a fibroblast cell line. In the presence of complement, sera from 28 (62%) DCM patients showed killing of the W1 cell line as compared to sera from 13 (30%) of ischemic patients ($p < 0.005$) and 3 (15%) normal subjects. Only one DCM patient showed killing of EA.hy 926 cell line, and one ischemic showed killing of the fibroblast cell line. These in vitro data suggest that a complement-dependent, antibody-mediated mechanism of damage to cardiac myocytes may contribute to the pathogenesis of DCM.

5.5. Autoantibodies to sarcolemmal Na-K-ATPase

A recent study, using porcine cerebral cortex Na-K-ATPase as an antigen in ELISA and as a substrate in enzyme activity measurement, tested sera from 100 DCM patients and 100 healthy individuals and found anti-Na-K-ATPase autoantibodies in 26% of DCM and 2% of normal subjects (Baba et al., 2002) (Table 3). Western blots showed that the antibodies recognized the α subunit, and 3H-ouabain bindings in the presence of patient IgG showed that dissociation constant was higher in DCM patients with antibodies than in those without, suggesting biologic activity for the antibody. Preliminary unpublished observations of these authors showed that the antibodies reacted with the α-3 and not the α-1 subunit isoform. By multiple regression analysis, the presence of anti-Na-K-ATPase autoantibodies was an independent predictor for the occurrence of ventricular tachycardia. Cardiac sudden death was independently predicted by the presence of antibodies, as well as poor systolic function. The authors speculated that these antibodies may lead to electrical instability, because of abnormal Ca^{2+} handling by reduced Na-K-ATPase activity, and delayed after-depolarizations via reverse-mode operation of the Na^{+}/Ca^{2+} exchanger, resulting from increased intracellular Na^{+} concentrations. Although this represents a tantalizing hypothesis, no definitive conclusions on the functional role of these antibodies can be drawn at present. It remains to be seen whether these antibodies are disease-specific for DCM, since no controls with heart failure from other etiologies were studied. It is worth noting that sarcolemmal Na-K-ATPase does not seem to fulfill strict criteria of organ-specific cardiac autoantigen: the α-1 subunit isoform is expressed in most tissues, the α-2 is predominant in skeletal muscle and can be detected in brain and heart, the α-3 is found in excitable tissues and the α-4 in testis (Urayama et al., 1989; Muller-Ehmsen et al., 2001). Similarly, the β-1 subunit isoform is fairly ubiquitous, whereas the β-2 and β-3 subunit isoforms are mostly found in skeletal muscle, neural tissues, lung, liver; in human heart, only α-1β-1, α-2β-1, α-3β-1 heterodimers are present, and are thought to be involved in the actions of cardiac glycosides (Schwinger et al., 1999).

5.6. Autoantibodies to mitochondrial and to extracellular matrix antigens

Using ELISA, autoantibodies against laminin, a large basement membrane glycoprotein, were found in 73–78% of myocarditis/DCM patients and 6% of normal subjects; the authors did not include ischemic heart disease controls, but they reported unpublished data indicating 25–35% prevalence in coronary artery disease (Wolff et al., 1989) (Table 3). Antibodies against distinct mitochondrial antigens, the M7 (Klein et al., 1984; Otto et al., 1998), the adenine nucleotide translocator (ANT) (Schultheiss and Bolte, 1985; Schultheiss et al., 1990) and the branched chain α-ketoacid dehydrogenase dihydrolipoyl transacylase (BCKD-E2) (Ansari et al., 1994) and other respiratory chain enzymes (Pohlner et al., 1997) have also been detected. The M7 antibodies, detected by ELISA, were of IgG class and were found in 31% of DCM patients, 13% of those with myocarditis, 33% of controls with hypertrophic cardiomyopathy, but not in control subjects with other cardiac disease, other immune-mediated disorders or in normal subjects (Klein et al., 1984) (Table 3). The test antigen was represented by different subcellular and submitochondrial beef heart preparations; sera were also tested on submitochondrial particles from pig kidney and rat liver. Using an indirect micro solid-phase radioimmunoassay (SPRIA) and ANT, a protein of the internal mitochondrial membrane, purified from beef heart, liver and kidney as antigen, anti-ANT antibodies were found in 57–91% of myocarditis/DCM sera, and in no controls with ischemic heart disease, or in normal subjects (Schultheiss and Bolte, 1985; Schultheiss et al., 1990) (Table 3). Mitochondrial antigens have generally been classified as nonorgan-specific (Bottazzo et al., 1986; Rose and Bona, 1993). However, the heart-specificity of the M7 antibodies was shown by absorption studies, whereas these were not performed with the ANT and the BCKD-E2 antibodies. Experimentally induced affinity-purified anti-ANT antibodies cross-reacted with calcium channel complex proteins of rat cardiac myocytes, induced enhancement of transmembrane calcium current and produced calcium-dependent cell lysis in the absence of complement (Schultheiss et al., 1988, 1990). The authors suggested that such enhancing effect of the antibodies might lead to impaired function of the ANT, imbalance of energy delivery and demand within the myocyte and subsequent cell death in vivo in patients. The presence of this mechanism of antibody-dependent cell lysis has not been shown using the antibodies present in patients' sera.

5.7. Blocking and stimulating autoantibodies to β-adrenergic receptors

Several groups have demonstrated antibodies against the β_1-adrenoceptor (Wallukat et al., 1991; Limas et al., 1989; Limas and Limas, 1991; Magnusson et al., 1990, 1994). Using a binding inhibition assay (inhibition of marked [^{3}H]dihydroalprenolol binding to rat cardiac membranes), a significant inhibitory activity, attributed to anti-β_1-adrenoceptor antibodies of IgG class, was found in 30–75% of DCM sera, 37% of ischemic or valvular heart disease controls and 18% of sera from normal subjects (Limas et al., 1989; Limas and Limas, 1991). Positive DCM sera were also found to immunoprecipitate β-adrenoceptors from solubilized cardiac membranes. Antibody-positive sera induced sequestration and endocytosis of β_1-receptors predominantly dependent on the β-receptor kinase, and selectively inhibited isoproterenol-sensitive adenylate cyclase activity (Limas et al., 1989; Limas and Limas, 1991). Magnusson et al. (1990), using as antigens synthetic peptides analogous to the sequences of the second extracellular loop of β_1- and β_2-adrenergic receptors by ELISA, found antibodies in 31% of DCM patients, 12% of normal subjects and in none of the controls with other cardiac disease. The antibodies from DCM sera exhibited inhibitory activity of isoproterenol binding to the β-adrenergic receptor.

Other studies showed that, when analyzed in a functional test system of spontaneously beating neonatal rat myocytes, antibody-positive DCM sera (Wallukat et al., 1991; Jahns et al., 1999, 2000) or the affinity purified β_1-receptor antibodies (Magnusson et al., 1994) increased the beating frequency of isolated myocytes in vitro. β_1-blocking drugs (propanolol, bisoprolol and metoprolol) inhibited the effect of the antibodies. These workers reported that the stimulating anti-β_1-receptor antibodies were present in 96% of myocarditis and 26–95% of DCM sera, 8–10% of controls with ischemic heart disease and 0–19% of normal subjects (Table 3). They also suggested that this antibody-mediated stimulation of the β_1-receptor, observed in vitro, could occur in vivo and account for the accelerated decline in ventricular systolic function in some myocarditis/DCM patients.

5.8. Autoantibodies to M_2-muscarinic receptors

Fu et al. (1993), using as antigen a synthetic peptide analogous to the 169–193 sequence of the second extracellular loop of human M2-muscarinic receptors and the ELISA method, showed anti-M2 antibodies in 39% of DCM sera and 7% of the normal subjects. The presence of these antibodies correlated with the presence of anti-β-receptor antibodies. A limitation of work involving the anti-receptor antibodies is that few disease controls have been studied. These receptors are not organ-specific cardiac autoantigens; in fact, their distribution is not restricted to the heart, and there are no cardiac-specific isoforms (Elalouf et al., 1993; Eglen et al., 1994).

5.9. Cardiac-specific antibodies in myocarditis/DCM: clinical correlates and potential functional role

The presence of organ- and disease-specific cardiac antibodies of IgG class against myosin and other unknown antigens in myocarditis/DCM patients supports the involvement of autoimmunity in at least one-third of patients (Caforio et al., 1990a; Neumann et al., 1990; Latif et al., 1993; Michels et al., 1994).

These antibodies were associated with shorter duration and minor severity of symptoms at diagnosis, as well as with greater exercise capacity (Caforio et al., 1990a, 1997b, 2001). In many patients who were antibody positive at diagnosis, these markers became undetectable at follow-up (Caforio et al., 1997b). These findings strongly suggest that cardiac-specific autoantibodies are early markers. The absence of antibodies at diagnosis in a proportion of patients could indicate that cell-mediated mechanisms are predominant, and/or that autoimmunity is not involved; since the pre-clinical stage in DCM may be prolonged, it might also relate to reduction of antibody levels with disease progression (Caforio et al., 1997b). These findings have been obtained using standard autoimmune serology techniques, in particular s-I IFL, ELISA and immunoblotting, and confirmed by several groups (Neumann et al., 1990; Latif et al., 1993; Michels et al., 1994; Limas et al., 1995). The low frequency of cardiac-specific antibodies in control patients with heart dysfunction not due to myocarditis/DCM (Caforio et al., 1990a; Caforio, 1994; Goldman et al., 1995) and the decrease in antibody titers in advanced DCM (Caforio et al., 1997b, 2001) suggest that these markers are not epiphenomena associated with tissue necrosis of various causes, but represent specific markers of immune pathogenesis. The role of inflammatory cytokines (e.g. the IL-2/sIL-2R system) as markers of T-lymphocyte activation in immune-mediated myocarditis/DCM and its relation to cardiac autoantibodies is a controversial issue (Limas et al., 1995; Caforio et al., 2001). In particular Limas et al. (1995) found that high titer anti-β_1-receptor antibodies were more common among DCM patients with abnormal sIL-2R serum levels. Others found no association between the cardiac-specific autoantibodies found by IFL and the anti-α-myosin antibodies detected by ELISA and sIL-2R levels (Caforio et al., 2001). sIL-2R may be related with distinct autoantibody specificities, e.g. in Graves' disease high sIL-2R was associated with anti-TSH receptor autoantibodies but was unrelated to the autoantibodies to intracellular antigens (anti-microsomal and anti-thyroglobulin) (Balazs and Farid, 1991). The same may apply to DCM, high sIL-2R being present in association with antibodies to extracellular, e.g. the anti-β_1-receptor, rather than intracellular antigens, e.g. α-myosin and the other cardiac-specific antigens involved in the IFL reaction. The cardiac-specific autoantibodies found by IFL and the anti-α-myosin antibodies detected by ELISA were found in similar proportions of patients with DCM and biopsy-proven myocarditis according to the Dallas criteria, included in the Myocarditis Treatment Trial (Mason et al., 1995), suggesting that conventional histology does not distinguish between patients with and without an ongoing immune-mediated process in myocarditis/DCM (Caforio et al., 1997a). The Myocarditis Treatment Trial failed to show an improvement in survival in biopsy-proven myocarditis with immunosuppressive therapy; however, no immunohistochemical or serological markers (e.g. increased HLA expression on endomyocardial biopsy and/or detection of cardiac-specific autoantibodies in the serum in the absence of viral genome in myocardial tissue) were used to identify those patients with immune-mediated pathogenesis in whom immunosuppression could have been beneficial (Mason et al., 1995). Interestingly, a recent randomized, placebo control study in DCM patients with HLA up-regulation on endomyocardial biopsy showed long-term benefit with immunosuppressive treatment (Wojnicz et al., 2001). Myocarditis/DCM patients with cardiac-specific autoantibodies should also be included in future trials of immunosuppressive therapy.

Myosin fulfilled the expected criteria for organ-specific autoimmunity, in that immunization with cardiac but not skeletal myosin reproduced, in susceptible mouse strains, the human disease phenotype of DCM (Neu et al., 1987; Smith and Allen, 1991). In this respect, less experimental data are available with other autoantigens. However, autoimmune diseases are often polyclonal, with production of autoantibodies to different autoantigens. Some of these autoantigens are involved earlier in disease and are more closely related to primary pathogenetic events compared to those, which play a role in secondary immunopathogenesis (Rose and Bona, 1993). Both experimental and clinical evidences, in particular the multiplicity of autoantibody specificities identified so far (Table 3), exist that this also applies to myocarditis/DCM. Myosin is an intracellular protein, thus there are two major hypotheses, which may be not mutually exclusive, to explain interruption of tolerance to this autoantigen.

These include molecular mimicry, since cross-reactive epitopes between cardiac myosin and infectious agents have been found, and myocyte necrosis due to viral infection or other tissue insults (Horwitz et al., 2000; Galvin et al., 2000; Rose, 2000). Both mechanisms would explain the association of viral infection with autoimmune myocarditis/DCM. Infection with Coxsackie B3 (CB3) virus triggers anti-myosin reactivity and autoimmune myocarditis in many mouse strains, and immunization with cardiac myosin induces disease in the same susceptible strains (Neu et al., 1987; Smith and Allen, 1991). In some strains, such as Balb/c mice, CB3 virus-induced or myosin-induced myocarditis is T cell-mediated (Smith and Allen, 1991), whereas in other strains, such as DBA/2 mice, it is an antibody-mediated disease (Kuan et al., 2000). The same may apply to humans, so that the anti-myosin antibodies may be directly pathogenic in some (Lauer et al., 2000) but not all patients with myocarditis/DCM (Caforio et al., 1997b) according to different immunogenetic backgrounds, isotype (Kuan et al., 2000) and/or subclass specificity of these antibodies (Warraich et al., 1999).

In relation to the proposed functional role of antibodies not against myosin, e.g. the anti-receptor and some of anti-mitochondrial antibodies (Table 3) in man, passive transfer of the myocarditis/DCM phenotype to genetically susceptible animals by antibody-positive patients' sera would provide conclusive evidence for antibody-mediated pathogenesis. Nonantigen-specific IgG adsorption has recently been used in DCM patients with high titer antibodies to the β_1-receptor, and it has been suggested that it has beneficial clinical effects, accompanied by undetectable antibody titers during follow-up (Muller et al., 2000). This does not imply a direct pathogenic effect of the anti-β_1-receptor antibodies. The adsorption technique used was nonantigen-specific; in addition, in antibody-mediated disorders the antibody titers rise again at the end of plasmapheresis. However, the authors have recently provided new evidence in favor of the possibility that the beneficial effect of immunoadsorption is related to removal of pathogenic cardiodepressant autoantibodies of IgG3 subclass, although no conclusion is possible on the potential pathogenic role of a specific autoantibody (e.g. β_1-receptor antibody) (Schimke et al., 2001; Felix et al., 2002; Staudt et al., 2002). It may be that this technique has a favorable immunomodulatory/immunosuppressive effect; in addition, IgG substitution performed after immunoadsorption to avoid infective complications of unselective IgG depletion may have contributed to the observed hemodynamic improvement (Mann, 2001; Gullestad et al., 2001); randomized studies are warranted. This does not undermine the possible role of any of the described antibodies (Table 3) as predictive markers. Subjects classified as negative for one antibody may be positive for another and combined testing may be advantageous. To this end, standardization of nomenclature and protocols for antibody detection and exchange of sera among laboratories currently assessing the individual antibodies will be useful.

In conclusion, several groups have shown that a subset of patients with myocarditis/idiopathic DCM and their symptom-free relatives has circulating heart-reactive autoantibodies. These autoantibodies are directed against multiple antigens, some of which are strictly expressed in the myocardium (e.g. organ-specific for the heart), others are expressed in heart and skeletal muscle (e.g. muscle-specific). Distinct autoantibodies have also different prevalence in disease and normal controls (e.g. by IFL the organ-specific antibodies are disease-specific for DCM, some of the muscle-specific antibodies are not). Different antibody techniques detect one (e.g. ELISA for myosin or for anti-receptor antibodies) or more antibody specificities (e.g. indirect IFL), thus they cannot be used interchangeably as screening tools. Antibody frequency in DCM vs. controls is expected to be different using distinct techniques; at present it is unknown whether the same subset (30–40%) of patients produce more than one antibody or different patient groups develop autoimmunity to different antigens. Antibodies of IgG class, which are shown to be cardiac and disease-specific for myocarditis/DCM, can be used as reliable markers of autoimmune pathogenesis for identifying patients, in whom immunosuppression and/or immunomodulation therapy may be beneficial, and their relatives at risk. Some of these autoantibodies may also have a functional role in patients, as suggested by in vitro data as well as by preliminary clinical observations, but further work is needed to clarify this important issue.

6. Idiopathic tachy and bradyarrhythmias

Idiopathic AV conduction blocks or other bradyarrhythmias may be seen in association with organ-specific or nonorgan-specific conditions. This led earlier investigators to hypothesize potential immune pathogenetic mechanisms. Cardiac conducting tissue antibodies (CCTA) were first reported by s-I IFI-S in patients with chronic AV block (Fairfax and Doniach, 1976). The antibodies were of IgG class, complement fixing and with titers between 1/10 and 1/80. More recently, stimulating antibodies against β_1- and β_2-adrenoceptors were found by ELISA in patients with primary electrical cardiac abnormalities, in particular conduction disease or tachyarrhythmia (Chiale et al., 1995). There are nonorgan-specific autoantibodies, which may be associated with cardiac CDs, such as the anti-SSA/Ro anti-nRNP specificities (Scott et al., 1983), but these are covered in another chapter.

6.1. Cardiac conducting tissue antibodies

The s-I IFL substrate for CCTA detection was ox heart false tendon (Fairfax and Doniach, 1976; Villecco et al., 1983; Obiassi et al., 1987). This tissue was used because it is well known that in ox heart, the false tendon contains the right bundle branch block (RBBB) and in ungulates, Purkinje cells are easily distinguishable from ordinary working myocardial cells by light microscopy. The presence of Purkinje cells was also confirmed on tissue sections by histochemical reactions for myosin ATPase and phosphorilase. Cryostat-cut sections were incubated with sera diluted 1/10, and fluorescein-labeled anti-human IgG, A, M and C3 antisera were used for CCTA detection. In the study by Obiassi et al., CCTA-positive sera stained only Purkinje cells.

Fairfax and Doniach (1976) found CCTA in 8.6% of patients with idiopathic AV block, 4.5% of those with blocks of known cause and 4.2% of healthy controls (Table 2).

CCTA were also found in 76% rheumatoid arthritis (RA) patients with RBBB and 20% of those without RBBB, but were rare in RBBB without RA (Villecco et al., 1983) (Table 2).

Obiassi et al. (1987) subsequently reported CCTA reacting only with Purkinje cells in 14–21% of patients with connective tissue disease (systemic lupus erythematosus, AR, Sjogren syndrome, progressive systemic sclerosis) and AV blocks, 30% of patients implanted with permanent pace-makers for nonischemic AV blocks, 34.5% of those with idiopathic block at or below the His bundle and 11% of normal subjects.

6.2. Stimulating autoantibodies to β-adrenergic receptors

Chiale et al. (1995), using as antigens synthetic peptides analogous to the sequences of the second extracellular loop of β_1- and β_2-adrenergic receptors by ELISA, found stimulating anti-β_1-antibodies at higher frequency in patients with DCM (38%) and in idiopathic VA (47.6%) compared to both normal (19%) and cardiomyopathy controls (6.2%) (Table 2). Conversely the antibody frequency in patients with CD (28.5%) or primary atrial arrhythmia (AA) (13.6%) was similar to that seen in normal and cardiomyopathy controls. In addition, they reported a higher frequency of anti-β_2-antibodies in VA (23.8%) compared to cardiopathic (3%) but not the healthy control subjects (14.7%). The authors suggest that the agonist- or catecholamine-like effects mediated by these antibodies may play a role in facilitating the occurrence of VA and the development of chronic myocardial dysfunction and DCM. However, prospective studies are needed to determine whether or not these antibodies are predictive markers of DCM development in patients with idiopathic arrhythmia and normal systolic function.

7. Systemic arterial hypertension

Systemic arterial hypertension is a syndrome of heterogeneous etiology and pathogenesis. An increased frequency of anti-heart autoantibodies to several antigens has recently been reported, suggesting that autoimmune mechanisms might be involved in selected patient subgroups.

7.1. Anti-heart autoantibodies by s-I IFL

Caforio et al. (1991) reported organ-specific anti-heart autoantibodies in 17% of sera from patients with autoimmune polyendocrinopathy, in the absence of symptoms and ECG and/or echocardiographic evidence of cardiac dysfunction (Table 2). However, a higher frequency of systemic arterial hypertension was found among antibody-positive patients. The authors concluded that the antibodies might represent markers of an autoimmune form of hypertension, although prospective studies were needed to confirm their hypothesis.

7.2. Stimulating autoantibodies to α_1-adrenergic receptors

Fu and Herlitz (1994)), using as antigens synthetic peptides analogous to the sequences of the second extracellular loop of α_1-adrenergic receptor by ELISA, found stimulating anti-α_1-antibodies of mainly IgM isotype in 4 (12%) of 33 normal controls, 3 (20%) of 15 patients with malignant essential hypertension and 7 (64%) of 11 with secondary malignant hypertension (Table 2). The patients' antibodies caused a decrease in tritiated prazosin binding sites and an increase in heart beating frequency of neonatal cultured rat cardiomyocytes; antibodies purified from the controls had no effect. These workers concluded that these autoantibodies had agonist-like activity, although it remained to be further investigated whether they were merely markers of a subgroup of patients with malignant hypertension or had a pathogenetic role.

Luther et al. (1997) subsequently showed that when analyzed in a functional test system of spontaneously beating neonatal rat myocytes, the Ig fractions of sera from 24 (44%) patients with primary hypertension and 3 (12%) normotensive controls contained antibodies against α_1-adrenergic receptor (Table 2). The autoantibodies increased the beating frequency of isolated myocytes in vitro, an effect that was blocked by α_1-adrenergic antagonists. Since the functional characteristics of the autoantibodies showed no desensitization phenomena, the authors suggested that they might play a role in increasing vascular resistance and promoting cardiac hypertrophy in primary hypertension.

7.3. Stimulating autoantibodies to the angiotensin receptor (AT1)

Fu et al. (2000), using ELISA, studied the presence of autoantibodies against G-protein-coupled cardiovascular receptors in malignant essential hypertension ($n = 14$), secondary malignant hypertension due to renovascular disease ($n = 12$), renovascular disease without malignant hypertension ($n = 11$) and normotensive healthy blood donors ($n = 35$). They found stimulating anti-angiotensin 1-receptor (AT1) antibodies in 14, 33, 18 and 14% of patients with malignant essential hypertension, secondary malignant hypertension, renovascular disease and normotensives, respectively (Table 2); no antibodies to bradykinin (B2) or angiotensin II subtype 2 (AT2) receptors.

Wallukat et al. (1999) analyzed in a functional test system of spontaneously beating neonatal rat myocytes, the Ig fractions of sera from 25 preeclamptic patients and compared them with those of 12 normotensive pregnant women and 10 pregnant patients with primary hypertension. Antibodies were detected by the chronotropic response to AT1 receptor-mediated stimulation of the rat myocytes coupled with receptor-specific antagonists. Ig from all preeclamptic patients, but not from controls, stimulated the AT1 receptor; this activity decreased after delivery. Affinity-column purification, peptide inhibition and Western blot experiments identified this activity as due to agonistic IgG antibodies against the second extracellular AT1 receptor loop. Confocal microscopy of vascular smooth muscle cells showed colocalization of purified patient IgG and AT1 receptor antibody. It was subsequently shown that these antibodies induce vascular cells to express tissue factor and stimulate NADPH oxidase (Dechend et al., 2000, 2003). These data suggest that they may contribute to the pathogenesis of preeclampsia (Roberts, 2000).

Key points

Myocarditis/idiopathic DCM:

- At present, criteria for involvement of organ-specific autoimmunity, according to Rose and Witebsky, are fulfilled in a subset of patients with myocarditis/idiopathic DCM, but not in other cardiovascular diseases in which circulating cardiac autoantibodies are found.
- A subset of patients with myocarditis/idiopathic DCM and their symptom-free relatives has circulating heart-reactive autoantibodies. These autoantibodies are directed against multiple antigens, some of which are only expressed in the heart (organ-specific), others are expressed in heart and only some skeletal muscle fibers (partially heart-specific) or react with heart and skeletal muscle (muscle-specific).
- Distinct autoantibodies have different frequency in disease and normal controls (e.g. by IFL, the organ-specific antibodies are disease-specific for myocarditis/DCM, some of the muscle-specific antibodies are not). Different antibody techniques detect one (e.g. ELISA for myosin or for anti-receptor antibodies) or more antibody specificities (e.g. indirect IFL), thus they cannot be used interchangeably as screening tools. Antibody frequency in DCM vs. controls is expected to be different using distinct techniques.
- It is currently unknown whether the same subset of patients produce more than one antibody or different patient groups develop autoimmunity to different antigens. Antibodies of IgG class, which are shown to be cardiac and disease-specific for myocarditis/DCM, can be used as reliable markers of autoimmune pathogenesis for identifying patients, in whom immunosuppression and/or immunomodulation therapy may be beneficial, and their relatives at risk.
- Some of these autoantibodies may also have a functional role in patients, as suggested by in vitro data as well as by preliminary clinical observations, but further work is needed to clarify this important issue.

Other cardiovascular conditions:

- Other cardiovascular conditions in which circulating autoantibodies against heart autoantigens or molecules involved in the cardiovascular system are found include: the post-pericardiotomy and post-myocardial infarction (Dressler) syndromes, rheumatic carditis, idiopathic brady or tachyarrhythmias, systemic arterial hypertension, and atherosclerosis (not discussed in this chapter).
- Research in this area is underway and is expected to clarify the potential role of the antibodies as diagnostic and/or prognostic markers as well as their possible functional activity.

References

Anderson, J.L., Carlquist, J.F., Lutz, J.R., et al. 1984. HLA A, B, and DR typing in idiopathic dilated cardiomyopathy: a search for immune response factors. Am. J. Cardiol. 53, 1326.

Ansari, A.A., Neckelmann, N., Villinger, F., et al. 1994. Epitope mapping of the branched chain α-ketoacid dehydrogenase dihydrolipoyl transacylase (BCKD-E2) protein that reacts with sera from patients with idiopathic dilated cardiomyopathy. J. Immunol. 153, 4754.

Aretz, H.T., Billingham, M.E., Edwards, W.E., et al. 1985. Myocarditis: a histopathologic definition and classification. Am. J. Cardiol. Pathol. 1, 1.

Baba, A., Yoshikawa, T., Ogawa, S. 2002. Autoantibodies against sarcolemmal Na-K-ATPase: possible upstream targets of arrhythmias and sudden death in patients with dilated cardiomyopathy. J. Am. Coll. Cardiol. 40, 1153.

Baig, M.K., Goldman, J.H., Caforio, A.L.P., et al. 1998. Familial dilated cardiomyopathy: cardiac abnormalities are common in asymptomatic relatives and may represent early disease. J. Am. Coll. Cardiol. 31, 195.

Balazs, C.Z., Farid, N.R. 1991. Soluble IL-2 receptor in sera of patients with Graves' disease. J Autoimmun. 4, 681.

Bauer, H., Waters, T.J., Talano, J.V. 1972. Antimyocardial antibodies in patients with coronary heart disease. Am. Heart J. 83, 612.

Bessen, D., Jones, K.F., Fischetti, V.A. 1989. Evidence for two distinct classes of streptococcal M protein and their relationship to rheumatic fever. J. Exp. Med. 169, 269.

Betterle, C., Spadaccino, A.C., Pedini, B. 1997. Autoanticorpi nelle malattie autoimmuni del muscolo scheletrico, della giunzione neuro-muscolare e del cuore. In: C. Betterle (Ed.), Gli autoanticorpi. Manuale-Atlante a colori di diagnostica. Piccin, Padova, p. 313.

This is a detailed review of the immunological methods used for detection of anti-heart autoantibodies, their relative advantages and disadvantages, as well as technical pitfalls. Examples of the various IFL patterns are also given.

Bottazzo, G.F., Todd, I., Mirakian, R., et al. 1986. Organ-specific autoimmunity. A 1986 overview. Immunol. Rev. 94, 137.

Caforio, A.L.P. 1994. Role of autoimmunity in dilated cardiomyopathy. Br. Heart J. 72, S30.

Caforio, A.L.P., McKenna, W.J. 1996. Recognition and optimum treatment of myocarditis. Drugs 52, 515.

Caforio, A.L.P., Bonifacio, E., Stewart, J.T., et al. 1990a. Novel organ-specific circulating cardiac autoantibodies in dilated cardiomyopathy. J. Am. Coll. Cardiol. 15, 1527.
This is the first description of organ-specific, partially organ-specific and skeletal muscle cross-reactive anti-heart autoantibodies, by standard indirect IFL and absorption, in sera from patients with dilated cardiomyopathy. Examples of these IFL patterns are given.

Caforio, A.L.P., Stewart, J.T., Bonifacio, E., et al. 1990b. Inappropriate major histocompatibility complex expression on cardiac tissue in dilated cardiomyopathy. Relevance for autoimmunity? J. Autoimmun. 3, 187.

Caforio, A.L.P., Wagner, R., Jaswinder, S.G., et al. 1991. Organ-specific cardiac antibodies: serological markers for systemic hypertension in autoimmune polyendocrinopathy. Lancet 337, 1111.
This is the first description of organ-specific, partially organ-specific and skeletal muscle cross-reactive anti-heart autoantibodies, by standard indirect IFL and absorption, in sera from patients with autoimmune polyendocrinopathy, in association with systemic arterial hypertension.

Caforio, A.L.P., Grazzini, M., Mann, J.M., et al. 1992. Identification of α and β cardiac myosin heavy chain isoforms as major autoantigens in dilated cardiomyopathy. Circulation 85, 1734.
This study demonstrates, using immunoblotting, that, similar to the animal model of autoimmune myocarditis, α and β cardiac myosin heavy chain isoforms are autoantigens recognized by the circulating anti-heart autoantibodies detected by IFL in patients with dilated cardiomyopathy.

Caforio, A.L.P., Keeling, P.J., Zachara, E., et al. 1994. Evidence from family studies for autoimmunity in dilated cardiomyopathy. Lancet 344, 773.
This is the first description of organ-specific anti-heart autoantibodies, by standard indirect IFL, in sera from asymptomatic relatives of dilated cardiomyopathy patients, from both familial and non familial pedigrees. The autoantibodies were associated with echocardiographic features of early disease.

Caforio, A.L.P., Goldman, J.H., Haven, A.J., et al. 1997a. Circulating cardiac autoantibodies as markers of autoimmunity in clinical and biopsy-proven myocarditis. Eur. Heart J. 18, 270.

Caforio, A.L.P., Goldman, J.H., Baig, K.M., et al. 1997b. Cardiac autoantibodies in dilated cardiomyopathy become undetectable with disease progression. Heart 77, 62.

Caforio, A.L.P., Goldman, J.H., Baig, K.M., et al. 2001. Elevated serum levels of soluble interleukin-2 receptor, neopterin and β-2 microglobulin in idiopathic dilated cardiomyopathy: relation to disease severity and autoimmune pathogenesis. Eur. J. Heart Fail. 3, 155.

Caforio, A.L.P., Mahon, N.J., Tona, F., et al. 2002. Circulating cardiac autoantibodies in dilated cardiomyopathy and myocarditis: pathogenetic and clinical significance. Eur. J. Heart Fail. 4, 411.

Camp, F.T., Hess, E.V., Conway, G., et al. 1969. Immunologic findings in idiopathic cardiomyopathy. Am. Heart J. 77, 610.

Chiale, P.A., Rosembaum, M.B., Elizari, M.V., et al. 1995. High prevalence of antibodies against β_1- and β_2-adrenoceptors in patients with primary electrical cardiac abnormalities. J. Am. Coll. Cardiol. 26, 864.

Dajani, A.S., Ayoub, E.M., Bierman, F.Z., et al. 1992. Guidelines for the diagnosis of rheumatic fever: Jones criteria, updated 1992. JAMA 268, 2069.

Dale, J.B., Beachey, E.H. 1986. Sequence of myosin cross-reactive epitopes of streptococcal M protein. J. Exp. Med. 164, 1785.

Dechend, R., Homuth, V., Wallukat, G., et al. 2000. AT1 receptor antibodies from preeclamptic patients cause vascular cells to express tissue factor. Circulation 101, 2382.

Dechend, R., Viedt, C., Muller, D.N., et al. 2003. AT1 receptor agonistic antibodies from preeclamptic patients stimulate NADPH oxidase. Circulation 107, 1632.

Dressler, W. 1956. A post-myocardial infarction syndrome: preliminary report of a complication resembling idiopathic recurrent benign pericarditis. JAMA 160, 1379.

Dressler, W. 1959. The post-myocardial infarction syndrome. A report of forty-four cases. Arch. Intern. Med. 103, 28.

Eglen, R.M., Reddy, H., Watson, N., et al. 1994. Muscarinic acetylcholine receptor subtypes in smooth muscle. Trends Pharmacol. Sci. 15, 114.

Elalouf, J.M., Buhler, J.M., Tessiot, C., et al. 1993. Predominant expression of beta 1-adrenergic receptor in the thick ascending limb of rat kidney: absolute mRNA quantitation by reverse transcription and polymerase chain reaction. J. Clin. Invest. 91, 264.

Engle, M.A., McCabe, J.C., Ebert, P.A., et al. 1974. The postpericardiotomy syndrome and anti-heart antibodies. Circulation 49, 401.

Escaned, J., Ahmad, R.A., Shiu, M.F. 1992. Pleural effusion following coronary perforation during balloon angioplasty: an unusual presentation of the postpericardiotomy syndrome. Eur. Heart J. 13, 716.

Fairfax, J.A., Doniach, D. 1976. Autoantibodies to cardiac conducting tissue and their characterization by immunofluorescence. Clin. Exp. Immunol. 23, 1.
This is the first description of cardiac conducting tissue autoantibodies, by standard indirect IFL.

Felix, S.B., Staudt, A., Landsberger, M., et al. 2002. Removal of cardiodepressant antibodies in dilated cardiomyopathy by immunoadsorption. J. Am. Coll. Cardiol. 39, 646.
This study provides new evidence in favour of the possibility that the beneficial effect of immunoadsorption in dilated cardiomyopathy is related to removal of cardiodepressant antibodies.

Felsh, G. 1966. The anti-globulin consumption test in rheumatic carditis. Dtsch Med. Wochenschr. 91, 2197.

Fletcher, G.F., Wenger, N.K. 1968. Autoimmune studies in patients with primary myocardial disease. Circulation 37, 1032.

Fu, L.X., Herlitz, H. 1994. Functional autoimmune epitope on α1-adrenergic receptors in patients with malignant hypertension. Lancet 344, 1660.

Fu, L.X., Magnusson, Y., Bergh, C.H., et al. 1993. Localization of a functional autoimmune epitope on the muscarinic acetylcholine receptor-2 in patients with idiopathic dilated cardiomyopathy. J. Clin. Invest. 91, 1964.

This is the first description of anti-muscarinic acetylcholine receptor-2 autoantibodies in dilated cardiomyopathy.

Fu, L.X., Herlitz, H., Schultze, W., et al. 2000. Autoantibodies against the angiotensin receptor (AT1) in patients with hypertension. J. Hypertens. 18, 945.

Galvin, J.E., Hemric, M.E., Ward, K., et al. 2000. Cytotoxic mAb from rheumatic carditis recognizes heart valves and laminin. J. Clin. Invest. 106, 217.

Goldman, J.H., Keeling, P.J., Warraich, R.S., et al. 1995. Autoimmunity to α-myosin in a subset of patients with idiopathic dilated cardiomyopathy. Br. Heart J. 74, 598.

Gullestad, L., Aass, H., Fjeld, J.G. et al. 2001. Immunomodulating therapy with intravenous immunoglobulin in patients with chronic heart failure. Circulation 103, 220.

Heine, W.I., Friedman, H., Mandell, M.S., et al. 1966. Antibodies to cardiac tissue in acute ischemic heart disease. Am. J. Cardiol. 77, 798.

Hess, E.V., Fink, C.W., Taranta, A., et al. 1964. Heart muscle antibodies in rheumatic fever and other diseases. J. Clin. Invest. 43, 886.

Horwitz, M.S., La Cava, A., Fine, C., et al. 2000. Pancreatic expression of interferon-γ protects mice from lethal coxsackievirus B3 infection and subsequent myocarditis. Nat. Med. 6, 693.

Itoh, K., Ohkumi, H., Kimura, E., et al. 1969. Immuno-serological studies on myocardial infarction and postmyocardial infarction syndrome. Jpn. Heart J. 10, 485.

Jahns, R., Boivin, V., Siegmund, C., et al. 1999. Autoantibodies activating human β1-adrenergic receptors are associated with reduced cardiac function in chronic heart failure. Circulation 99, 649.

Jahns, R., Boivin, V., Krapf, T., et al. 2000. Modulation of β1-adrenoceptor activity by domain-specific antibodies and heart-failure associated autoantibodies. J. Am. Coll. Cardiol. 36, 1280.

Jones, T.D. 1944. The diagnosis of rheumatic fever. JAMA 126, 481.

Kaplan, M.H., Dallenbach, F.D. 1961. Immunologic studies of heart tissue. III. Occurrence of bound gamma globulin in auricular appendages from rheumatic hearts. Relationship to certain histopathologic features of rheumatic heart disease. J. Exp. Med. 113, 1.

Kaplan, M.H., Frengley, D.J. 1969. Autoimmunity to the heart in cardiac disease. Current concepts of the relation of autoimmunity to rheumatic fever, postcardiotomy and postinfarction syndromes and cardiomyopathies. Am. J. Cardiol. 24, 459.

Kaplan, M.H., Svec, K.H. 1964. Immunologic relation of streptococcal and tissue antigens. III. Presence in human sera of streptococcal antibody cross-reactive with heart tissue. Association with streptococcal infection, rheumatic fever, and glomerulonephritis. J. Exp. Med. 119, 651.

Kaplan, M.H., Meyeserian, M., Kushner, I. 1961. Immunologic studies of heart tissue. IV. Serologic reactions with human heart tissue as revealed by immunofluorescent methods: isoimmune, Wassermann, and autoimmune reactions. J. Exp. Med. 113, 17.

Kaplan, M.H., Bolande, R., Rakita, L., et al. 1964. Presence of bound immunoglobulins and complement in the myocardium in acute rheumatic fever. N. Engl. J. Med. 271, 637.

This fascinating series of seminal papers by Kaplan MH, et al., contains the most relevant early experimental and clinical observations in the field of organ-specific autoimmunity and cardiovascular disease. It provides historical perspective and inspires very modern working hypotheses for researchers in this area.

Kirsner, A.B., Hess, E.V., Fowler, N.O. 1973. Immunologic findings in idiopathic cardiomyopathy: a prospective serial study. Am. Heart J. 86, 625.

Klein, R., Maisch, B., Kochsiek, K., et al. 1984. Demonstration of organ specific antibodies against heart mitochondria (anti-M7) in sera from patients with some forms of heart diseases. Clin. Exp. Immunol. 58, 283.

This is the first description of organ specific antibodies against heart mitochondria (anti-M7) in sera from patients with some forms of heart diseases.

Kleinsorge, H., Dornbusch, S., Romer, R. 1960. Autoimmunization bei entzundlichen und degenerativen Herz krankungen. Int. Arch. Allergy 16, 200.

Krisher, K., Cunningham, M.W. 1985. Myosin: a link between streptococci and heart. Science 227, 413.

This is a very important paper providing evidence for molecular mimicry between myosin and streptococcal antigens.

Kuan, A.P., Zuckier, L., Liao, L., et al. 2000. Immunoglobulin isotype determines pathogenicity in antibody-mediated myocarditis in naïve mice. Circ. Res. 86, 281.

Latif, N., Baker, C.S., Dunn, M.J., et al. 1993. Frequency and specificity of antiheart antibodies in patients with dilated cardiomyopathy detected using SDS-PAGE and western blotting. J. Am. Coll. Cardiol. 22, 1378.

Latif, N., Smith, J., Dunn, M.J., et al. 1994. Complement-mediated cytotoxic activity of anti-heart antibodies present in the sera of patients with dilated cardiomyopathy. Autoimmunity 19, 99.

Lauer, B., Schannwell, M., Kuhl, U., et al. 2000. Antimyosin autoantibodies are associated with deterioration of systolic and diastolic left ventricular function in patients with chronic myocarditis. J. Am. Coll. Cardiol. 35, 11.

Ledford, D.K., Espinoza, L.R. 1987. Immunologic aspects of cardiovascular disease. JAMA 20, 2974.

Limas, C.J., Limas, C. 1991. β-Receptor antibodies and genetics in dilated cardiomyopathy. Eur. Heart J. 12 (Suppl. D), 175.

Limas, C.J., Goldenberg, I.F., Limas, C. 1989. Autoantibodies against β-adrenoceptors in idiopathic dilated cardiomyopathy. Circ. Res. 64, 97.

This is the first description of antibodies against β-adrenoceptors in sera from patients with dilated cardiomyopathy.

Limas, C.J., Goldenberg, I.F., Limas, C. 1995. Soluble interleukin-2 receptor levels in patients with dilated cardiomyopathy.

Correlation with disease severity and cardiac autoantibodies. Circulation 91, 631.

Luther, H.P., Homuth, V., Wallukat, G. 1997. α_1-adrenergic receptor antibodies in patients with primary hypertension. Hypertension 29, 678.

Magnusson, Y., Marullo, S., Hoyer, S., et al. 1990. Mapping of a functional autoimmune epitope on the β-adrenergic receptor in patients with idiopathic dilated cardiomyopathy. J. Clin. Invest. 86, 1658.

Magnusson, Y., Wallukat, G., Waagstein, F., et al. 1994. Autoimmunity in idiopathic dilated cardiomyopathy: characterization of antibodies against the β_1-adrenoceptor with positive chronotropic effect. Circulation 89, 2760.

These two papers describe the anti-β_1-adrenoceptor antibodies with positive chronotropic effect, that are detected in sera from patients with dilated cardiomyopathy.

Mahon, N.G., Madden, B., Caforio, A.L.P., et al. 2002. Immunohistochemical evidence of myocardial disease in apparently healthy relatives of patients with dilated cardiomyopathy. J. Am. Coll. Cardiol. 39, 455.

Maisch, B., Berg, P., Kochsiek, K. 1979. Clinical significance of immunopathological findings in patients with post-pericardiotomy syndrome: relevance of antibody pattern. Clin. Exp. Immunol. 38, 189.

Maisch, B., Deeg, P., Liebau, G., et al. 1983a. Diagnostic relevance of humoral and cytotoxic immune reactions in primary and secondary dilated cardiomyopathy. Am. J. Cardiol. 52, 1071.

Maisch, B., Deeg, P., Liebau, G., et al. 1983b. Diagnostic relevance of humoral and cell-mediated immune reactions in patients with viral myocarditis. Clin. Exp. Immun. 48, 533.

Mann, D.L. 2001. Autoimmunity, immunoglobulin adsorption and dilated cardiomyopathy: has the time come for randomized clinical trials? J. Am. Coll. Cardiol 38, 184.

Mason, J.W., O'Connell, J.B., Herskowitz, A., et al. 1995. A clinical trial of immunosuppressive therapy for myocarditis. N. Engl. J. Med. 333, 269.

Michels, V.V., Moll, P.P., Rodeheffer, R.J., et al. 1994. Circulating heart autoantibodies in familial as compared with nonfamilial idiopathic dilated cardiomyopathy. Mayo Clin. Proc. 69, 24.

Muller, J., Wallukat, G., Dandel, M., et al. 2000. Immunoglobulin adsorption in patients with idiopathic dilated cardiomyopathy. Circulation 101, 385.

Muller-Ehmsen, J., Juvvadi, P., Thmpson, C.B., et al. 2001. Ouabain and substrate affinities of human Na-K-ATPase α-1β-1, α-2β-1, α-3β-1 when expressed separately in yeast cells. Am. J. Physiol. Cell. Physiol. 281, C1355.

Neu, N., Rose, N.R., Beisel, K.W., et al. 1987. Cardiac myosin induces myocarditis in genetically predisposed mice. J. Immunol. 139, 3630.

Neumann, D.A., Burek, C.L., Baughman, K.L., et al. 1990. Circulating heart-reactive antibodies in patients with myocarditis or cardiomyopathy. J. Am. Coll. Cardiol. 16, 839.

Nicholson, G.C., Dawkins, R.L., McDonald, B.L., et al. 1977. A classification of anti-heart antibodies: differentiation between heart-specific and heterophile antibodies. Clin. Immunol. Immunopathol. 7, 349.

This is a detailed description of the IFL patterns given by anti-heart autoantibodies, as well by non cardiac or muscle specific antibodies which could be misclassified as anti-heart. Examples of the various IFL patterns are also shown.

Obiassi, M., Brucato, A., Meroni, P.L., et al. 1987. Antibodies to cardiac Purkinje cell: further characterization in autoimmune diseases and atrioventricular heart block. Clin. Immunol. Immunopathol. 42, 141.

Otto, A., Stahle, I., Klein, R., et al. 1998. Anti-mitochondrial antibodies in patients with dilated cardiomyopathy (anti-M7) are directed against flavoenzymes with covalently bound FAD. Clin. Exp. Immunol. 111, 541.

Peters, R.W., Scheinman, M.M., Raskin, S., et al. 1980. Unusual complications of epicardial pacemakers. Am. J. Cardiol. 45, 1088.

Pohlner, K., Portig, I., Pankuweit, S., et al. 1997. Identification of mitochondrial antigens recognized by antibodies in sera of patients with idiopathic dilated cardiomyopathy by two-dimensional gel electrophoresis and protein sequencing. Am. J. Cardiol. 80, 1040.

Portig, I., Pankuweit, S., Maisch, B. 1997. Antibodies against stress proteins in sera of patients with dilated cardiomyopathy. J. Mol. Cell. Cardiol. 29, 2245.

Richardson, P., McKenna, W.J., Bristow, M., et al. 1996. Report of the 1995 World Health Organization/International Society and Federation of Cardiology Task Force on the definition and classification of cardiomyopathies. Circulation 93, 841.

Roberts, J.M. 2000. Angiotensin-1 receptor autoantibodies. A role in the pathogenesis of preeclampsia? Circulation 101, 2335.

Robinson, J.H., Kehoe, M.A. 1992. Group A streptococcal M proteins: virulence factors and protective antigens. Immunol. Today 13, 362.

This is a very accurate paper reviewing recent evidence for molecular mimicry between heart and streptococcal antigens.

Rose, N.R. 2000. Viral damage or 'molecular mimicry'—placing the blame in myocarditis. Nat. Med. 6, 631.

These are very important review papers from leading figures in the autoimmunity field.

Rose, N.R., Bona, C. 1993. Defining criteria for autoimmune diseases (Witebsky's postulates revisited). Immunol. Today 14, 426.

Schimke, I., Muller, J., Priem, F., et al. 2001. Decreased oxidative stress in patients with idiopathic dilated cardiomyopathy one year after immunoglobulin adsorption. J. Am. Coll. Cardiol. 38, 178.

Schultheiss, H.P., Bolte, H.D. 1985. Immunological analysis of auto-antibodies against the adenine nucleotide translocator in dilated cardiomyopathy. J. Mol. Cell. Cardiol. 17, 603.

Schultheiss, H.P., Ulrich, G., Janda, I., et al. 1988. Antibody mediated enhancement of calcium permeability in cardiac myocytes. J. Exp. Med. 168, 2105.

These two papers contain the first description of autoantibodies against the ANT and first in vitro evidence that such antibodies may have a functional role.

Schultheiss, H.P., Kuhl, U., Schwimmbeck, P., et al., 1990. Biomolecular changes in dilated cardiomyopathy. In: G. Baroldi, F. Camerini, J.F. Goodwin (Eds.), Advances in Cardiomyopathies, p. 221.

Schwinger, R.H.G., Wang, J., Frank, K., et al. 1999. Reduced sodium pump α1-, α3-, β1-isoform protein levels and Na,K-ATPase activity but unchanged Na/Ca exchanger protein levels in human heart failure. Circulation 99, 2105.

Scott, J.S., Maddison, P.J., Taylor, P.V., et al. 1983. Connective-tissue disease, antibodies to ribonucleoptrotein, and congenital heart block. N. Engl. J. Med. 309, 209.

Smith, S.C., Allen, P.M. 1991. Myosin-induced myocarditis is a T cell-mediated disease. J. Immunol. 147, 2141.

Staudt, A., Bohm, M., Knebel, F., et al. 2002. Potential role of autoantibodies belonging to the immunoglobulin G-3 subclass in cardiac dysfunction among patients with dilated cardiomyopathy. Circulation 106, 2448.
This paper contains recent evidence in favour of a functional role for autoantibodies of IgG-3 subclass in dilated cardiomyopathy.

Urayama, O., Shutt, H., Sweadner, J. 1989. Identification of three isozyme proteins of the catalytic subunit of the Na,K-ATPase in rat brain. J. Biol. Chem. 264, 8271.

Van der Geld, H. 1964. Anti-heart antibodies in the postcardiotomy and postmyocardial infarction syndrome. Lancet II, 617.

Villecco, A.S., De Liberali, E., Bianchi, F.P., et al. 1983. Antibodies to cardiac conduction tissue and abnormalities of cardiac conduction in rheumatoid arthritis. Clin. Exp. Immunol. 53, 536.

Wallukat, G., Morwinski, M., Kowal, K., et al. 1991. Antibodies against the β-adrenergic receptor in human myocarditis and dilated cardiomyopathy: β-adrenergic agonism without desensitization. Eur. Heart J. 12 (Suppl. D), 178.

Wallukat, G., Homuth, V., Fischer, T., et al. 1999. Patients with preeclampsia develop agonist autoantibodies against the angiotensin AT1 receptor. J. Clin. Invest. 103, 945.

Warraich, R.S., Dunn, M.J., Yacoub, M.H. 1999. Subclass specificity of autoantibodies against myosin in patients with idiopathic dilated cardiomyopathy: proinflammatory antibodies in dilated cardiomyopathy patients. Biochem. Biophys. Res. Commun. 259, 255.

Witebsky, E., Rose, N.R., Terplan, K., et al. 1957. Chronic thyroiditis and autoimmunization. JAMA 164, 1439.

Wojnicz, R., Nowalany-Kozielska, E., Wojciechowska, C., et al. 2001. Randomized, placebo controlled study for immunosuppressive treatment of inflammatory dilated cardiomyopathy. Two-year follow-up results. Circulation 104, 39.
This paper provides new evidence in favour of efficacy of immunosuppression in patients with dilated cardiomyopathy, selected on the basis of positive immunohistochemical markers of immune activation on endomyocardial biopsy.

Wolff, P.G., Kuhl, U., Schultheiss, H.P. 1989. Laminin distribution and autoantibodies to laminin in dilated cardiomyopathy and myocarditis. Am. Heart J. 117, 1303.

Zabriskie, J.B. 1967. Mimetic relationships between group A streptococci and mammalian tissues. Adv. Immunol. 7, 147.

Zabriskie, J.B., Hs, K.C., Seegal, B.C. 1970. Heart-reactive antibody associated with rheumatic fever: characterization and diagnostic significance. Clin. Exp. Immunol. 7, 147.

Zitnan, D., Bosmanski, K. 1966. Antimyocardial serum factors in rheumatic fever detected by the immunofluorescence method. Acta Rheum. Scand. 12, 267.

Zweiman, B., Arnason, B.G.W. 1987. Immunologic aspects of neurological and neuromuscolar diseases. JAMA 258, 2970.

Handbook of Systemic Autoimmune Diseases, Volume 1
The Heart in Systemic Autoimmune Diseases
A. Doria and P. Pauletto, editors

CHAPTER 3

Non-organ Specific Autoimmunity Involvement in Cardiovascular Disease

Piersandro Riboldi[a], Maria Gerosa[a], Angela Tincani[b], Pier Luigi Meroni[*,a]

[a]*Allergy, Clinical Immunology and Rheumatology Unit, Department of Internal Medicine, University of Milan, IRCCS Istituto Auxologico Italiano, Via L. Ariosto, 13, 20145 Milan, Italy*
[b]*Department of Rheumatology and Clinical Immunology, Spedali Civili, Brescia, Italy*

1. Introduction

Cardiac involvement is one of the main complications that substantially contribute to the morbidity and mortality of patients suffering from systemic autoimmune diseases (Moder et al., 1999; Riboldi et al., 2002). Such an involvement has been recognized since the beginning of the 20th century, but in the last decades newly recognized clinical entities have been detailed.

All anatomical heart structures can be affected by several pathogenic mechanisms as summarized in Table 1. This chapter will focus on humoral non-organ specific autoimmune pathogenic mechanisms affecting different anatomical cardiac structures in patients suffering from systemic autoimmune diseases.

2. Valvular involvement

2.1. Libman–Sacks endocarditis

Libman–Sacks 'atypical verrucous endocarditis' is the most characteristic and classic cardiac lesion in Systemic Lupus Erythematosus (SLE). The valve lesions appear as single or multiple verrucous vegetations adherent to the underlying endocardium and more frequently found near the edge of the valves, on both surfaces, on the rings and commisures, and less frequently on the chordae tendinae, papillary muscles, atrial and ventricular mural endocardium. Libman–Sacks vegetations are characterized by: (a) an outer exudative zone of fibrin, nuclear debris and haematoxylin body deposition; (b) a middle zone of fibroblast and capillary proliferation; and (c) an inner zone of neovascularization occasionally accompanied by mononuclear cell infiltration. Deposits of immunoglobulins and complement were reported in the inner zone and granular immune deposits were also found at the base of the valve and along the valve leaflet. These findings have been suggested to represent the result of immune complex deposition that is thought to play a major pathogenic role in inducing the lesions (Quismorio, 1997).

The end-stage of Libman–Sacks verrucous endocarditis is a fibrous plaque, sometimes with focal calcification (Mandell, 1987). If the lesions are extensive enough, their healing may be accompanied by marked scarring, thickening, and deformity of the valve, which ultimately leads to valve dysfunction (Bulkley and Roberts, 1975; Mandell, 1987). Valve involvement is rarely responsible for severe haemodynamic changes, but can be complicated by thromboembolic disease and/or infective endocarditis.

* Corresponding author.
E-mail address: pierluigi.meroni@unimi.it (P.L. Meroni).

DOI: 10.1016/S1571-5078(03)01003-1

Table 1
Heart involvement by non-organ specific autoimmunity

Anatomical structure	Pathogenic mechanisms	Clinical setting
Valves	AutoAbs, IC, thrombosis	APS, SLE
Myocardium	AutoAbs, IC, CMI, thrombosis	SLE, SS, RA, SSc, APS
Pericardium	AutoAbs, IC	SLE, SSc, RA
Conductive Tissue	AutoAbs	NLS, SSc
Cardiac arteries	AutoAbs, IC, CMI, atherosclerosis	SLE, RA, DM, APS

AutoAbs, auto-antibodies; IC, immune-complexes; CMI, cell-mediated immunity; SS, Sjogren syndrome; DM, dermatomyositis.

2.2. Anti-phospholipid antibodies (aPL) and cardiac valvulopathy

Transthoracic and transoesophageal echocardiographic studies found a high prevalence of heart valve abnormalities in patients suffering from the primary anti-phospholipid antibody syndrome (PAPS) (Lockshin et al., 2003). On the other hand it is still debated whether the heart involvement in SLE patients with aPL is comparable or even higher than in SLE patients without the antibodies (Lockshin et al., 2003). Moreover, anecdotal reports on a thrombus over a histologically normal mitral valve (Nickele et al., 1994) and myxoid aortic valve degeneration (Galve et al., 1992) in patients with aPL have been published. Altogether these findings suggest a possible role for aPL in endocardial damage leading to valve lesions. Valve abnormalities associated with aPL are similar to those previously reported in SLE, varying from minimal thickening and/or vegetations to severe valve distortion and dysfunction (Lockshin et al., 2003).

An immune complex-mediated injury was initially hypothesized to be the first insult to the valve as also reported in Libman–Sacks endocarditis. Actually, deposits of immunoglobulins and complement, but not serum albumin have been found in the sub-endothelial connective tissue. The immune complex deposition apparently induces a mild inflammatory process that ends into vascular proliferation, fibroblast influx, fibrosis and calcification—all events that have also been described in the classical Libman–Sacks verrucous endocarditis (Ziporen et al., 1996).

The same authors (Ziporen et al., 1996) have evaluated by immunohistochemical methods the cardiac valves derived from patients with secondary and primary APS. Deposits of immunoglobulins and co-localized complement components (C1q, C3c and C4 with granular appearance) were observed in macroscopically or microscopically altered valves. The pattern of deposition was alike in all the valves, appearing as a distinct, sub-endothelial, ribbon-like layer along the surface of valve leaflets or cusps. This finding seems to be specifically related to the APS, as it was not seen in any of the normal or altered control valves. Using an anti-idiotypic monoclonal antibody to human anti-cardiolipin (aCL) IgG, the authors also found that immunoglobulin deposits were mainly due to IgG displaying aCL activity. The aCL specificity of the deposited antibodies was further confirmed by investigating the antibody specificity of the immunoglobulins eluted from the valve tissues. It is as yet unknown whether the sub-endothelial aCL deposition represents a primary event or is due to another unknown initiating insult.

However, because the formation of circulating immune complexes containing aPL is not apparently implicated in the pathogenesis of the other APS manifestations, it has been suggested that aPL might react with 'planted' antigens. Actually, aPL were reported to be able to bind endothelial cells mainly through the recognition of beta2-glycoprotein I (β2GPI) expressed on their surface membranes (Del Papa et al., 1995; Simantov et al., 1995). In vitro and in vivo experimental models did show that aPL binding to endothelial cells might induce several biological effects that could account for the appearance of a pro-inflammatory and a pro-coagulant endothelial phenotype (Meroni et al., 2001a). The aPL thrombogenic potential may also be exerted by interfering with the functions of already activated platelets, monocytes, and plasma proteins involved in blood coagulation and fibrinolysis (Meroni et al., 2001a). These mechanisms might theoretically contribute to the initial valve lesions.

Histological findings in the lesioned valve tissues from APS patients appear to display peculiar characteristics in comparison with those encountered in the thrombotic lesions usually occurring in the syndrome. In fact, the characteristic histopathological lesion in APS is a thrombotic vascular occlusion without clear signs of inflammation (Ford et al., 1994). In contrast, mild inflammatory changes were observed in the affected valves from patients with secondary (Leung et al., 1990; Jouhikainen et al., 1994) as well as primary APS (Pope et al., 1991; Ziporen et al., 1996). Interestingly, Pope et al. (1991) reported decreased total complement levels with low C3 and C4 in 11 out of 14 patients with APS and valvular heart disease, even though only three out of those 11 patients met the diagnostic criteria for SLE while others were apparently suffering from the primary APS. These findings were suggested to represent an additional fact in favour of the role of immune complexes in the pathogenesis of the heart valve lesions.

Being that endothelial cells are a target for aPL, their involvement in the pathogenesis of the valvular disease was recently investigated by Afek et al. (1999). Sixteen valves from 10 patients with APS were studied as compared to control valves. Interestingly, an increase in $\alpha_3\beta_1$ integrin endothelial expression together with immunoglobulin deposition on the affected valves was observed, while this was not the case in the control valves which displayed only a thin sub-endothelial band of collagen IV. The authors suggested a possible 'cause–effect' relationship between antibody deposition and the induction of a pro-adhesive endothelial phenotype.

On the whole, these findings seem to suggest a true pathogenic role for aPL in the development of valvular lesions and are against the hypothesis that these antibodies represent an epiphenomenona merely due to an immune response against antigens exposed on valves damaged by other causes. It has been hypothesized that the primary event is the aPL binding to valvular endothelial cells, followed by cell activation/damage that eventually ends in the appearance of a pro-inflammatory and pro-coagulant phenotype. This might play a pivotal role in favouring superficial thrombosis, sub-endocardial mononuclear-cell infiltration, and eventually, fibrosis or calcification.

Anti-phospholipid antibodies are now considered pathogenic auto-antibodies, but they are apparently unable to induce thrombotic manifestations per se. In this regard, a *two-hit hypothesis* was suggested: aPL (*first hit*) increases the risk of thrombotic events that occur in the presence of another thrombophilic condition (*second hit*). Such a hypothesis is in line with the experimental findings in murine models and might explain why patients persistently positive for aPL display thrombotic events only occasionally (Meroni and Riboldi, 2001). In this regard, the selective endothelial vulnerability of one section of the vascular tree rather than another or, alternatively, involvement of the valvular endocardium might be related to anatomic, cellular, and molecular localization of the *second hit*.

3. Cardiac arteries

3.1. Lesson from experimental animal models

Involvement of cardiac arteries is a common feature in patients suffering from SLE as well as in mice that spontaneously develop 'SLE-like' disease. For example, NZB/NZW F_1 mice display myocardial infarcts with hyaline thickening of small arteries, and about one-half of the MRL *lpr/lpr* mice develop acute necrotizing polyarteritis primarily involving coronary and renal arteries. Moreover, the high prevalence of myocardial infarctions in MRL *lpr/lpr* mice has been related to small vessel vasculopathy rather than to inflammation of medium-sized arteries (Hahn, 1997). Palmerston North (PM) mice is an additional SLE animal model characterized by a widespread necrotizing vasculitis of the small and medium arteries (Hahn, 1997). The main histopathological findings in these animals are suggestive of immune complex-mediated vascular damage.

At variance, the (NZW × BXSB) F_1 mice is the most interesting experimental animal model of accelerated degenerative coronary artery disease, quite comparable to that found in SLE patients (Hashimoto et al., 1992). In fact, up to 50% of these mice die at around 24 weeks of age because of extensive myocardial infarctions mainly due to small coronary artery involvement (Hashimoto et al., 1992). Interestingly, BXSB and the (NZW × BXSB) F_1 mice are also found positive for β2GPI-dependent aPL, suggesting that thrombotic events in addition to immune complex deposition might be responsible for such manifestations.

3.2. Atherosclerotic involvement

Epidemiological studies showed an increase of cardio- and cerebro-vascular events in patients suffering from systemic autoimmune diseases, such as SLE and Rheumatoid Arthritis (RA). Moreover, autopsy studies have pointed out that an accelerated atherosclerotic process is largely responsible for such manifestations (Salmon and Roman, 2001; Thiagarajan, 2001; Van Doornum et al., 2002).

Although it has been initially considered a bland lipid storage disease, atherosclerosis is now suggested as representing a process closely related to inflammation. Substantial advances in basic and experimental science have actually underlined the pivotal role of inflammatory mechanisms in induction, progression, and plaque rupture (Libby et al., 2002). Interestingly, accelerated atherosclerosis in systemic autoimmune diseases appears to be, at least in part, independent of the conventional risk factors and much closer to the chronic inflammatory status of these diseases (Libby et al., 2002). The immune system plays a key role in the pathogenesis of atherosclerosis by involving effectors of both innate and acquired immunity (Hansson et al., 2002).

The pathogenesis of atherosclerosis in systemic autoimmune diseases will be extensively addressed in another chapter "Atherosclerosis and Autoimmunity of the present book". It is, however, useful to mention the role of several differing autoantibodies in the atherosclerotic process. According to the 'oxidation hypothesis', low-density lipoproteins (LDL) are retained in the sub-endothelium and undergo oxidation. These modified lipids are thought to be responsible for 'triggering' inflammatory responses in macrophages and vascular wall cells. Epitopes generated by the LDL oxidation have been implicated as targets for autoantibodies. Some anti-oxidized LDL (ox-LDL) antibodies can enhance ox-LDL uptake by macrophages, most likely through involvement of the Fcγ receptors (FcγR) rather than via the usually employed scavenger receptor (CD36). Such an increased uptake was suggested as playing a role in experimental murine models of accelerated atherosclerosis, probably by favouring foam cell formation and macrophage activation. In line with this finding, several groups have found an association between raised anti-ox-LDL, antibody levels and premature atherosclerosis (Sherer and Shoenfeld, 2002). However, recent findings have shown that reduction of anti-ox-LDL, antibodies as well as animal immunization with ox-LDL or with bacterial antigens able to induce antibodies cross-reacting with the ox-LDL themselves, may induce a protective rather than an aggravating effect on the atherosclerotic process (Binder et al., 2003; Rose and Afanasyeva, 2003). It has been suggested that different sub-populations of anti-ox-LDL antibodies do exist and, in particular, that in addition to pathogenic antibodies, protective antibodies may also be found.

Interestingly, β2GPI was found to bind ox-LDL and to inhibit their uptake by macrophages, thus displaying some protection against atherosclerosis; however, the binding of anti-β2GPI antibodies to the ox-LDL/β2GPI complexes makes their engulfment by macrophages even more efficient, thus raising the possibility for an additional pathogenic mechanism for atherosclerosis closely linked to a well-known autoantibody family (Matsuura et al., 2002). Moreover, anti-β2GPI antibodies, being able to directly react with their antigens expressed on the endothelial cell membranes and to induce a pro-inflammatory and a pro-coagulant endothelial phenotype, have also been thought to play a role in early steps of the atherosclerotic process (Meroni et al., 2001a).

Finally, raised plasma levels of antibodies against the heat shock protein (HSP) 65 have been associated with sonographic-documented carotid atherosclerosis in humans. Immunization with HSP65 has been found to be able to accelerate atherosclerotic lesions both in rabbits and mice (Wick et al., 2001). Interestingly, interleukin (IL)-4 knockout mice displayed less fatty streak formation than wild type animals when immunized with HSP65 (George et al., 2000). These data underline the potential role of a cytokine profile that favours the humoral immune responses (Th2 type) in atherosclerosis.

Recently Liuzzo et al. (1999, 2000) reported increased levels of an unusual subset of T cells, $CD4^{+}CD28^{null}$, in up to 65% of patients with unstable but not in stable angina patients. This lymphocyte subpopulation was originally described in patients with RA and was found to be associated with extra-articular (mainly vascular) manifestations of the disease. Such a subpopulation represents the main cellular source for interferon (IFN)-γ that is increased in unstable angina and responsible for monocyte/macrophage activation, particularly through the up-regulation of FcγRI (CD64). This finding identifies an additional link between cytokine secretion and effector mechanisms related to antibody processing, such as FcγR.

3.3. Coronary artery involvement in primary vasculitis

Kawasaki disease (KD) is one of the major causes of heart disease in children, especially in Japan and North America. Even if the disease is self-limited, without prompt treatment, about 20–30% of patients develop coronary artery abnormalities due to an inflammatory arteritis, with subsequent formation of coronary aneurysms (Freeman and Shulman, 2001; Lehman, 2001).

KD is a medium-sized vessel vasculitis with pathologic feature closely related to infantile polyarteritis (Lehman, 2001). Circulating immune complexes have been demonstrated and reported to be a predictor of the disease; accordingly, the pathogenesis of the vasculitis was related to an inflammatory process triggered by their deposition. However, still uncharacterized are the antibodies and antigens responsible. The recent demonstration of the presence of oligoclonally expanded IgA-secreting plasma cells in the vascular walls of KD patients strongly supports the view that the immune response in KD is antigen-driven in contrast with the previous hypothesis of a response to a super-antigen (Rowley et al., 2001).

Both anti-neutrophil cytoplasm antibodies (ANCA) and anti-endothelial cell antibodies (AECA) have been reported in KD patients. However, while ANCA are rarely found, AECA have been described by several groups in up to 70 % of the patients (Meroni et al., 2001b). AECA are apparently good candidates for pathogenic mechanisms: (i) their presence correlates with disease activity, being more frequently detectable during the acute phase of the disease; (ii) in vitro experimental models showed the ability of AECA to display a complement-dependent cytotoxic activity against endothelial cell monolayers (Meroni et al., 2001b). Moreover, Grunebaum et al. (2002) have recently reported that $F(ab)_2$ fragments of IgG and IgM-AECA from KD patients were able to induce a pro-inflammatory and pro-adhesive phenotype in human umbilical vein endothelial cells (HUVEC). The same authors showed that active immunization of naïve Balb/C mice with human KD-AECA Ig induced the appearance of murine AECA as a result of the idiotypic network manipulation. The murine AECA displayed the same in vitro pro-inflammatory activity of the original KD-AECA human Ig and the mice developed proteinuria and IgG deposition in the renal mesangium. It has been suggested that AECA might be the initial insult to the endothelium, eventually triggering a vessel wall inflammatory process.

KD is characterized by a systemic inflammation, especially during the acute phase, and high plasma levels of pro-inflammatory cytokines have been reported in these patients (Freeman and Shulman, 2001; Lehman, 2001). Interestingly, the AECA mediated endothelial complement-dependent cytotoxicity was reported to take place on cytokine-activated endothelial cells only, suggesting that endothelial activation and neo-antigen expression or antigen up-regulation might be pathogenic mechanisms (Meroni et al., 2001b).

However, in spite of the above-mentioned findings, no association between the AECA presence and titres was found with coronary artery involvement in KD patients (Meroni et al., 2001b). Moreover, even in the recent experimental in vivo idiotypic model, no histological or immunofluorescence evidence for cardiac vasculitis could be found (Grunebaum et al., 2002).

Alternative pathogenic mechanisms potentially responsible for the vessel wall damage were also reported: (i) local vessel infiltration of pro-adhesive activated macrophages (Furukawa et al., 1992; Koga et al., 1998; Katayama et al., 2000); and (ii) high plasma levels of vascular endothelial growth factor (VEGF) (Maeno et al., 1998). Serum VEGF levels in acute KD, and particularly in infants who developed coronary artery lesions, were actually much higher than in the control infectious diseases. Since VEGF stimulates nitric oxide production and increases vascular permeability, it might be involved in vascular damage and remodelling as well as in inducing the sub-endothelial oedema and endothelial cell gap formation found in the skin of acute KD patients.

Heart vessel involvement may also occur in the context of other primary vasculitides, particularly in polyarteritis nodosa (PAN) and Churg–Strauss syndrome (CSS). While autopsy demonstration of such involvement was reported in up to 64% of the cases (for example in CSS patients), clinical manifestations are much less common (Raza et al., 2001). The pathogenic mechanisms responsible for the cardiac vessel damage have not been investigated in detail, but it has been suggested that immune complex deposition may play a major role.

4. Heart conduction tissue

Complete heart block (CHB) is the most serious manifestation of the Neonatal Lupus Syndrome (NLS), a congenital syndrome which affects infants born to mothers who carry anti-SSA/Ro and anti-SSB/La autoantibodies.

Transplacental transfer of the maternal IgG autoantibodies has been strongly suggested as representing a key pathogenic mechanism, although there are still some open questions (Buyon and Clancy, 2003). Table 2 summarizes the facts in favour as well as those against a direct pathogenic role of anti-SSA/Ro and anti-SSB/La autoantibodies in CHB.

Although the topic will be detailed in another chapter of the book, it is useful to point out that these autoantibodies are thought to mediate fetal myocardial damage through two main pathogenic mechanisms. Once bound to their respective antigens (mainly expressed on the surface blebs of apoptotic myocardiocytes) these autoantibodies can opsonize the apoptotic cells thus favouring their uptake by macrophages and the induction of a local inflammatory and pro-fibrotic process (Buyon and Clancy, 2003). Such a hypothesis is in line with the histopathological signs of inflammation and fibrosis reported in the affected cardiac tissues in some cases (Meckler and Kapur, 1998). In addition, there is evidence from both in vitro and in vivo experimental models that anti-SSA/Ro and anti-SSB/La IgG antibodies can directly affect the function of Ca^{2+} cell membrane channels (Buyon and Clancy, 2003). Since ionic currents across the cell membrane play a pivotal role in the excitation–contraction phenomena, such interference might explain the CHB peculiar electrophysiological abnormalities (Buyon and Clancy, 2003).

Electrocardiographic abnormalities, other than those found in CHB, have been reported in association with anti-SSA/Ro antibodies, such as bradycardia, atrio-ventricular (AV) blocks of varying degrees and prolongation of the QT interval (Brucato et al., 2000; Gordon et al., 2001; Cimaz et al., 2000). Incomplete AV blocks and QT prolongation are the abnormalities which point to much closer and direct involvement of the cardiac conduction tissue. The latter abnormality, in particular, is thought to be of clinical relevance because it can favour malignant ventricular arrhythmias that increase the risk of sudden infant death

Table 2
Pathogenic role of anti-SSA/Ro and anti-SSB/La autoantibodies in CHB: facts in favour and against

In favour	Against
Presence of maternal autoAbs in foetal/neonatal circulation	Few babies of anti-SSA/SSB positive mothers are affected
Elution of anti-SSA/Ro Abs from cardiac tissues of affected foetuses	Discordance of CHB manifestation in twins
Identification of anti-SSB/La idiotypes a neonate with CHB	CHB is exceptional in adult patients positive for anti- SSA/Ro-SSB/La Abs
Complete AV block in pups of mice passively injected with anti-SSA/Ro 52 Abs	
Anti-SSA/Ro IgG inhibits L-type Ca^{2+} channel in rat and rabbit heart, in vitro	

(Schwartz et al., 1998). QT internal prolongation was initially found in children born to anti-SSA/Ro positive mothers with a prevalence up to 40%; an ongoing multicenter study, however, did confirm such a prevalence (Meroni et al., personal communication). At variance with classic CHB, the QT interval prolongation was found to be transient, since it normalized within the first year of life. Interestingly, a close relationship between QT interval normalization and the disappearance of the maternal anti-SSA/Ro antibodies form the neonatal circulation was recently reported (Cimaz et al., 2003). Although the pathogenetic mechanisms involved in the QT prolongation are not yet known, the close association with the presence of anti-SSA/Ro antibodies does suggest a pivotal role for these antibodies. As hypothesized for the pathogenesis of CHB it is likely that interference of the autoantibodies with myocardial Ca^{2+} channels might be important.

5. Myocardial tissue

5.1. Myocardial tissue involvement and aPL

Since the recognition of the APS, a variety of cardiac manifestations have been associated with aPL. Besides coronary thrombotic events and accelerated atherosclerosis (which are detailed in another chapter "Atherosclerosis and Autoimmunity of the present book") and the well-known valvulopathy, a large variety of both systolic and diastolic dysfunctions has been described in primary and secondary APS, even in the presence of normal valves and coronary arteries (Leung et al., 1990; Airoldi et al., 1996; Espinola-Zavaleta et al., 1999; Tektonidou et al., 2001; Cervera et al., 2002). Antiphospholipid antibodies have been associated with small thrombi in intra-myocardial arterioles and have been reported as causative factors of the diastolic dysfunction (Murphy and Leach, 1989; Leung et al., 1990; Tektonidou et al., 2001). Autopsy examination of the heart of patients with secondary APS have shown micro-vascular thrombosis of small arterioles of the myocardium with no evidence of vessel wall inflammation (Brown et al., 1988; Greisman et al., 1991). This intra-myocardial occlusive vasculopathy could lead to diastolic abnormalities through asymptomatic myocardial ischaemia. Moreover, post-mortem examination of patients with catastrophic APS has shown multiple thrombosis within the intra-myocardial arteries (Asherson et al., 1998). Comparable histological alterations could be hypothesized in APS patients presenting with acute or sub-acute ischaemic myocardial events, with normal major epicardial arteries at angiography. Few cases of heart involvement during the post-partum period characterized by cardiomyopathy with impaired left ventricular function and persistent positivity for aPL have been also reported (Kochenour et al., 1987; Hochfeld et al., 1994; Kupfermic et al., 1994; Airoldi et al., 1996). Although immunoglobulin and complement deposition was found at the myocardial biopsy in some patients, the main pathogenic mechanism beyond such manifestations is likely to be related to the thrombophilic activity of aPL.

5.2. Myocarditis in SLE

Clinical evidence of a direct myocardial involvement in SLE is uncommon, while at autopsy SLE myocarditis is recognized more frequently than those reported in clinical series (Moder et al., 1999). Post-mortem examination of cardiac specimens and endomyocardial biopsies has shown immune complex deposition, lymphocyte and plasma cell perivascular infiltration and fibrinoid necrosis (Quismorio, 1997). Immunofluorescence in several cases demonstrated granular deposits of immunoglobulins and C3 in perivascular areas (Bidani et al., 1980). The pathogenesis of these lesions is represented in most cases by complement activation secondary to immune complex deposition. Complement activation leads to the formation of anaphylatoxins C5a and C3a that enhance the inflammatory process and the generation of the lytic membrane attack complex (MAC) (Walport, 2001). In a subgroup of patients, positive for anti-RNP autoantibodies, myocarditis may be associated with inflammatory skeletal myositis (Borenstein et al., 1978).

6. Endocardium

Endocardial fibroelastosis (EFE) is a rare and poorly understood disease of the endo-myocardium.

The pathologic features consist of collagen and elastin deposition, ventricular hypertrophy, and diffuse endocardial thickening. Its a etiopathogenesis remains unclear, but it has been suggested that EFE may be secondary to an autoimmune process (Nield et al., 2002a). In line with this hypothesis, an association with maternal anti-SSA/Ro and anti-SSB/La antibodies and CHB has been well documented (Silverman et al., 1995).

A recent study has reported an immunohistochemical analysis on foetuses and children with EFE and CHB associated with maternal anti-SSA/Ro and/or anti-SSB/LA antibodies. The analysis was performed on autopsy specimens, explanted hearts or endomyocardial biopsies in four cases and in five controls. All the cases showed a dense and diffuse IgG infiltrate across myocardial and AV nodal tissue, while three also showed IgM deposition and multiple foci of infiltrating T cells. Control hearts displayed diffuse deposition of IgG, but no IgM or T cell infiltrates. The fact that EFE occurred in these babies despite adequate ventricular pacing was thought to be against the hypothesis that EFE may be a phenomenon attributable to long-standing heart block, bradycardia, and congestive heart failure. In addition, the immunohistological findings favour a foetal immune response against the self endomyocardium (Nield et al., 2002a). The same group has recently reported three cases of isolated EFE associated with maternal anti-SSA/Ro and anti-SSB/La antibodies in the absence of CHB. The immunohistochemical analysis demonstrated a pattern similar to that of CHB-associated EFE, with diffuse areas of IgG deposition, milder IgM deposition, $CD8^+$ T cell and occasional B cell infiltrates in the myocardium. The TUNEL staining was negative indicating the absence of apoptosis in the cardiac tissue (Nield et al., 2002b).

Taken together, these data suggest that endomyocardial damage in these patients is closely associated with maternal anti-SSA/Ro and anti-SSB/La antibodies crossing the transplacental barrier in utero. In a subgroup of foetuses and infants the initial damage mediated by the maternal autoantibodies could be perpetuated by an ongoing foetal immune response to the myocardium, ultimately leading to fibroelastosis.

7. Pericardium

Pericarditis and pericardial effusion are the most frequent cardiac manifestations in systemic autoimmune diseases. Immune complex deposition is the main pathogenic mechanism at least in SLE, SLE-like diseases and some vasculitides. In scleroderma (SSc) no obvious pathogenic mechanism has been substantiated. More likely, the explanation may be that pericardial effusions in this disease have a haemodynamic origin, linked to the frequently associated pulmonary hypertension.

Acknowledgements

This study has been in part supported by Ricerca Corrente IRCCS Istituto Auxologico Italiano 2002-03 (to PLM).

Key points

- Cardiac involvement is one of the main complications that contribute to the morbidity and mortality of patients suffering from systemic autoimmune diseases.
- Basically all the anatomical cardiac structures can be affected by different humoral non-organ autoimmune processes.
- Heart valves can be damaged by circulating immune complexes in the classical Libman-Sachs endocarditis or by in situ formed complexes in the APS.
- Accelerated atherosclerosis sustained by the systemic inflammation linked to the underlying disease states as well as by different autoantibodies is mainly responsible for coronary artery involvement.
- Heart vessels can be also affected by the vasculitic process in systemic vasculitides and by the aPL-associated thrombotic vasculopathy.
- Anti-SSA/Ro and anti-SSB/La antibodies display a pathogenic role in damaging the heart conduction tissue (NLS) or the endo-myocardial tissue (EFE).

References

Afek, A., Shoenfeld, Y., Manor, R., Goldberg, I., Ziporen, L., George, J., Polak-Charcon, S., Amigo, M.C., Garcia-Torres, R., Segal, R., Kopolovie, J., 1999. Increased endothelial cell expression of alpha-3-beta1 integrin in cardiac valvulopathy in the primary (Hughes) and secondary antiphospholipid syndrome. Lupus 8, 502.
The paper reports the first demonstration of the association between Ig deposits and endothelial activation in lesioned heart valves from APS patients.

Airoldi, M.L., Eid, O., Tosetto, C., Meroni, P.L., 1996. Post-partum dilated cardiomyopathy in antiphospholipid positive woman. Lupus 5, 247.

Asherson, R.A., Cervera, R., Piette, J.C., Font, J., Lie, J.T., Burcoglu, A., Lim, K., Munoz-Rodriguez, F.J., Levy, R.A., Boue, F., Rossert, J., Ingelmo, M., 1998. Catastrophic antiphospholipid syndrome. Clinical and laboratory features of 50 patients. Medicine 77, 195.

Bidani, A.K., Roberts, J.L., Schwartz, M.M., Lewis, E.J., 1980. Immunopathology of cardiac lesions in fatal systemic lupus erythematosus. Am. J. Med. 69, 849.

Binder, C.J., Horkko, S., Dewan, A., Chang, M.K., Kieu, E.P., Goodyear, C.S., Shaw, P.X., Palinski, W., Witztum, J.L., Silverman, G.J., 2003. Pneumococcal vaccination decreases atherosclerotic lesion formation: molecular mimicry between *Streptococcus pneumoniae* and oxidized LDL. Nature Med. 9, 736.
The paper pointed out the existence of different sub-populations of anti-oxLDL antibodies with protective or facilitating activity against atherosclerosis.

Borenstein, D.G., Fye, W.B., Arnett, F.C., Stevens, M.B., 1978. The myocarditis of systemic lupus erythematosus: association with myositis. Ann. Intern. Med. 89, 619.

Brown, J.H., Doherty, C.C., Allen, D.C., Morton, P., 1988. Fatal cardiac failure due to myocardial microthrombi in systemic lupus erythematosus. BMJ 296, 1505.

Brucato, A., Cimaz, R., Catelli, L., Meroni, P.L., 2000. Anti-Ro associated sinus bradycardia in newborns. Circulation 102, 388.

Bulkley, B.H., Roberts, W.C. 1975. The heart in systemic lupus erythematosus and the changes induced in it by corticosteroid therapy: a study of 36 necropsy patients. Am. J. Med. 58, 243.

Buyon, J.P., Clancy, R.M. 2003. Neonatal lupus: review of proposed pathogenesis and clinical data from the US-based research registry for neonatal lupus. Autoimmunity 36, 41.
Extensive and up-dated review on the pathogenic mechanisms involved in Neonatal Lupus.

Cervera, R., Piette, J.C., Font, J., Khamashta, M.A., Shoenfeld, Y., Camps, M.T., Jacobsen, S., Lakos, G., Tincani, A., Kontopoulou-Griva, I., Galeazzi, M., Meroni, P.L., Derksen, R.H., de Groot, P.G., Gromnica-Ihle, E., Baleva, M., Mosca, M., Bombardieri, S., Houssiau, F., Gris, J.C., Quere, I., Hachulla, E., Vasconcelos, C., Roch, B., Fernandez-Nebro, A., Boffa, M.C.,Hughes, G.R., Ingelmo, M., 2002. Antiphospholipid syndrome: clinical and immunologic manifestations and patterns of disease expression in a cohort of 1000 patients. Arthritis Rheum. 46, 1019.

Cimaz, R., Stramba-Badiale, M., Brucato, A., Catelli, L., Panzeri, P., Meroni, P.L., 2000. QT interval prolongation in asymptomatic anti-SSA/Ro-positive infants without congenital heart block. Arthritis Rheum. 43, 1049.

Cimaz, R., Meroni, P.L., Brucato, A., Fesslova, V., Panzeri, P., Goulene, K., Stramba-Badiale, M., 2003. Concomitant disappearance of electrocardiographic abnormalities and of acquired maternal autoantibodies during the first year of life in infants who had QT interval prolongation and anti-SSA/Ro positivity without congenital heart block at birth. Arthritis Rheum. 48, 266.

Del Papa, N., Guidali, L., Spatola, L., Bonara, P., Borghi, M.O., Tincani, A., Balestrieri, G., Meroni, P.L., 1995. Relationship between anti-phospholipid and anti-endothelial cell antibodies, III: beta sub 2 glycoprotein I mediates the antibody binding to endothelial membranes and induces the expression of adhesion molecules. Clin. Exp. Rheumatol. 13, 179.

Espinola-Zavaleta, N., Vargas-Barron, J., Colmenares-Galvis, T., Cruz-Cruz, F., Romero-Cardenas, A., Keirns, C., Amigo, M.C., 1999. Echocardiographic evaluation of patients with primary antiphospholipid syndrome. Am. Heart J. 137, 973.

Ford, S.E., Kennedy, L., Ford, P.M. 1994. Clinicopathologic correlations of antiphospholipid antibodies: an autopsy study. Arch. Pathol. Lab. Med. 118, 491.

Freeman, A.F., Shulman, S.T. 2001. Recent developments in Kawasaki disease. Curr. Opin. Infect. Dis. 14, 357.

Furukawa, S., Matsubara, T., Yabuta, K. 1992. Mononuclear cell subsets and coronary artery lesion in Kawasaki disease. Arch. Dis. Child. 67, 706.

Galve, E., Ordi, J., Barquinero, J., Evangelista, A., Vilardell, M., Soler-Soler, J., 1992. Valvular heart disease in the primary antiphospholipid syndrome. Ann. Intern. Med. 116, 293.

George, J., Shoenfeld, Y., Gilburd, B., Afek, A., Shaish, A., Harats, D., 2000. Requisite role for interleukin-4 in the acceleration of fatty streaks induced by heat shock protein 65 or *Mycobacterium tuberculosis*. Circ Res. 23, 1203.

Gordon, P.A., Khamashta, M.A., Hughes, G.R., Rosenthal, E., 2001. Increase in the heart rate-corrected QT interval in children of anti-Ro-positive mothers, with a further increase in those with siblings with congenital heart block: comment on the article by Cimaz et al. Arthritis Rheum. 44, 242.

Greisman, S.G., Thayaparan, R.S., Godwin, T.A., Lockshin, M.D., 1991. Occlusive vasculopathy in systemic lupus erythematosus. Arch. Intern. Med. 15, 389.

Grunebaum, E., Blank, M., Cohen, S., Afek, A., Kopolovic, J., Meroni, P.L., Youinou, P., Shoenfeld, Y., 2002. The role of anti-endothelial cell antibodies in Kawasaki disease-in vitro and in vivo studies. Clin. Exp. Immunol. 130, 233.
The paper reports original in vivo and in vitro experimental models that supports the pathogenic role of AECA in the Kawasaki disease.

Hahn, B.H. 1997. Animal models of systemic lupus erythematosus. In: D.J. Wallace, B.H. Hahn (Eds.), Dubois' Lupus Erythematosus. Williams & Wilkins, Baltimore, p. 339.

Hansson, G.K., Libby, P., Schonbeck, U., Zhon-Qun, Y., 2002. Innate and adaptive immunity in the pathogenesis of atherosclerosis. Circ. Res. 91, 281.

Hashimoto, Y., Kawamura, M., Ichikawa, K., Suzuki, T., Sumida, T., Yoshida, S., Matsuura, E., Ikehara, S., Koike, T., 1992. Anticardiolipin antibodies in NZW BXSB F1 mice. A model of antiphospholipid syndrome. J. Immunol. 149, 1063.

Hochfeld, M., Druzin, M.L., Maia, D., Wright, J., Lambert, R.E., McGuire, J., 1994. Pregnancy complicated by primary antiphospholipid antibody syndrome. Obstet. Gynecol. 83, 804.

Jouhikainen, T., Pohjola-Sintonen, S., Stephansson, E. 1994. Lupus anticoagulant and cardiac manifestations in systemic lupus erythematosus. Lupus 3, 167.

Katayama, K., Matsubara, T., Fujiwara, M., Furukawa, S., 2000. CD14 + CD16 + monocyte subpopulation in Kawasaki disease. Clin. Exp. Immunol. 121, 566.

Kochenour, N.K., Branch, D.W., Rote, N.S., Scott, J.R., 1987. A new postpartum syndrome associated with antiphospholipid antibodies. Obstet. Gynecol. 69, 460.

Koga, M., Ishihara, T., Takahashi, M., Umezawa, Y., Furukawa, S., 1998. Activation of peripheral blood monocytes and macrophages in Kawasaki disease: ultrastructural and immunohistochemical investigation. Pathol. Int. 48, 512.

Kupfermic, M.J., Lee, M.J., Green, D., Peacemen, A.M., 1994. Severe post-partum pulmonary, cardiac and renal syndrome associated with antiphospholipid antibodies. Obstet. Gynecol. 83, 806.

Lehman, T.J.A. 2001. The vasculitic diseases of childhood. In: R.A. Asherson, R. Cervera (Eds.), Vascular Manifestations of Systemic Autoimmune Diseases. CRC Press, Boca Raton, FL, pp. 393.

Extensive review on the different organ involvement in the Kawasaki disease.

Leung, W.H., Wong, K.L., Lau, C.P., Wong, C.K., Cheng, C.H., 1990. Association between antiphospholipid antibodies and cardiac abnormalities in patients with systemic lupus erythematosus. Am. J. Med.
89, 411.

Libby, P., Ridker, P.M., Maseri, A. 2002. Inflammation and atherosclerosis. Circulation 105, 1135.

Liuzzo, G., Kopecky, S.L., Frye, R.L., Fallon, M.O., Maseri, A., Goronzy, J.J., Weyand, C.M., 1999. Perturbation of the T-cell repertoire in patients with unstable angina. Circulation 100, 2135.

Liuzzo, G., Goronzy, J.J., Yang, H., Kopecky, S.L., Holmes, D.R., Frye, R.L., Weyand, C.M., 2000. Monoclonal T-cell proliferation and plaque instability in acute coronary syndromes. Circulation 102, 2883.

Lockshin, M., Tenedios, F., Petri, M., McCarty, G., Forastiero, R., Krilis, S., Tincani, A., Erkan, D., Khamashta, M.A., Shoenfeld, Y., 2003. Cardiac disease in the antiphospholipid syndrome: recommendations for treatment. Committee consensus report. Lupus 12, 518.

Consensus report on the heart involvement in primary and secondary APS.

Maeno, N., Takei, S., Masuda, K., Akaike, H., Matsuo, K., Kitajima, I., Maruyama, I., Miyata, K., 1998. Increased serum levels of vascular endothelial growth factor in Kawasaki disease. Pediatr. Res. 44, 596.

Mandell, B.F. 1987. Cardiovascular involvement in systemic lupus erythematosus. Semin. Arthritis Rheum. 17, 126.

Matsuura, E., Kobayashi, K., Kasahara, J., Yasuda, T., Makino, H., Koike, T., Shoenfeld, Y., 2002. Anti-beta 2-glycoprotein I autoantibodies and atherosclerosis. Int. Rev. Immunol. 21, 51.

Meckler, K.A., Kapur, R.P. 1998. Congenital heart block and associated cardiac pathology in neonatal lupus syndrome. Pediatr. Dev. Pathol. 1, 136.

Meroni, P.L., Riboldi, P. 2001. Pathogenetic mechanisms mediating antiphospholipid syndrome. Curr. Opin. Rheumatol. 13, 377.

Meroni, P.L., Raschi, E., Testoni, C., Tincani, A., Balestrieri, G., 2001a. Antiphospholipid antibodies and the endothelium. Rheum. Dis. N. Am. 27, 587.

Meroni, P.L., Del Papa, N., Raschi, E. 2001b. Anti-endothelial cell antibodies. In: R.A. Asherson, R. Cervera (Eds.), Vascular Manifestations of Systemic Autoimmune Diseases. CRC Press, Boca Raton, FL, p. 107.

Extensive review on the prevalence and the diagnostic and prognostic value of AECA in different pathological conditions.

Moder, K.G., Miller, T.D., Tazelaar, H.D. 1999. Cardiac involvement in systemic lupus erythemathosus. Mayo Clin. Proc. 74, 75.

Murphy, J.J., Leach, I.H. 1989. Findings at necropsy in the heart of a patient with anticardiolipin syndrome. Br. Heart J. 62, 61.

Nickele, G.A., Foster, P.A., Kenny, D. 1994. Primary antiphospholipid syndrome and mitral valve thrombosis. Am. Heart J. 128, 1245.

Nield, L.E., Silverman, E.D., Smallhorn, J.F., Taylor, G.P., Mullen, J.B., Benson, L.N., Hornberger, L.K., 2002a. Endocardial fibroelastosis associated with maternal anti-Ro and anti-La antibodies in the absence of atrioventricular block. J. Am. Coll. Cardiol. 40, 796.

Nield, L.E., Silverman, E.D., Taylor, G.P., Smallhorn, J.F., Mullen, J.B., Silverman, N.H., Finley, J.P., Law, Y.M., Human, D.G., Seaward, P.G., Hamilton, R.M., Hornberger, L.K., 2002b. Maternal anti-Ro and anti-La antibody-associated endocardial fibroelastosis. Circulation 105, 843.

The paper reports for the first time the occurrence of endocardial fibroelastosis in the presence of maternal anti-SSA/Ro and anti-SSB/La antibodies but without CHB.

Pope, J.M., Canny, C.L.B., Bell, D.A. 1991. Cerebral ischemic events associated with endocarditis, retinal vascular disease, and lupus anticoagulant. Am. J. Med. 90, 299.

Quismorio, F.P. Jr. 1997. Cardiac abnormalities in systemic lupus erythematosus. In: D.J. Wallace, B.H. Hahn (Eds.), Dubois' Lupus Erythematosus. Williams & Wilkins, Baltimore, p. 653.

Extensive review on the heart involvement in SLE.

Raza, K., Carruthers, D.M., Bacon, P.A. 2001. In: R.A. Asherson, R. Cervera (Eds.), Vascular Manifestations of Systemic Autoimmune Diseases. CRC Press, Boca Raton, FL, p. 213.

Extensive review on the different organ involvement in systemic autoimmune vasculitis.

Riboldi, P., Gerosa, M., Luzzana, C., Catelli, L., 2002. Cardiac involvement in systemic autoimmune diseases. Clin. Rev.

Allergy Immunol. 23, 237.
Review paper on the cardiac involvement in systemic autoimmune diseases.

Rose, N., Afanasyeva, M. 2003. Autoimmunity: busting the atherosclerotic claque. Nature Med. 9, 641.

Rowley, A.H., Shulman, S.T., Spike, B.T., Mask, C.A., Baker, S.C., 2001. Oligoclonal IgA response in the vascular wall in acute Kawasaki disease. J. Immunol. 15, 1334.

Salmon, J.E., Roman, M.J. 2001. Accelerated atherosclerosis in systemic lupus erythematosus: implications for patient management. Curr. Opin. Rheumatol. 13, 341.

Schwartz, P.J., Stramba-Badiale, M., Segantini, A., Austoni, P., Bosi, G., Giorgetti, R., Grancini, F., Marni, E.D., Perticone, F., Rosti, D., Salice, P., 1998. Prolongation of the QT interval and the sudden infant death syndrome. N. Engl. J. Med. 338, 1709.

Sherer, Y., Shoenfeld, Y. 2002. Atherosclerosis. Ann. Rheum. Dis. 61, 97.
Updated commentary on the different immune-mediated mechanisms involved in the pathogenesis of atherosclerosis.

Silverman, E.D., Buyon, J., Laxer, R.M., Hamilton, R., Bini, P., Chu, J.L., Elkon, K.B., 1995. Autoantibody response to the Ro/La particle may predict outcome in neonatal lupus erythematosus. Clin. Exp. Immunol. 100, 499.

Simantov, R., LaSala, J.M., Lo, S.K., Gharavi, A.E., Samaritano, L.R., Salmon, J.E., Silverstein, R.L., 1995. Activation of cultured vascular endothelial cells by antiphospholipid antibodies. J. Clin Invest. 96, 2211.

Tektonidou, M.G., Ioannidis, J.P., Moyssakis, I., Boki, K.A., Vassiliou, V., Vlachoyiannopoulos, P.G., Kyriakidis, M.K., Moutsopoulous, H.M., 2001. Right ventricular diastolic dysfunction in patients with anticardiolipin antibodies and antiphospholipid syndrome. Ann. Rheum. Dis. 60, 43.

Thiagarajan, P. 2001. Atherosclerosis, autoimmunity, and systemic lupus erythematosus. Circulation 104, 1876.
Extensive review on the accelerated atherosclerosis in SLE.

Van-Doornum, S., McColl, G., Wicks, I.P. 2002. Accelerated atherosclerosis. An extraarticular feature of rheumatoid arthtritis? Arthritis Rheum. 46, 862.
Review paper on the premature atherosclerosis in RA.

Walport, M.J. 2001. Complement (Second of two parts). N. Engl. J. Med. 344, 1140.

Wick, G., Perschinka, H., Millonig, G. 2001. Atherosclerosis as an autoimmune disease: an update. Trends Immunol. 22, 665.

Ziporen, L., Goldberg, I., Arad, M., Hojnik, M., Ordi-Ros, J., Afek, A., Blank, M., Sandbank, Y., Vilardell-Tarres, M., de Torres, I., Weinberger, A., Asherson, R.A., Kopolovic, Y., Shoenfeld, Y., 1996. Libman–Sacks endocarditis in the antiphospholipid syndrome: Immunopathogenic findings in deformed heart valves. Lupus 5, 196.

Handbook of Systemic Autoimmune Diseases, Volume 1
The Heart in Systemic Autoimmune Diseases
A. Doria and P. Pauletto, editors

CHAPTER 4

Pathogenesis of Anti-SSA/Ro-SSB/La Associated Congenital Heart Block

Robert M. Clancy*, Jill P. Buyon

Department of Medicine, Division of Rheumatology, New York University Medical Center, Hospital for Joint Diseases, 301 East 17th Street, New York, NY 10003, USA

1. Introduction

Autoantibody associated congenital heart block (CHB) is a passively acquired autoimmune disease in a fetus, which is strongly associated with maternal antibodies to the intracellular ribonucleoproteins SSA/Ro and/or SSB/La (anti-Ro/La). It is a widely held view that these maternal autoantibodies, which are transferred across the placenta into the fetal circulation, actually cause CHB and are not merely disease markers. However, the molecular mechanism explaining their pathogenesis is not completely defined. In fact, CHB occurs in only 2% of offspring born to mothers with anti-Ro/La antibodies suggesting that there might be a subset of pathogenic antibodies as well as fetal factors, which contribute to disease expression. CHB is one of several fetal/neonatal autoimmune diseases in pregnancy, which include transient myasthenia gravis and alloimmune thrombocytopenia. However, these two latter diseases stand in striking contrast to CHB with regard to the target antigen and its surface accessibility to the cognate maternal autoantibody, and the time course of clinical manifestations. In transient myasthenia gravis (TMG) and neonatal alloimmune thrombocytopenia (NAIT), symptoms parallel the half-life of IgG immunoglobulins and abate coincident with the clearance of the maternal antibodies from the neonatal circulation. In contrast to these transient diseases, CHB, at least third degree, is permanent, and progressive deterioration in myocardial function can occur after the circulating maternal antibodies are no longer detectable in the child. Moreover, in some neonates of anti-Ro/La positive-mothers, subclinical disease can be initially present (first degree block) and months later deteriorate to more advanced degrees of block (second and third degree). This suggests that the antibody insult leading to fibrosis can be variable, kept in check in most fetuses, and in others rapid and relentless. Accordingly, the Abs are necessary but insufficient to cause CHB. In this review, the capacity of maternal Abs to initiate an inflammatory cellular response in the target tissue and promote fibrosis is addressed, and the following highlighted: (1) to define the molecular pathways for macrophages which engulf apoptotic cells in CHB; (2) to identify how macrophage derived TGFβ fits into the pathogenic mechanism for CHB and (3) to summarize our current progress on the identification of fetal susceptibility genes in CHB. Regarding the latter, an emphasis on genes encoding immune response products such as HLA Class II molecules is giving way to those encoding cytokines and growth factors such as TGFβ. It is envisioned that a genetic approach will provide a haplotype chip in which the expression of a collection of gene products with defined SNPs will predict the child of an anti-Ro (or other pathogenic antibody)

*Corresponding author.
E-mail addresses: bobdclancy@aol.com (R.M. Clancy), jbuyonic@aol.com (J.P. Buyon).

DOI: 10.1016/S1571-5078(03)01004-3

mother at greatest risk for the development of CHB. In addition, a discussion of current progress and future plans for the development of an animal model of CHB is provided. A clear understanding of the pathogenesis, which includes a molecular description of the fine specificity of maternal anti-Ro/La antibodies and of fetal susceptibility genes, will yield new diagnostic tools and therapies to aid in the management of CHB.

2. Background: molecularly defined pathways for macrophages which engulf apoptotic cells in health and disease

Even though an enormous number of cells are continuously undergoing apoptosis in tissues of higher organisms, these dying cells are rarely observed in vivo due to their efficient engulfment and degradation by phagocytic cells such as macrophages. Under the best of circumstances, clearance of apoptotic cells by macrophages should proceed in the absence of an exuberant inflammatory response. However, in a model of passively acquired autoimmunity; anti-SSA/Ro-associated CHB (Clancy et al., 2002) macrophages, during phagocytosis of dying cells, paradoxically activate immune responses and contribute to excessive tissue injury. One of the proposed hypotheses to explain the pathogenicity of maternal anti-Ro/La antibodies is that apoptosis of fetal cardiac conducting cells and/or working myocytes results in translocation of intracellular Ro to the cell surface where it can be bound by cognate autoantibodies (described in detail, below). Macrophages, which encounter this alternative 'meal' will use different 'utensils' or macrophage receptors to remove the opsonized apoptotic cardiocytes than the ones, which they use during physiological removal of apoptotic cells. Macrophage receptors (or utensils) are reviewed (below) with an emphasis on a pro-fibrotic response by activated macrophages. The fibrotic replacement of the atrioventricular node ingestion of apoptotic cells and subsequent secretion of TGFβ by well-intended macrophages depends in part on the presentation of the 'meal' and the 'utensil' used for eating (Fig. 1).

2.1. The disposal of dying cells in health

Apoptosis, or programmed cell death, is a process crucial in developing tissues including the fetal heart (Savill, 1997). Over the last few years, receptors for apoptotic cells have been identified on the surface of the phagocyte. A key concept when describing these phagocyte receptors is that the interaction between macrophage receptors clearing apoptotic cells involves the so-called pattern recognition molecules of the innate immune system. The aggregation of glycoproteins and phospholipids is either directly recognized by macrophage receptors (PSR, CD14, SRA, lectin like receptor) or indirectly recognized by receptors (MER, CD36, CD91) secondary to the binding of collectins. The 'collectins', extracellular soluble proteins (GAS-6, Thrombospondin-1, calreticulin) bind to 'cryptic sites' which are present in apoptotic but not normal cells. These direct or indirect recognition processes are thought to be low affinity, high avidity systems whose effectiveness is markedly enhanced by local aggregation (Gregory, 2000; Platt et al., 1998; Savill and Fadok, 2000).

Recently, a phosphatidylserine receptor (PSR) (Fadok et al., 2000) was cloned. It interacts with phosphatidylserine on apoptotic cells in a stereospecific interaction and is widely expressed in different tissues and cells (Henson et al., 2001). This broad distribution of the PSR supports the observation that most tissue cells, as well as professional phagocytes, can ingest apoptotic cells. In addition, Gas-6 is a soluble protein that can recognize and bind phosphatidylserine on apoptotic cells (Nakano et al., 1997) and Gas-6 could act as a bridging molecule to bind the macrophage receptor Mer (Scott et al., 2001). Interestingly, mer-/- mice show a marked defect in removal of apoptotic cells in the thymus. Other phosphatidylserine-binding membrane proteins include the scavenger receptors (see below and Rigotti et al. (1995), Shiratsuchi et al. (1999), Svensson et al. (1999), Fukasawa et al. (1996), and Tait and Smith (1999)). And the list includes the scavenger receptor of A class (SRA), which is best known as the acetylated LDL receptor. However, although murine macrophages rely on the class A scavenger receptor to recognize and uptake apoptotic thymocytes, mice with a genetic deletion of the

	MEAL	UTENSILS
	Apoptotic cell Recognition ligand:	Macrophage receptors:
HEALTHY CONTROL	**Phosphatidyserine, C1q, Tsp-1, Gas-6, ABC1**	**Pattern recognition by diverse collection of low affinity high avidity receptors**
CHB	**Maternal antibodies bound to SSA/Ro, SSB/La; Fc portion of IgG**	**Specific recognition By FcγR1, FcγRIIA and FcγRIIIA**

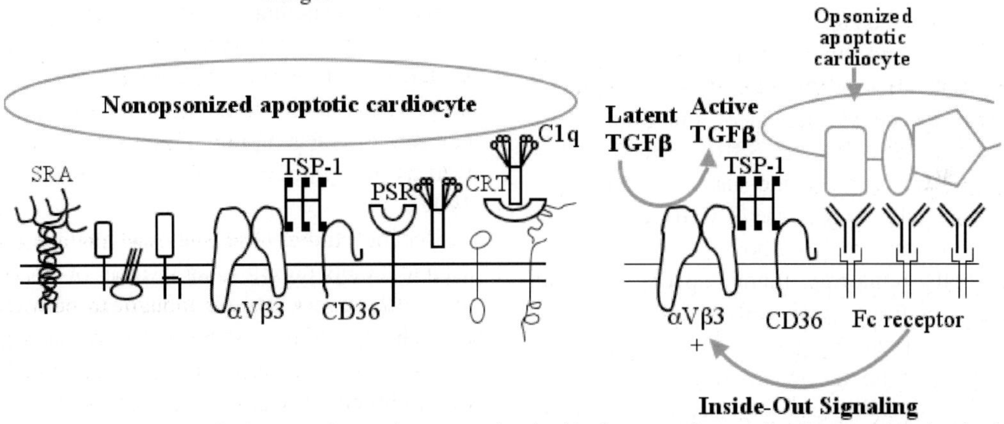

Figure 1. Schematic which distinguish between phagocytic receptors involved in clearance of apoptotic cells versus those involved in removal of 'opsonized' apoptotic cells (e.g. anti-Ro/La bound to apoptotic cardiocytes).

receptor cleared apoptotic cells in vivo with normal efficiency (Platt et al., 1996).

The vitronectin receptor composed of the alphaV/-beta3 integrins interacts with class B scavenger receptor CD36 via a bridge of thrombospondin, a protein of the extracellular matrix. Interestingly, the Drosophila relative of mammalian CD36, croquemort (crq) has been molecularly and genetically characterized (Franc et al., 1996). CRQ is specifically expressed in embryonic macrophages that are capable of removing dying cells. While chromosomal deletion of the crq1 locus do not impact their ability to engulf bacteria, macrophages in these embryos fail to phagocytose apoptotic corpses (Franc et al., 1999).

CD91, also known as α2 macroglobulin receptor or LDL-related receptor protein is a large, transmembrane molecule which binds indirectly to phosphatidylserine. In addition, CD91 binds and internalizes heat-shock proteins, which are released from damaged cells (Binder et al., 2000, 2001; Misra et al., 1999; Basu et al., 2001). It has also been suggested to bind calreticulin (Basu et al., 2001; Basu and Srivastava, 1999). Perhaps the calreticulin seen on cells in vitro all came from damaged cells in the culture, with subsequent binding to surface 'receptors' such as CD91.

As noted above, the first study of apoptotic cell recognition suggested the involvement of a lectin (Duvall et al., 1985). The uptake of apoptotic lymphocytes by activated macrophages can be inhibited by PS and *N*-acetylglucosoamine, suggesting the involvement of lectin-like receptors, while the integrin binding peptide RGDS and cationic amino acids and sugars have little blocking ability. More recently, the complement protein C1q was reported to bind to blebs on apoptotic keratinocytes (Korb and Ahearn, 1997) and to localized sites on other apoptotic cell types (Ogden et al., 2001).

CD14 represents an interesting candidate for apoptotic cell recognition. This soluble or glycophosphoinositide-linked protein is involved in the appropriate interaction of lipopolysaccharides with

Toll-like receptor 4. It has been implicated in recognition of apoptotic cells, particularly apoptotic lymphocytes. The counter-ligand on the apoptotic cell has been suggested to be ICAM3 (Moffatt et al., 1999), which is upregulated or exposed on apoptotic lymphocytes through an unknown mechanism.

2.2. *The disposal of dying cells in disease*

While in clearance of dying cells in the midst of healthy tissue relied on aggregation in apoptotic blebs of carbohydrate and lipids, it is noteworthy that cellular protein also redistributes during apoptosis. For example, the deoxyribonucleo- and ribonucleo-binding proteins SSA/Ro and SSB/La (Ro/La; discussed below) are found on the surface of apoptotic but not normal cells. In the case of CHB, anti-Ro/La antibodies (i.e. maternal antibodies) binds to the apoptotic cells rendering them 'opsonized' and the clearance of these dying cells is altered due to the interaction of the Fc portion of the opsonized immunoglobulin with the macrophage receptor, Fc receptors. The signaling pathway leading to phagocytosis in macrophages via FcR has been extensively studied. They involve specific recognition involving two major classes of Fcγ receptors: receptors that activate effector functions and receptors that inhibit these functions. FcRs that mediate phagocytosis in human macrophages fall within the activation class and include FcγR1, FcγRIIA and FcγRIIIA. In addition, macrophages also express FcγRIIb, an inhibitory receptor that does not participate in phagocytosis. Most of the activation type FcRs associate with the Fc receptor common *g* chain, which contains an immunoreceptor tyrosine based activation motif (ITAM). In contrast, FcγRIIB is a single-chain molecule that contains an immunoreceptor tyrosine based inhibitory motif (ITIM) in its cytoplasmic domain.

In CHB, we speculate that Fc dependent signal transduction pathway facilitates the fibrosis promoting activity of Thrombospondin-1. Under normal circumstances where there is clearance of dying cells in the midst of healthy tissue, thrombospondin 1 is one of several low affinity, high avidity proteins. In contrast, in CHB, thrombospondin 1 is a bridge protein between the integrin alphaV/beta3 (αVβ3) and CD36. Interestingly, a key to the activity by this trio is the alphaV/beta3, which is regulated by inside-out signaling. PSR dependent signaling versus Fc signaling involves a switch of αVβ3 from off to on. For example, we recently evaluated for surface expression of the activation epitope of αVβ3 using the mAb LIBS1 (Ginsberg et al., 1990). Macrophages cultured with opsonized apoptotic cardiocytes expressed a stimulated phenotype, supported by a threefold increase in active αVβ3 integrin. The inside out signaling resulting in αVβ3 leads to a profribosing activity of Thrombospondin-1 demonstrated with three profibrosing actions: (1) Thrombospondin-1 converts latent TGFβ to active TGFβ, (2) active TGFβ upregulates its own synthesis as well as the synthesis of TSP-1 (Yehualaeshet et al., 1999).

Recent studies have shown that macrophages secrete TGFβ during phagocytosis of nonopsonized apoptotic targets. This is consistent with the notion that this cytokine is required to accelerate the resolution of inflammation as apoptotic cells are being purged (Huynh et al., 2002; Fadok et al., 2000). However, Brown and colleagues, by including macrophages from healthy donors and evaluating clearance of both nonopsonized and opsonized aptoptotic cells (IgG bound to mimic Fcγ-mediated uptake). have uncovered yet another perspective to this complicated biologic balancing act of keeping inflammation in check.

As Brown et al. (2003) suggests "quantitative and kinetic balance of pro and anti-inflammatory mediators produced locally determines the safe outcome of many tissue processes and contributes to immunological homeostasis". Notable in Fig. 4 of their paper, TGFβ secretion by healthy donor-macrophages increased from undetectable levels to approximately 150 pg/ml when incubated with non-opsonized apoptotic neutrophils but increased to approximately 600 pg/ml when incubated with opsonized apoptotic neutrophils. While the significance of this finding might not be immediately intuited, it is notable that excessive and prolonged production of TGFβ can result in tissue fibrosis (Sporn et al., 1986). The observations by Brown and coworkers can in part be explained by the capacity of thrombospondin-1 pathway to sustain the secretion of TGFβ.

3. Pathogenesis: evidence of a distinct pathogenic mechanism for CHB compared to other fetal/neonatal diseases in pregnancy

The manifestations of the disease often wane as the neonate blood levels of the pathogenic antibody decrease and/or when the fetal antigen is no longer expressed by the neonate. In some diseases such as, neonatal alloimmune thrombocytopenia (NAIT) and Transient Myasthenia Gravis (TMG), the pathogenic antibody assumes a prominent pathogenic role. However, in others such as Autoimmune Associated CHB, while the pathogenic antibody is a necessary factor to the disease, other factors such as roles of apoptosis and of macrophages to clear cell corpses are equally important. Moreover, the capacity of the placenta to transport maternal IgG as well as a contribution by fetal genetic factors are necessary to further define the pathogenesis.

Our description begins with a subgrouping of FcRs into two general classes—those involved in effector functions (above) and those that transport immunoglobulins across epithelial barriers including those involved as the pathogenic antibody traverses the placenta via the IgG transport system. The anatomy of the placenta displays multiple stratums; the chorion, the allantois and the amnion. The chorion plays a central role in IgG transport and features of its anatomy include two layers of cells; the outer syncytiotrophoblast cells and the inner trophoblast. Each layer of the chorion is involved in immunoglobulin transport. For example, the transportation of IgG through the syncytiotrophoblast cell layer is mediated by a particular MHC Class I-like Fc receptor, FcR neonatal/β_2m (FcRn/β_2m). Once across the syncytiotrophoblast, IgG enters the villus interstitium via bulk fluid flow. At this site, it must pass the endothelial-like trophoblast cells. Early studies, in the passage of IgG and IgG-coated red blood cells showed that the villus trophoblast expressed receptors specific for FcγRII (CD32), the most abundant receptor in the FcγR family. The FcγRII2b isoform is predominantly expressed by trophoblast cells, and it has been suggested to be involved in IgG transport to the fetus' circulation (Lyden et al., 2001). Interestingly, maternal IgG must crosslink FcRn/β_2m, an absolute requirement for transport (Kolonin et al., 2002) and the cell surface density of FcRn/β_2m does not reach a functional level until 13–15 wk of gestation. This in part, is consistent with the clinical fact that symptoms of fetal/neonatal autoimmunity in pregnancy do not develop until late in first trimester of pregnancy. In addition, if maternal IgG is subgrouped as protective and fetal-reactive, the IgG transport will engage the good IgG with the bad. If the pool of fetal-reactive IgG can be diluted with an IV administration of human IgG, then the transport of fetal reactive IgG will be diminished accordingly.

3.1. Pathogenic antibody in NAIT, TMG and CHB

Three milestones in the research roadmap are the identification of the pathogenic antibody, the identification this antibody in the fetal circulation and the molecular characterize the candidate antigens in target fetal tissues. In NAIT, recent studies have identified the cognate maternal autoantibodies in the fetal circulation and they have defined the fetal platelet antigens inherited from the father (Bussel, 2001; Friedman and Aster, 1985). The parental antigen incompatibility involves five major human platelet antigens (HPA) systems. HPA-1, a surface platelet protein, which expresses a paternally inherited polymorphism involving a change from cytosine to thymine at position 196 in Exon 1 of platelet glycoprotein IIIA, is the most common HPA, causing approximately 78% of proven cases (Wiener et al., 2000; Dettke et al., 2001). Platelet antigens are fully expressed as early at the 19th week of gestation and the depletion of fetal platelets occurs in utero. This is an example of passive acquired autoimmunity where both the antigen, the surface protein glycoprotein IIIA on platelets and the cognate maternal anti-platelet glycoprotein IIIA are present in the fetal circulation (Table 1). A depletion of platelets ensues by a mechanism involving complement and the reticuloendothelial systems via a Fc dependent mechanism (Fromont et al., 1992). The fetus/neonate is at risk for demise due to intracranial bleeding. In the short term the platelet count is restored by an infusion of maternal platelets, which lack the paternal HPA, and therefore, are not depleted by maternal anti-platelet glycoprotein IIIA. Eventually,

Table 1
Differentiation of fetal/neonatal autoimmune diseases

	Fetal/neonatal autoimmune disease in pregnancy		
	TMG	NAIT	CHB
Antibody	IgG	IgG	IgG
Target	Neuromuscular junction	GPIIb/IIIa	SSA-Ro/SSB-La
Cellular location	Surface	Surface	Nuclear
Function	Interrupt?	Clearance by RES Ab-ag-complement	Heart block
Time of disease	In utero/transient	In utero/transient	In utero/permanent
Therapy of neonate	Neostigmine	Platetet infusion	Pacemaker
Sex	M + F	M + F	M + F

TMG: Transient Myasthenia Gravis; NAIT: Neonatal Alloimmune Thrombocytopenia; CHB: autoantibody associated Congential Heart Block.

maternal anti- platelet antibody decrease and the neonatal platelets are regenerated leading to the restoration of normal platelet counts and function.

TMG is manifested by a lack of movement and joint contractures in utero and it is caused by the binding of a blocking antibody to the nicotinic acetylcholine receptor (AChR) at the neuromuscular junctions (Polizzi et al., 2000; Riemersma et al., 1996; Kolonin et al., 2002). AChR, a member of the superfamily of pentameric ligand-gated ion channels, mediates chemical synaptic transmission (Table 1). The skeletal muscle type, found at the neuromuscular junctions is comprised of five subunits; initially $(\alpha_1)_2\beta_2\gamma\delta$ during the embryonic stage. During neonatal maturation, the pentamer's γ-subunit is downregulated; and substituted by ε to form the adult AChR heteropentamer $(\alpha_1)_2\beta_2\varepsilon\delta$. During pregnancy, there is a transplacental passage of the mother's peripheral blood IgG antibodies specific to the AChR. In myasthenia gravis, the mother's disease, there is involvement of the antibody IgG1/k, which attacks the main immunogenic region (MIR) on the AChR alpha subunit. However, in fetal disease, a reactivity involves anti-γ subunit-IgG Ab targeting the γ-subunit of the fetal AChR. Recent studies have also shown that this antibody has a blocking action. For example, antibody titers (IgG) in cord blood were shown to inhibit the acetylcholine induced currents of fetal but not adult acetylcholine receptor expressed in Xenopus oocytes. Moreover, anti-γ-chain of the neonatal AChR were found in the serum of the mother and neonate. Six weeks after birth, the sera levels were sampled again. The mothers sera contained anti-γ chain of AChR while the serum from the infant offered negligible titer levels. Interestingly, the infant's symptoms had also completely disappeared. The latter is consistent with the complete recovery of function following the regeneration of the neuromuscular junction.

In contrast, to the tissue injuries in NAIT and TMG which are transitory, the manifestation of CHB is the permanent loss of conduction tissue at the AV groove, a specialized tissue which provides the electrical conduction between atrial and ventricular tissues. Four ribo/deoxyribonuclear proteins SSA/Ro 60 kDa, SSA/Ro 52 kDa, SSA/Ro 52 kDa beta and SSB/La 48 kDa, which bind RNA or DNA are implicated in disease. SSA/Ro 60 kDa and SSB/La directly binds a spectrum of RNAs, while SSA/Ro 52 kDa and SSA/Ro 52 kDa beta are putative transcriptional factors (Chan et al., 1986; Ben-Chetrit et al., 1989; Ben-Chetrit et al., 1988). The latter, a variant transcript encoding exon-4 deficient 52 beta Ro (which as a weight of 45 kDa) is disproportionately expressed in the fetal heart at 22 wk gestation when compared to other tissues and hearts at various ages (Chan et al., 1995). In contrast, 48 kDa La, 60 kDa Ro, and 52 kDa Ro are ubiquitously expressed. Anti-Ro/La antibodies are present in cord blood of CHB mothers. Moreover, in a twin study where the twins were discordant for CHB, there was a decrease in levels of anti-Ro in the cord of the affected infant, indicating that there may be increased binding of this antibody to target organs in affected infants (Harley et al., 1985).

In consideration of surface binding, one hypothesis is that apoptosis might result in translocation of intracellular antigens to the external leaflet of the membrane. Casciola-Rosen et al. (1994) first demonstrated, by confocal microscopy, the presence of SSA/Ro and SSB/La in surface blebs of apoptotic keratinocytes. Applicability of apoptosis to the pathogenesis of CHB is supported by several observations. It is a selective process of physiological cell deletion in embryogenesis and normal tissue turnover, plays an important role in shaping morphological and functional maturity (Ucker, 1991; Hale et al., 1996) and affects scattered single cells rather than tracts of contiguous cells (Takeda et al., 1996). Perhaps a novel view of apoptosis is that it facilitates the placing of target autoantigens in a position to be recognized by previously generated antibodies. In autoimmune associated CHB, the newly accessible antigen is not 'inducing' an immune response (i.e. immunogenic) but rather becomes a target of cognate maternal autoantibodies already present in the fetal circulation (i.e. antigenic).

Our laboratory initially addressed apoptosis in vitro using cultured human fetal cardiocytes. Incubation of 4-day cultured human fetal cardiocytes with 0.5 μM staurosporine or 0.3 mM 2,3-dimethoxy-1,4-naphthoquinone (DMNQ) induced the characteristic morphologic changes of apoptosis, internucleosomal cleavage of DNA and the signature 85 kDa cleavage fragment of poly ADP-ribose polymerase (PARP) (Miranda-Carus et al., 1998). Apoptosis could also be induced by culturing the cells on poly(2)-hydroxyethylmethacrylate (pHEMA) (Clancy et al., 2002). The surface expression of 48 kDa SSB/La, 52 and 60 kDa SSA/Ro was demonstrated by confocal microscopy and scanning electron microscopy using affinity-purified antibodies to each of the respective antigens (Miranda-Carus et al., 1998, 2000).

Tran et al. (2002a,b) have recently identified physiologic apoptosis, translocation of SSB/La, and binding of anti-SSB/La antibodies in the developing murine heart. We have extended this in vivo work and examined cardiac sections from several available autopsies. As assessed by TUNEL (FITC and immunoperoxidase detection), apoptosis was increased in available sections including septal tissue (containing the conduction system), right ventricle and left ventricle from two fetuses (20 and 22 wk gestational age) dying with CHB as well as age-matched normal abortuses from elective termination. Notably, apoptotic cardiocytes were not present in contiguous tracts but rather were diffusely scattered between nonapoptotic cells (Fig. 2, Panel A).

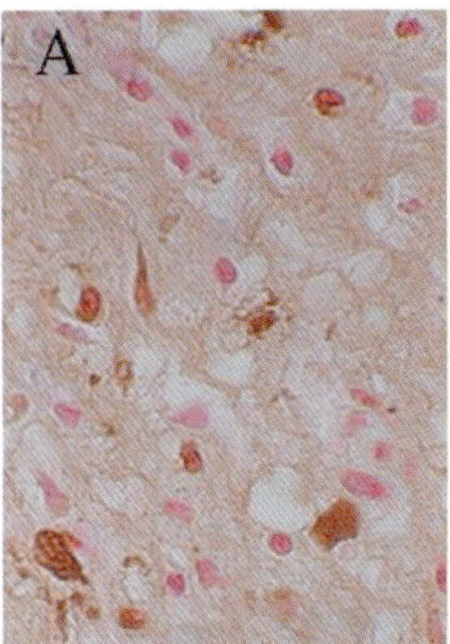

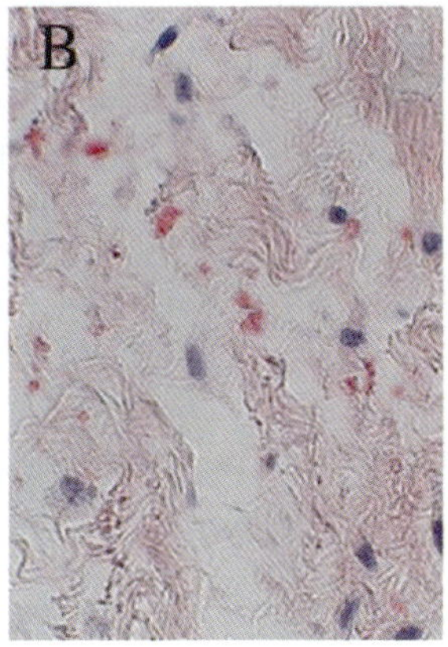

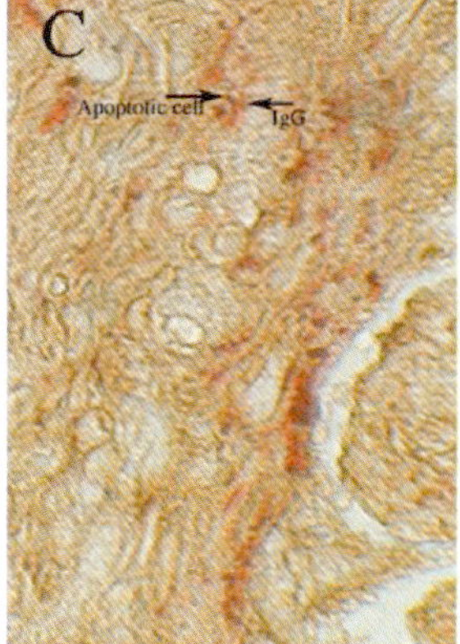

Figure 2. Histological evidence of increased apoptosis and deposition of human IgG in conduction tissue of a 20-wk fetus with CHB. Panel A shows a longitudinal section through the septal tissue of a 20-wk fetus with CHB, counterstained with hematoxylin and eosin. Apoptotic cells are identified by TUNEL peroxidase and are scattered among healthy cells. In Panel B, the same tissue section is stained with alkaline phosphatase conjugated to anti-human IgG. In Panel C, the same tissue section was double-stained with TUNEL peroxidase and alkaline phosphatase conjugated to anti-human IgG to demonstrate colocalization of apoptosis and IgG, respectively.

Apoptosis was most pronounced in the septal regions. Furthermore, human IgG was colocalized to the apoptotic cells (Fig. 2, Panel C). Although apoptosis had not been previously examined, earlier studies have shown deposition of IgG in the hearts from two infants dying of CHB and hydrops (29 and 30 wk gestation, respectively) in several areas of the heart including the conduction system (Litsey et al., 1985; Lee et al., 1987). The authors reported that, in some areas, 'IgG appeared to outline cells' (Lee et al., 1987).

Regarding the specificity of the anti-SSA/Ro-SSB/La antibodies is the fetal heart uniquely susceptible? Dieude et al. (2002) have recently reported (confirmed in our laboratory as well) that lamin B1 is redistributed during apoptosis but, unlike SSA/Ro or SSB/La, is not bound by cognate antibodies. These findings support discordance in the final cellular destination of translocated nuclear autoantigens during the process of apoptosis. In the case of lamin B1, physiologic non-inflammatory clearance of apoptotic cells should proceed uneventfully even in the presence of circulating cognate antibodies. However, in CHB, the maternal anti-SSA/Ro-SSB/La antibodies result in opsonization and inflammatory/fibrotic sequelae. Even if it turns out that SSA/Ro-SSB/La are not absolutely unique in this regard, there may be other factors such as complement binding of certain antigens or degradation of antigens that facilitate clearing without further sequelae. Establishing the fact that at least one other nuclear autoantigen is not surface-bound during apoptosis of human fetal cardiomyocytes is a step forward.

The consequences of antibody-bound (opsonized) apoptotic cardiocytes were initially explored in vitro using a coculturing system (Miranda-Carus et al., 2000). Macrophages coincubated with these opsonized cells secreted increased levels of TNFα over basal conditions or coculture with apoptotic cardiocytes incubated with IgG from a healthy control. Other investigators have also demonstrated that phagocytosis of opsonized apoptotic cells is proinflammatory (Fadok et al., 1998; Manfredi et al., 1998), an example of which is the observation that ingestion of apoptotic cells bound by anticardiolipin antibodies results in the release of TNFα from cocultured macrophages (Manfredi et al., 1998). Histologic studies confirmed the in vitro coculturing model. Giant cells and macrophages (frequently seen proximal to IgG) were present in septal regions as well as areas of thickened fibrous subendocardium, most apparent in the two fetuses dying before 23 wk. These studies extend previous reports of a mononuclear cell infiltration in the myocardium of a fetus dying in utero at 18 wk of gestation (Herreman, 1985) and the demonstration of patchy lymphoid aggregates throughout the myocardium of an infant delivered at 30 wk and dying in the immediate postnatal period (Lee et al., 1987).

Macrophages potentially contribute to several aspects of the pathologic process mediated by maternal autoantibodies (as described above). Although the pathways of clearance and cytokine secretion may vary, these scavengers phagocytose both nonopsonized and opsonized apoptotic cells. Concomittently or alternatively, macrophages may present antigen to lymphocytes (perhaps those of either maternal or fetal origin), further contributing to an inflammatory process. Furthermore, macrophages may provide a critical link between inflammation and ultimate scarring by secretion of alkaline phosphatases resulting in increased calcification (Tintut et al., 2002). In fact, macrophages could be seen contained in areas of calcification, particularly in the early cases. However, in a term neonate with CHB who died at birth, macrophages were less abundant and not associated with calcified areas, suggesting a diminished role in inflammation as the pathologic process evolves.

Perhaps CHB occurs as a consequence of unresolved scarring of the AV node secondary to the transdifferentiation of cardiac fibroblasts to unchecked proliferating myofibroblasts (scarring phenotype in which smooth muscle actin (SMAc) is expressed). Histologic support for this hypothesis was provided by the detection of myofibroblasts in all the affected CHB fetuses regardless of the timing of death relative to detection. As expected, myofibroblasts were located in areas of fibrosis. In the 20-wk CHB fetus, clusters of macrophages in close proximity to myofibroblasts were present in scar tissue near the AV groove as well as the thickened fibrous subendocardium (Fig. 3). Sections from the septum of the 22-wk CHB fetus showed myofibroblasts associated with extensive fibrous matrix and marked calcification in the inferior portion of the atrial wall where the AV node is likely to reside. In the term

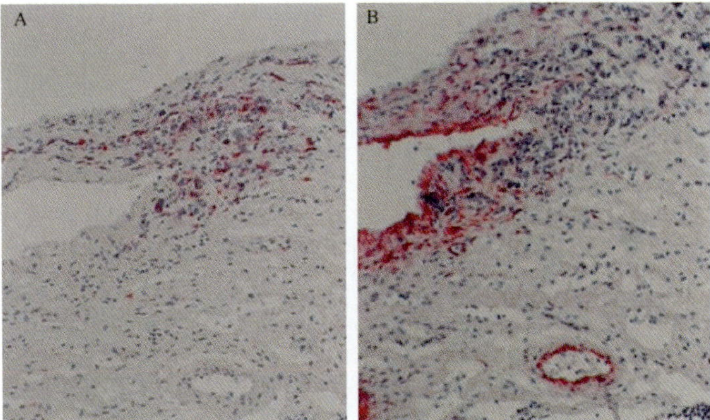

Figure 3. Proximity of macrophages and myofibroblasts in the septum of the heart from a 20-wk fetus with CHB. Panels A and B are longitudinal sections through the septum of a 20-wk CHB heart. Tissue was first incubated with anti-CD68 (macrophage; Panel A) or anti-SMAc (myofibroblast and blood vessel smooth muscle cells; Panel B), and then stained with alkaline phosphatase.

neonate dying at birth of CHB, myofibroblasts were observed in areas of scar. In contrast, these cells were not observed in either septal or ventricular tissue from the control 22 and 23-wk abortuses and a term neonate dying of noncardiac causes. For the 20 and 22-wk CHB hearts, there was a strong positive correlation between the absolute number of macrophages and the content of myofibroblasts.

The functional implication of the cellular colocalization demonstrated on the histologic sections was examined by in vitro studies in which cultured human fetal cardiac fibroblasts, exposed to supernatants obtained from macrophages incubated with opsonized apoptotic cardiocytes, markedly increased the expression of the myofibroblast marker SMAc (scarring phenotype) (Clancy et al., 2002). The addition of neutralizing anti-TGFβ antibodies to the 'opsonized' supernatant blocked expression of SMAc, supporting a potential role of TGFβ in the final pathologic cascade to scarring.

An important future direction of this work relates to the identification of signal transduction molecules using the supernatants derived from our in vitro model of CHB. Myofibroblasts are key cells in the formation of granulation tissue in healing wounds, but there is evidence that abnormal persistence of these cells may lead to fibrotic lesions in several internal organs, including the heart. In support of this hypothesis, when macrophages from normal controls are co-incubated with sera from mothers of CHB infants and apoptotic fetal cardiocytes, the supernatant gains the ability to cause proliferation but blocks transdifferentiation, whereas TGFβ1 itself has the opposite effects. These supernatants also induced NFkB in fibroblasts, which is a critical regulator of chronic inflammatory disease. Transfection of dominant negative forms of Rac into fibroblasts in this system inhibited myofibroblast formation, implicating the Rho family of proteins in the downstream pathway. In other systems, TGFβ receptor kinase substrates known as SMADs have also been shown to translocate to the nucleus to act as transcription factors in a pathway believed to promote fibrosis in diseases such as sceroderma. While it is often assumed that fibrosis is simply the end result of an inflammatory insult, a recently published pathologic description of Lyme carditis associated with second-degree heart block prompts a reappraisal of the elements of tissue injury, response, and ultimate repair or scar in the human heart. Right ventricular biopsy revealed mononuclear cells around the myocardial microvasculature and within the endocardium (Hajjar and Kradin, 2002). Despite prolonged inflammation (second-degree heart block was present for 8 wk), the cascade to fibrosis was not irrevocably programmed, since the block resolved following antibiotic therapy. This absence of permanent injury stands in strong contrast to the rapid progression to scarring seen in autoantibody-associated CHB. The expression of specific combinations of cytokines may ultimately provide the explanation.

3.2. Roles by the L-type calcium channel α_{IC} and the 5-HT_4 receptor as putative antigens in CHB

In 1997, an important paper was published which demonstrated arrhythmogenicity of IgG and anti-52-kDa SSA/Ro affinity-purified antibodies from mothers of children with CHB (Boutjdir et al., 1997). To assess the effect of IgG fractions and affinity-purified antibodies on conduction and heart rate, electrocardiogram (EKG) recordings were obtained from whole human fetal hearts, aged 18–24 wk. Baseline EKGs were recorded after a stabilization period of 30–45 min. Perfusion of the heart for 27 min with purified anti-52 kDa SSA/Ro antibodies from three mothers whose children had CHB resulted in bradycardia associated with widening of the QRS-complex that could represent bundle branch block or an intraventricular defect in the conducting system. The average increase in R–R and P–P interval corresponded to 32 and 30%, respectively. At 33 min of perfusion, complete AV block was diagnosed with the presence of only P waves and missing QRS complexes. Reperfusion of the heart with antibody-free Tyrode's solution for 48 min resulted in partial and slow recovery. In contrast, IgG from four control mothers did not have any measurable effect on AV conduction. These findings were further characterized by studying the effects of IgG fractions and affinity-purified anti-52 kDa SSA/Ro antibodies on whole cell L-type ICa recorded by the patch clamp technique (Hamill et al., 1981). IgG from two mothers whose children had CHB, but not from three control mothers, inhibited peak ICa at all voltages tested. The average inhibition at 0 mV was 59%. Similarly, affinity-purified anti-52 kDa SSA/Ro antibodies from three CHB-mothers inhibited peak ICa by 56% at 0 mV. Accordingly, inhibition of ICa by the autoantibodies in isolated myocytes further supports the contribution of Ca^{2+} channels to the conduction abnormalities observed in the whole heart.

The biophysical properties by which the autoantibodies inhibited whole cell ICa were then investigated at the single channel level using the cell-attached configuration of the patch-clamp method (Hamill et al., 1981). Barium currents were recorded through Ca^{2+} channels as described (Chen et al., 1996). Bath application of affinity-purified anti-52 kDa SSA/Ro antibody from two CHB-mothers produced a significant decrease in the Ca^{2+} channel activity and the ensemble average current. The ensemble average currents decreased from 0.23 pA to 0.13 (−43%, $p < 0.02$). Similar inhibition was obtained with IgG from two CHB-mothers, but no significant effect was observed with IgG from three control mothers. Analysis of single channel kinetics indicated that this inhibition was the result of shorter open times and longer closed times, which could also explain the basis of the whole cell ICa inhibition by the autoantibody. The effect of the affinity-purified antibody and IgG from mothers whose children have CHB was less pronounced in the cell-attached than the whole-cell recordings, suggesting involvement of a diffusible cytosolic constituent in mediating the response to autoantibodies. These studies confirmed two earlier publications, both in animal models, indirectly invoked arrhythmogenic effects of anti-SSA/Ro-SSB/La antibodies. Alexander et al. (1992) reported that superfusion of newborn rabbit ventricular papillary muscles with IgG-enriched fractions from sera containing anti-SSA/Ro-SSB/La antibodies specifically reduced the plateau phase of the action potential consistent with an alteration of calcium influx. Garcia et al. (1994) using isolated adult rabbit hearts, showed that IgG fractions from women with anti-SSA/Ro-SSB/La antibodies induced conduction abnormalities and reduced the peak slow inward current (ICa) in patch-clamp experiments of isolated rabbit ventricular myocytes. Since conduction in the AV node is essentially dependent on calcium electrogenesis, AV block would be expected to result from treatments leading to reduction of the ICa in ventricular myocytes. The L-type calcium channel is mainly responsible for ICa in ventricular myocytes and for the propagation of the action potential in the AV node.

We have closely followed the work of Dr Boutjdir and his colleagues over the past several years and it is fascinating that the L-type calcium channel may have a direct or potentially indirect role in the pathogenesis of CHB. One of the important projects we have recently worked on was driven by our interest in the concept that maternal antibodies to one or all components of the Ro/La system directly bind the L-type calcium channel. To accomplish this we obtained the full-length insert of the L-type calcium channel α_{IC}

(CaV1.2, a generous gift of Drs Klugbauer and Hofmann, Germany). The cDNA plasmid was transfected into HEK 293 cells and treatment resulted in transient expression of the L-type calcium channel based on immunoreactivity by anti-cardiac Type α_{IC} (Alomone labs). However, we were unable to observe reactivity of the L-type calcium channel with an IgG fraction of sera obtained from a Ro/La positive mother with a CHB child (lanes 7, 8; Fig. 4).

This result suggested that at least under the conditions tested the L-type calcium channel may not be directly recognized by anti-Ro/La antibodies; hence, an indirect effect remains possible.

Recently, crossreactivity between one or any of the SSA/Ro-SSB/La components and a cardiac receptor may provide a molecular explanation for pathogenicity; this hypothesis is supported by a report of Eftekhari et al. (2000). Antibodies reactive with the serotoninergic 5-hydroxytryptamine $(5\text{-HT})_{4A}$ receptor, cloned from human adult atrium, also bind 52 kDa SSA/Ro. Moreover, affinity-purified 5-HT$_4$ antibodies antagonized the serotonin-induced L-type calcium channel activation in human atrial cells. Two peptides in the C terminus of 52 kDa SSA/Ro, aa365–382 and aa380–396, were identified that shared some homology with the 5-HT$_4$ receptor. The former was recognized by sera from mothers of children with neonatal lupus and it was this peptide that was reported to be cross-reactive with peptide aa165–185, derived from the second extracellular loop of the 5-HT$_4$ receptor (Eftekhari et al., 2000). These findings are of particular importance, since over 75% of serum from mothers of children with CHB contain antibodies to 52 kDa SSA/Ro as detected by ELISA, immunoblot and immunoprecipitation (Buyon et al., 1993; Julkunen et al., 1993). Following this exciting lead, our laboratory addressed whether the 5-HT$_4$ receptor is a target of the immune response in mothers whose children have CHB. Initial experiments demonstrated mRNA expression of the 5-HT$_4$ receptor in the human fetal atrium. Electrophysiologic studies established that human fetal atrial cells express functional 5-HT$_4$ receptors. Sera from 116 mothers enrolled in the Research Registry for Neonatal Lupus and whose children have CHB were evaluated. Ninety-nine (85%) of these maternal sera contained antibodies to SSA/Ro, 84% of which were reactive with the 52 kDa SSA/Ro component by immunoblot. Of the total 116 sera, none were reactive with the peptide spanning aa165–185 of the serotoninergic receptor when background reactivity with albumin was eliminated (Buyon et al., 2002). Accordingly, these results suggest that antibodies to the 5-HT$_4$ receptor do not contribute to the pathogenesis of CHB.

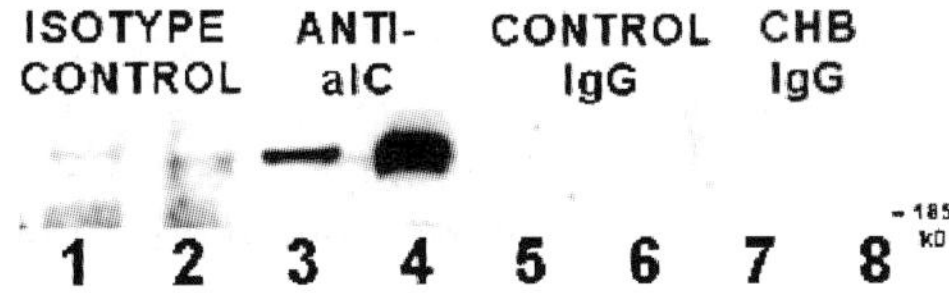

Figure 4. Western blot detection of the L-type calcium channel aIC in transfected HEK 293 cells and human fetal heart cardiocytes. CaV1.2 L-type calcium channel was introduced into HEK293cells by the Fugene transfection method and in addition fetal human cardiocytes were isolated. Lysates of the former were run in lanes 1, 3, 5 and 7, and of the latter in lanes 2, 4, 6 and 8. Transfer to nitrocellulose was followed by an assessment of reactivity by isotype control, anti-L-type calcium channel (aIC), a healthy control IgG and IgG containing maternal antibodies to all components of the Ro/La system (CHB IgG). Ponceau red staining contained equivalent protein loading (not shown). The results are representative of five experiments.

Taken together, that anti-Ro/La binds to a surface cardiocyte protein to exert electrophysiological effects is an idea with some potential, providing that the work would be followed up with molecular studies.

3.3. Identification of fetal susceptibility genes in CHB

Damage to the cardiac conduction system occurs in a previously normal fetus and is presumed to arise from transplacental passage of these maternal antibodies. Despite the clear associations of these passively transferred autoantibodies with the irreversible development of heart block, only a fraction of the infants exposed actually develops cardiac disease. The frequency of anti-Ro antibody in the maternal population has been reported as 1/200 whereas the frequency of CHB is reported as 1:11,000 of live births (2% of anti-Ro positive population). However, this incidence dramatically increases to about 20% in subsequent pregnancies. The increased risk by women who already had a child with CHB implies that these women and/or CHB child are somehow different as a group from the members of the general anti-Ro positive population and thus, evaluation of candidate genes is an important first step in understanding CHB. The inflammatory/fibrosis cytokines as indicated by our in vitro model of CHB were also examined. The results of our initial genetic tests indicate that a high production genotype of TNFα and/or TGFβ and low activity variant of MCP (inactivates complement) are found more often in children with neonatal lupus (CHB in particular) than their unaffected siblings. Early in our studies, we also evaluated the contribution by the immune related product HLA Class II as a risk factor. This effort was an important focus since HLA molecules are highly polymorphic and these molecules play an important role in presenting peptides derived from Ro/La to T cells.

A focus of genetic studies on the major histocompatibility complex was previously evaluated for NAIT and TMG. For NAIT, HPA1 negative women who carry HLA-B8 and HLA DR3 have an increased risk of alloimmunization to the HPA1 antigen (Decary et al., 1991). Similarly, in TMG, Myasthenia Gravis mothers who have HLA-DQ8 and HLA-DR3 alleles, are associated with an increased risks of TMG (Degli-Esposti et al., 1992). Previous studies have evaluated the role of HLA type and mothers and their CHB children (Siren et al., 1999a,b; Miyagawa et al., 1997a,b). Siren et al. performed HLA typing on a series of 24 children with CHB (including one set of identical twins) and 45 mothers of children with CHB from Finland, and several suggestive associates were found. HLA-Cw3 was found in increased frequency in the children with CHB (18/23, 75%, $p = 0.001$) in comparison to population norms (27%). Class II genes were also implicated in Siren's study, but only maternal associations were found. Three class II alleles were enriched in the 45 mothers in the series: DRB1*03 (30/45, 67%, $p = 0.003$ vs normal of 16%), DQB1*0201 (30/44, 68%, $p = 0.002$ vs normal 21%) and DQA1*05 (32/44, 73%, $p = 0.003$ vs normal 29%). No class II allele was significantly enriched in the children. The authors also looked at allele sharing between mother and child and concluded that it was significantly elevated. Miyagawa et al. studied 26 Japanese women with anti-Ro antibody, and found that maternal HLA Class II types were associated with different fetal outcomes. For example, maternal DRB1*1101-DQA1*0501-DQB1*01 was associated with offspring bearing the cutaneous manifestation of neonatal lupus but free from heart block, whereas maternal HLADQB1*0602 was associated with CHB offspring free of rashes. Only maternal HLA types were found to differ significantly from the norms in this study, and the HLA type of CHB children was not correlated with outcome. In our laboratory DNA was isolated from 87 children (40 CHB, 18 rash, 29 unaffected siblings) and their 72 mothers (all anti-Ro +, 85% Caucasian) enrolled in the Research Registry for NL and we evaluated DRB1 with regard to both maternal and fetal disease. HLA-DRBI alleles were determined by a DNA-based technique, with PCR amplification using sequence specific oligonucleotide primers. Consistent with prior reports on HLA associations with anti-Ro/La Ab, 86% of mothers were DR2, DR3 or both (DR3/DR2), while a Caucasian control population was 55%. Interestingly, the DR3/DR2 was 80% of CHB-children and 72% of children with rash, and 66% of unaffected children. To specifically address maternal/fetal sharing of DRB1 per se in considering the potential pathogenetic role of maternal T cells, a cohort was selected that comprised the following dyads: 25 mother/child CHB, 11 mother/child rash, and 16 mother/child unaffected. Included were two mothers who each had two CHB-children, three mothers of two children with rash, and three mothers of two unaffected children and one with NL. Four of the 72 mothers were homozygous for DRB1 alleles, establishing unidirectional compatibility from the fetal perspective in five offsprings, which was equivalently distributed among the different groups (two CHB, one rash, two unaffected). Moreover, there were no differences among the groups in bidirectional compatibility; specifically, 1/25 CHB was DRB1 identical to the mother, 3/16 rash, and 2/18 unaffected. Results from this large cohort do not substantiate previous reports of increased DRB1 compatibility of CHB-children with their mothers. DR3/DR2 is a significant maternal risk factor and in addition, these studies support for the notion that the enriched HLA antigen is a risk factor for CHB or rash.

The association of DQA1*0501 with rash in the absence of heart block in this small Japanese series is in contrast to the data presented above by Siren in which DQA1*05 was associated with heart block in Finish mothers, suggesting there may be racial variation. Taken together, Class II molecules segregate with the mothers and not the children with CHB. In addition, the Ro + mothers have a similar profile of DRB1, namely enrichment of representation by DR2/DR3; Yet, the same mother can have one child with CHB and another with NL rash. Although nearly 100% of mothers will be found to have anti-Ro + Ab if their pregnancies are complicated by CHB, only 2% of anti-Ro + mothers when followed prospectively will have children with CHB. These studies indicate that HLA as well as the fine specificity of maternal antibody are necessary but not sufficient to cause CHB, and that fetal genetic factors likely play a role in fetal susceptibility. In addition, the fetal factors are less likely to be immune response genes. Rather, it indicates a focus on the inflammatory/fibrosis cytokine cascade (described below).

In a model of histopathology of CHB, macrophage secretion of TNFα was promoted by apoptotic fetal cardiocytes exposed to sera containing antibody to Ro and La. The gene encoding TNFα is located in the major histocompatibility complex class III region on chromosome 6. The gene is highly polymorphic. Recently, a biallelic polymorphism was found at position −308 within the human TNFα promoter. The common (wild-type) allele, −308G, also called TNF1, has a frequency of approximately 80% in Caucasians and 92% in African-Americans (Wilson et al., 1993). The rare allele, −308A, also called TNF2, accounts for the rest. The TNFα gene is linked to the HLA-DR locus, and whites but not blacks have a strong linkage disequilibrium between the −308A allele and HLA-DR3 (Wilson et al., 1993).

Several publications support the notion that the TNF2 polymorphism may serve a role as one of the fetal factors contributing to the pathogenesis of neonatal lupus. The haplotype containing the −308A allele has been shown in mitogen-activated peripheral blood lymphocytes and enriched monocyte cells to be associated with high TNFα production (Pociot et al., 1993). This is presumed to be due to increased binding of specific transcription factors to the area of the polymorphism. Accordingly, macrophages from a fetus with this specific allele might secrete more TNFα when phagocytosing opsonized apoptotic cardiocytes, thus increasing inflammation in the tissue. It is also of interest that higher TNFα serum levels have been demonstrated in whites with the HLA-DR3 allele (Bouma et al., 1996). Mothers of children with neonatal lupus are frequently DR3, which is not surprising since this HLA DR is strongly associated with anti-Ro/La antibodies (Werth et al., 2000). Thus it is quite likely that DR3 will also be present in many of the offspring who have the rare TNF2. The TNF2 allele, even if present in the mother (as might be predicted), would not cause cardiac problems since the adult heart does not express Ro/La on the cell surface. Significantly increased frequency of the −308A (high-producer) allele of TNFα was observed in all NL groups compared to controls.

There are other important candidates, including membrane cofactor protein (MCP; also known as CD46). It is expressed on a wide variety of cell types and it functions as a cofactor for factor I-mediated cleavage of C4b and C3b, thus preventing inadvertent formation of membrane attack complexes. With regard to the mechanism of tissue injury, consideration should be given to the possibility that protective molecules may be diminished on the surface of fetal cells. The tissue expression pattern of MCP has been studied by Buyon et al. in normal fetal tissues at the critical 19–24 wk gestational age, when cardiac conduction defects can first be detected in CHB fetuses (Gorelick et al., 1995). Immunoblots of organs from six fetuses (aged 19–24 wk) probed with rabbit anti-MCP antibodies revealed a band at 60 kDa in addition to the known 65 and 55 kDa isoforms which comprise the codominant allelic system of MCP. Five fetuses expressed the most common MCP polymorphism (predominance of the 65 kDa isoform, upper band α phenotype) in the kidney, spleen, liver and lung. In contrast, all hearts from these five fetuses demonstrated a different pattern in which there was a marked decrease in the intensity of the 65 kDa band and accentuation of the lower molecular weight bands. In a sixth fetus which expressed the second most common polymorphism (equal expression of the 65 and 55 kDa MCP isoforms, αβ phenotype), the heart was similar to the other tissues. Preferential expression of the MCP β isoform in five of six fetal hearts, irrespective of the phenotype of other organs, suggests tissue-specific RNA splicing or post-translational modification. The clinical significance of this tissue-specific phenotype is unknown at present but may provide an important clue to the susceptibility of the fetal heart to antibody-mediated damage. Transforming growth factor (TGF) β1 is a multifunctional cytokine which modulates the proliferation and differentiation of many cell types (Sporn et al., 1986). It is considered to play a critical role in fibrotic conditions. TGFβ activates gene transcription thereby increasing synthesis and secretion of collagen and other matrix proteins (Ignotz and Massague, 1986). It decreases the synthesis of proteolytic enzymes, such as collagenase, which degrade matrix proteins. The active form of TGFβ is a 25 kDa disulfide-linked dimer comprised of two identical chains of 112 amino acids, synthesized in a latent form as a protein containing 390 aa. The human gene encoding TGFβ is on chromosome 19q13, and the promoter region of this cytokine has been characterized (Kim et al., 1989). All positions are defined relative to the first major transcription start site (position +1). The first +840 bases are a nontranslated region and codon one begins at position +841. Awad et al. (1998) have identified five polymorphisms in the TGFβ gene: two in the promoter region at positions −800 and −509, one at position +72 in a nontranslated region, and two in the signal sequence at positions +869 and +915. The polymorphisms at positions +869 and +915, which change codon 10 (T or C, leucine → proline) and codon 25 (G or C, arginine → proline), are associated with interindividual variation in the levels of TGFβ1 production. For both polymorphisms, the allele encoding proline is associated with lower TGFβ synthesis in vitro and in vivo. In contrast, the homozygous Arg^{25} genotype has been associated with relatively high in vitro and in vivo TGFβ1 levels (Awad et al., 1998; El-Gamel et al., 1999). Stimulated lymphocytes of homozygous genotype (arginine/arginine) from control individuals produced significantly more TGFβ in vitro compared with heterozygous (arginine/proline) individuals. In patients requiring lung transplantation for a fibrotic lung condition, there was an increase in the frequency of the high-producer TGFβ allele (arginine) (Awad et al., 1998). This allele was also associated with allograft fibrosis in transbronchial biopsies when compared with controls and with nonallograft fibrosis (El-Gamel et al., 1999). Previous animal and human studies have shown that high TGFβ1 producers develop significantly more lung fibrosis in response to a number of inflammatory triggers such as radiation (Franko et al., 1997), chemotherapy (Phan and Kunkel, 1992) and lung transplantation (Nakamura et al., 1995). Patients with cystic fibrosis of the TGFβ high producer genotype for codon 10 had more rapid deterioration in lung function than those with a TGFβ1 low producer genotype (Arkwright et al., 2000). The genotype frequency of codon 10 in one group of 107 Caucasian controls in the United Kingdom for T/T, T/C, and C/C was 41, 48, and 11%, respectively. The genotype frequency of codon 25 for G/G, G/C, C/C was 81, 18, and 1%, respectively (Awad et al., 1998; Werth et al., 2000). In a separate cohort of 94 healthy controls, >95% Caucasian, for codon 10, T/T, T/C, C/C was 39.4, 45.7, 14.9%; for codon 25, G/G, G/C, C/C was 84, 16, 0% (Holweg et al., 2001). Of relevance, preliminary genotyping data suggest that children with CHB have a higher frequency of the fibrosis-promoting polymorphism at codon 10 of TGFβ than unaffected siblings (Backer et al., 2002). In contrast, there were no significant differences between controls and other NL groups. For the TGFβ polymorphism, Arg^{25} there were no significant differences between NL groups and controls.

In sum, available data substantiate the speculation that CHB results from unresolved wound healing subsequent to the transdifferentiation of cardiac fibroblasts into proliferating myofibroblasts, a pathologic process initiated by specific maternal Abs. AV nodal cells and perhaps the working myocardium may be particularly vulnerable to the myofibroblast, a critical 'fetal factor', ultimately leading to fibrosis. It is acknowledged that in vitro studies may represent an exaggerated model only applicable in the more severely affected fetuses. It seems reasonable to predict that there are both susceptibility and regulatory factors, such as fetal polymorphisms of cytokines, which could influence the extent of the proposed pathologic cascade to result in permanent third degree heart block. Focus on these latter candidates, as proposed herein, should provide insights into the pathogenesis of antibody-associated CHB and the rarity of irreversible injury.

3.4. Murine model of CHB

While clinical data leave little doubt regarding the association of anti-SSA/Ro and/or SSB/La antibodies with the development of CHB, and experimental data are beginning to suggest pathogenicity, efforts to establish an animal model have been limited. Kalush et al. reported that offspring of BALB/c mice immunized with the monoclonal anti-DNA idiotype 16/6 had conduction abnormalities (Kalush et al., 1994). Of 31 pups born to mothers with experimental SLE, eight had first degree heart block, two had second degree heart block, two had complete block, 10 had bradycardia, and two demonstrated widening of the QRS complex. None of these disorders could be detected in the 20 offspring of healthy control mice. One of the difficulties in interpreting these findings is that the immunized mothers synthesized a variety of autoantibodies including antibodies reactive with 16/6 Id, ss/dsDNA, Sm, RNP, cardiolipin, SSA/Ro and SSB/La. Accordingly, it is not possible to segregate out which specific antibody might be responsible for the arrhythmias detected in these pups. The electrocardiographic data are provocative; however, no histologic data were provided to assess the status of the SA or AV node, or the presence of myocarditis.

To further establish an antibody-specific murine model to correlate arrhythmogenic effects of maternal autoantibodies with the in vivo genesis of CHB, we have immunized female Balb/C mice with 100 μg of one of the following 6 × His human recombinant proteins purified by Ni^{2+} affinity chromatography: 48 kDa SSB/La, 60 kDa SSA/Ro, 52 kDa SSA/Ro (52α full-length), and 52β. Control animals were given the same injections with a Ni^{2+} affinity-purified polypeptide encoded by pET-28 alone. Following primary immunization in complete Freund's adjuvant and two boosters (50 μg) in incomplete Freund's adjuvant, high titer immune responses to the respective antigens were established by ELISA and immunoblot of recombinant antigens, and immunoprecipitation of $[^{35}S]$-methionine-labeled in vitro translation products. Sera from mice immunized with either 52α or 52β immunoprecipitated radiolabeled murine 52 kDa SSA/Ro, confirming that these mice were specifically reactive with the murine homologue. Moreover, immunoblot of a newborn murine heart demonstrated the presence of 52 kDa SSA/Ro. Mice were mated and boosters continued every 3 wk to ensure continued high titer antibody responses. EKGs were performed on all pups using standard limb leads at birth or within 2 days postpartum. Maternal antibodies to the primary immunogens were detected by ELISA in the pups.

Results are summarized in Table 2. Of 54 pups born to six fertile mice immunized with 60 kDa SSA/Ro, none had CHB; of 27 pups born to three fertile mice immunized with 48 kDa SSB/La, none had CHB. In contrast, of 78 pups born to five fertile mice immunized with 52α and 86 pups born to five fertile mice immunized with 52β, one and five pups, respectively, had complete AV block. Accordingly, this antibody-specific animal model provides strong preliminary evidence for a pathogenic role of antibodies reactive with 52 kDa SSA/Ro, particularly the 52β form, in the development of CHB. Moreover, analogous to the frequency of 1–5% given for women with SLE who have anti-SSA/Ro and/or SSB/La antibodies (Lee, 1993), this model suggests that additional factors promote disease expression.

Currently, we are exploiting the potential for genetic manipulation to exaggerate several fetal factors. Interestingly, based on the histological clues of abnormal apoptosis in CHB, we are evaluating

Table 2
Murine model of CHB

Immunogen	Mothers immunized (*N*)	Fertile (*N*)	AV block			
			Pups (*N*)	I (*N*)	II (*N*)	III (*N*)
48 kDa SSB/La	10	3	27	2	0	0
52α SSA/Ro	8	5	78	3	1	1
52β SSA/Ro	5	5	86	5	0	5[a]
60 kDa SSA/Ro	7	6	54	10	0	0
β-galactosidase	3	2	11	0	0	0
Vector	4	4	43	0	0	0

[a] One 52β-mother had three pups with CHB in the same litter; another mother had one CHB pup.

several apoptosis-related genes. Manipulation to attenuate apoptosis have been shown to have a critical role in animal models of autoimmune disease. For example, mutations in the Fas ligand (Fas-lpr) causes a murine form of lupus in many different strains, perhaps most severely in the MRL/lpr mouse. This mutation leads to down regulation of apoptosis, formation of autoantibodies, and eventually to inflammation of the skin and kidneys in these mice. Similar down-regulation of apoptosis could predispose to CHB at two levels. First as in the known animal model. Increasing the time course of apoptosis in the fetus could lead to prolonged exposure of Ro and La in apoptotic blebs on the surface of cells undergoing natural selection in the cardiac conduction pathway. This could allow more time for a critical interaction between antibody and antigen, leading to inflammation and scarring that might not otherwise have occurred.

An approach to exacerbate apoptosis relative to the normal heart and varied in different anatomical sections was also recently reported. For example, Nelson et al. (2000) have generated several lines of transgenic mice that express FasL specifically in the heart, where it is normally absent. The transgenic (Tg) mice appear to be phenotypically normal, with no signs of distress during normal activity. Autopsy of all organs revealed pathologic changes in the heart only. Histologic analysis of the Tg hearts expressing the highest levels of FasL demonstrated diffuse concentric hypertrophy and mild interstitial changes consisting of leukocyte infiltration (predominantly neutrophils), interstitial hypercellularity, and fibrosis. Unexpectedly there was no sign of cardiomyocyte necrosis or apoptosis in the 8–12 wk mice, however, neonatal or fetal hearts were not examined. Interestingly, TGFbeta1 protein was increased in Tg hearts compared to NTg hearts. The strength of this model is in the potential to increase apoptosis, resulting in increased accessibility of the antigens to maternal Abs.

An additional murine model with the potential to increase apoptosis is the Transgenic mice expressing TNFα in the cardiac myocyte. Feldman and colleagues have generated transgenic mice (FVB background) expressing TNFα in the heart. The transgene construct contains the mouse α-myosin heavy chain promoter with cDNA of mouse TNFα. A modified transgene was used to reduce the extent of TNFα overproduction by including AU-rich destabilizing sequences (Piecyk et al., 2000). The histology of the transgenic animals was easily distinguishable from age-matched control animals at all ages (6, 12, and 24 wk), and an evolution of histopathological changes developed over time. There was an increase and hypertrophy of interstitial cells, which appeared to consist mostly of histiocytes, fewer lymphocytes, and hypertrophied interstitial connective tissue cells. Apoptotic cell death in this population was evident both by routine light microscopy and by the TUNEL assay. There was also mild interstitial edema, an apparent increase in the production of matrix material, and focal interstitial fibrosis. The fibrosis in some animals was more pronounced near the endocardium. The interstitial changes were associated with mild myocyte hypertrophy and focal myocyte degeneration in the form of rare areas of single-cell dropout and occasional myocyte multinucleation.

Recently, transgenic Rac-ET mice were developed (FVB/N background) after inserting the expression of constitutively activated Rac1 (V12Rac1) under the control of the α-myosin heavy chain promoter (Sah et al., 1999). It was previously shown that Rac1 overexpression results in hypertrophy, which suggests that in general myocardial architecture responds to the same signals that induce cytoskeletal reorganization in nonmuscle cells. Interestingly, the deregulation of signaling by Rac1 and PAK, followed by loss of cellular adhesion, lead to myocyte impaired force transmission and decreased systolic function. There are two phenotypes: a lethal dilated cardiomyopathy and cardiac hypertrophy. In these survivors, there was marked elevation of activated PAK, a signaling molecule, which is downstream of Rac1. Interestingly, these differential pathologic effects suggest that different cardiac structures respond differently to activation of the Rac-1 pathway. The mice have no fertility problems. In sum, models yield enhanced apoptosis and increased expression of Ro/La antigens and the relationship between exaggerated apoptosis and CHB is currently under investigation.

4. Conclusions

In summary, immunohistological analyses of available cardiac sections from several cases of CHB/myocarditis with varying degrees of pathology parallel the results obtained exploiting in vitro coculturing systems. Physiologic apoptosis may initiate an inflammatory process via antibody binding and ingestion by macrophages, which not only fuels continued apoptosis but contributes to the transdifferentiation of cardiac fibroblasts to a scarring phenotype. The heart block of neonatal lupus is not only progressive (second to third-degree) but characteristically irreversible, despite brief exposure to autoantibodies and limited period of inflammation. This is underscored by the finding of extensive fibrosis even in the earliest deaths. Furthermore, persistence of this phenotype even after birth may be related to the progression of block seen in some infants postpartum (Askanase et al., 2002). Moreover, fibrosis of the AV node contradicts the paradigm that fetal wounds heal without scarring (Moulin et al., 2001). Disruption of healing may involve the continued presence of myofibroblasts, a consequence of protracted stimulation from the macrophages. Irreversible fibrotic replacement of normal tissue may be unique to heart block acquired in utero following autoantibody-initiated inflammation. Other inflammatory stimuli, as in Lyme disease, induce transient block (Hajjar and Kradin, 2002) arguing against the assumption that fibroblast transdifferentiation is merely a common final pathway of inflammation. It seems reasonable to predict that there are both susceptibility and regulatory factors, such as fetal polymorphisms of Fc receptors and cytokines, each of which could influence the extent of the proposed pathologic cascade to result in permanent third degree heart block. Dissecting the individual components in this fibrotic pathway should provide insights into the pathogenesis of antibody-associated CHB, the rarity of irreversible injury, and rationale for therapy.

Key points

- Distinguish between phagocytic receptors involved in clearance of apoptotic cells versus those involved in removal of 'opsonized' apoptotic cells (e.g. anti-Ro/La bound to apoptotic cardiocytes).
- Role by Fc receptors (FcRs) in CHB-Identify FcRs based on two general classes; those involved in clearance of opsonized apoptotic cells and those that transport immunoglobulins across epithelial barrier.
- The manifestations of NAIT and TMG are transient and parallel fetal/neonatal levels of pathogenic antibodies. Compared with these fetal/neonatal autoimmune diseases in pregnancy, CHB progresses despite clearance of maternal antibody in fetal/neonatal blood.
- Antigens for several fetal/neonatal autoimmune diseases in pregnancy (e.g. NAIT and TMG) are on the surface of target cells. In contrast, antigens in CHB are intracellular.
- Apoptosis is a phenomenon which fully explains specificity of anti-SSA/Ro and anti-SSB/La antibodies.
- In vitro and in vivo studies of the relationship between antiRo/La and CHB have led to the hypothesis that transdifferentiation of cardiac fibroblasts leads to scarring of the AV node. TGFβ plays a central role in fibrosis.
- Report of preliminary findings on the contribution of fetal factors and CHB indicate that the genes from the fetal perspective are less likely to immune response genes (HLA) while inflammatory/fibrosis cytokine cascade may be an important contributor to disease associated genes.
- The current progress toward developing a murine model of CHB is summarized and genetic manipulation in mice to exaggerate fetal factors is identified as an important future direction.

Acknowledgements

We thank Dr Nathalie Berg who performed many of the experiments described in the section involving the transfection experiments of the L-type calcium channel. The basic research into the pathogenesis of CHB is possible due to the support by research grants: NIH Grant No. AR-42455 to J.P.B., and NIAMS Contract #NO1AR42220 (Research Registry for Neonatal Lupus), and in part by NIH Grant No. AR48409 (to RMC).

References

Alexander, E., Buyon, J.P., Provost, T.T., et al. 1992. Anti-Ro/SS-A antibodies in the pathophysiology of congenital heart block in neonatal lupus syndrome, an experimental model. In vitro electrophysiologic and immunocytochemical studies. Arthritis Rheum. 35, 176.

Arkwright, P.D., Laurie, S., Super, M., et al. 2000. TGF-beta(1) genotype and accelerated decline in lung function of patients with cystic fibrosis. Thorax 55, 459.

Askanase, A.D., Friedman, D.M., Copel, J., et al. 2002. Spectrum and progression of conduction abnormalities in infants born to mothers with anti-SSA/Ro-SSB/La antibodies. Lupus 11, 145.

Awad, M.R., El-Gamel, A., Hasleton, P., et al. 1998. Genotypic variation in the transforming growth factor-beta1 gene: association with transforming growth factor-beta1 production, fibrotic lung disease, and graft fibrosis after lung transplantation. Transplantation 66, 1014.

Backer, C., Yin, X., Chandrashekhar, S., et al. 2002. Increased frequency of the high produce genotype TT (codon 10) of TGF beta in congenital heart block and TNF2 allele in families with neonatal lupus. Arthritis Rheum. 46 (Suppl.), S261, Abstract.

Basu, S., Srivastava, P.K. 1999. Calreticulin, a peptide-binding chaperone of the endoplasmic reticulum, elicits tumor- and peptide-specific immunity. J. Exp. Med. 189, 797.

Basu, S., Binder, R.J., Ramalingam, T., et al. 2001. CD91 is a common receptor for heat shock proteins gp96, hsp90, hsp70, and calreticulin. Immunity 14, 303.

Ben-Chetrit, E., Chan, E.K., Sullivan, K.F., et al. 1988. A 52-kD protein is a novel component of the SS-A/Ro antigenic particle. J. Exp. Med. 167, 1560.

Ben-Chetrit, E., Gandy, B.J., Tan, E.M., et al. 1989. Isolation and characterization of a cDNA clone encoding the 60-kD component of the human SS-A/Ro ribonucleoprotein autoantigen. J. Clin. Invest. 83, 1284.

Binder, R.J., Han, D.K., Srivastava, P.K. 2000. CD91: a receptor for heat shock protein gp96. Nat. Immunol. 1, 151.

Binder, R.J., Karimeddini, D., Srivastava, P.K. 2001. Adjuvanticity of alpha 2-macroglobulin, an independent ligand for the heat shock protein receptor CD91. J. Immunol. 166, 4968.

Bouma, G., Xia, B., Crusius, J.B., et al. 1996. Distribution of four polymorphisms in the tumour necrosis factor (TNF) genes in patients with inflammatory bowel disease (IBD). Clin. Exp. Immunol. 103, 391.

Boutjdir, M., Chen, L., Zhang, Z.H., et al. 1997. Arrhythmogenicity of IgG and anti-52-kD SSA/Ro affinity-purified antibodies from mothers of children with congenital heart block. Circ. Res. 80, 354.

Brown, J.R., Goldblatt, D., Buddle, J., et al. 2003. Diminished production of anti-inflammatory mediators during neutrophil apoptosis and macrophage phagocytosis in chronic granulomatous disease (CGD). J. Leukoc. Biol. 73, 591.
This study demonstrated that when macrophages release excessive amounts of TGFbeta when engulfing opsonized apoptotic cells (IgG bound to mimic Fcgamma-mediated uptake).

Bussel, J.B. 2001. Alloimmune thrombocytopenia in the fetus and newborn. Semin. Thromb. Hemost. 27, 245.

Buyon, J.P., Winchester, R.J., Slade, S.G., et al. 1993. Identification of mothers at risk for congenital heart block and other neonatal lupus syndromes in their children. Comparison of enzyme-linked immunosorbent assay and immunoblot for measurement of anti-SS-A/Ro and anti-SS-B/La antibodies. Arthritis Rheum. 36, 1263.

Buyon, J.P., Clancy, R., Di Donato, F., et al. 2002. Cardiac 5-HT(4) serotoninergic receptors, 52 kD SSA/Ro and autoimmune-associated congenital heart block. J. Autoimmun. 19, 79.

Casciola-Rosen, L.A., Anhalt, G., Rosen, A. 1994. Autoantigens targeted in systemic lupus erythematosus are clustered in two populations of surface structures on apoptotic keratinocytes. J. Exp. Med. 179, 1317.

Chan, E.K., Francoeur, A.M., Tan, E.M. 1986. Epitopes, structural domains, and asymmetry of amino acid residues in SS-B/La nuclear protein. J. Immunol. 136, 3744.

Chan, E.K., Di Donato, F., Hamel, J.C., et al. 1995. 52-kD SS-A/Ro: genomic structure and identification of an alternatively spliced transcript encoding a novel leucine zipper-minus autoantigen expressed in fetal and adult heart. J. Exp. Med. 182, 983.

Chen, L., el-Sherif, N., Boutjdir, M. 1996. Alpha 1-adrenergic activation inhibits beta-adrenergic-stimulated unitary Ca2 + currents in cardiac ventricular myocytes. Circ. Res. 79, 184.

Clancy, R.M., Askanase, A.D., Kapur, R.P., et al. 2002. Transdifferentiation of cardiac fibroblasts, a fetal factor in anti-SSA/Ro-SSB/La antibody-mediated congenital heart block. J. Immunol. 169, 2156.
This study provides an in vitro model of CHB with a focus on the relationship between maternal autoantibodies and the transdifferentiation of fibroblast to myofibroblasts.

Decary, F., L'Abbe, D., Tremblay, L., et al. 1991. The immune response to the HPA-1a antigen: association with HLA-DRw52a. Transfus. Med. 1, 55.

Degli-Esposti, M.A., Andreas, A., Christiansen, F.T., et al. 1992. An approach to the localization of the susceptibility genes for generalized myasthenia gravis by mapping recombinant ancestral haplotypes. Immunogenetics 35, 355.

Dettke, M., Dreer, M., Hocker, P., et al. 2001. Human platelet antigen-1a antibodies induce the release of the chemokine RANTES from human platelets. Vox Sang 81, 199.

Dieude, M., Senecal, J.L., Rauch, J., et al. 2002. Association of autoantibodies to nuclear lamin B1 with thromboprotection in systemic lupus erythematosus: lack of evidence for a direct role of lamin B1 in apoptotic blebs. Arthritis Rheum. 46, 2695.
Although SSA/Ro is a nuclear proteins which under apoptotic conditions is accessible to maternal antibody, this property cannot be generalized to all nuclear proteins. This study showed that lamin B1 is redistributed during apoptosis but is not bound by cognate antibodies.

Duvall, E., Wyllie, A.H., Morris, R.G. 1985. Macrophage recognition of cells undergoing programmed cell death (apoptosis). Immunology 56, 351.

Eftekhari, P., Salle, L., Lezoualc'h, F., et al. 2000. Anti-SSA/Ro52 autoantibodies blocking the cardiac 5-HT4 serotoninergic receptor could explain neonatal lupus congenital heart block. Eur. J. Immunol. 30, 2782.

El-Gamel, A., Awad, M.R., Hasleton, P.S., et al. 1999. Transforming growth factor-beta (TGF-beta1) genotype and lung allograft fibrosis. J. Heart Lung Transpl. 18, 517.

Fadok, V.A., Bratton, D.L., Konowal, A., et al. 1998. Macrophages that have ingested apoptotic cells in vitro inhibit proinflammatory cytokine production through autocrine/paracrine mechanisms involving TGF-beta, PGE2, and PAF. J. Clin. Invest. 101, 890.

Fadok, V.A., Bratton, D.L., Rose, D.M., et al. 2000. A receptor for phosphatidylserine-specific clearance of apoptotic cells. Nature 405, 85.

In this study, the cloning of a phosphatidylserine receptor (PSR), which stereospecifically interacts with phosphatidylserine is reported. The expression of PSR is not restricted to leukocytes and it is widely expressed by different nonprofessional phagocytic cells.

Franc, N.C., Dimarcq, J.L., Lagueux, M., et al. 1996. Croquemort, a novel Drosophila hemocyte/macrophage receptor that recognizes apoptotic cells. Immunity 4, 431.

Franc, N.C., Heitzler, P., Ezekowitz, R.A., et al. 1999. Requirement for croquemort in phagocytosis of apoptotic cells in Drosophila. Science 284, 1991.

Franko, A.J., Sharplin, J., Ghahary, A., et al. 1997. Immunohistochemical localization of transforming growth factor beta and tumor necrosis factor alpha in the lungs of fibrosis-prone and 'non-fibrosing' mice during the latent period and early phase after irradiation. Radiat. Res. 147, 245.

Friedman, J.M., Aster, R.H. 1985. Neonatal alloimmune thrombocytopenic purpura and congenital porencephaly in two siblings associated with a 'new' maternal antiplatelet antibody. Blood 65, 1412.

Fromont, P., Bettaieb, A., Skouri, H., et al. 1992. Frequency of the polymorphonuclear neutrophil Fc gamma receptor III deficiency in the French population and its involvement in the development of neonatal alloimmune neutropenia. Blood 79, 2131.

Fukasawa, M., Adachi, H., Hirota, K., et al. 1996. SRB1, a class B scavenger receptor, recognizes both negatively charged liposomes and apoptotic cells. Exp. Cell Res. 222, 246.

Garcia, S., Nascimento, J.H., Bonfa, E., et al. 1994. Cellular mechanism of the conduction abnormalities induced by serum from anti-Ro/SSA-positive patients in rabbit hearts. J. Clin. Invest. 93, 718.

Ginsberg, M.H., Frelinger, A.L., Lam, S.C., et al. 1990. Analysis of platelet aggregation disorders based on flow cytometric analysis of membrane glycoprotein IIb–IIIa with conformation-specific monoclonal antibodies. Blood 76, 2017.

Gorelick, A., Oglesby, T., Rashbaum, W., et al. 1995. Ontogeny of membrane cofactor protein: phenotypic divergence in the fetal heart. Lupus 4, 293.

Gregory, C.D. 2000. CD14-dependent clearance of apoptotic cells: relevance to the immune system. Curr. Opin. Immunol. 12, 27.

Hajjar, R.J., Kradin, R.L. 2002. Case records of the Massachusetts General Hospital. Weekly clinicopathological exercises. Case 17-2002. A 55-year-old man with second-degree atrioventricular block and chest pain. N. Engl. J. Med. 346, 1732.

Hale, A.J., Smith, C.A., Sutherland, L.C., et al. 1996. Apoptosis: molecular regulation of cell death. Eur. J. Biochem. 236, 1.

Hamill, O.P., Marty, A., Neher, E., et al. 1981. Improved patch-clamp techniques for high-resolution current recording from cells and cell-free membrane patches. Pflugers Arch. 391, 85.

Harley, J.B., Kaine, J.L., Fox, O.F., et al. 1985. Ro (SS-A) antibody and antigen in a patient with congenital complete heart block. Arthritis Rheum. 28, 1321.

In this twin study, there were twins, who were discordant for CHB. There was a decrease in levels of anti-Ro in the cord of the affected infant, indicating that there may be increased binding of this antibody to target organs in affected infants.

Henson, P.M., Bratton, D.L., Fadok, V.A. 2001. The phosphatidylserine receptor: a crucial molecular switch? Nat. Rev. Mol. Cell Biol. 2, 627.

Herreman, G.G.N. 1985. Maternal connective tissue disease and congenital heart block. N. Engl. J. Med. 312, 1329 (letter).

Holweg, C.T., Baan, C.C., Niesters, H.G., et al. 2001. TGF-beta1 gene polymorphisms in patients with end-stage heart failure. J. Heart Lung Transpl. 20, 979.

Huynh, M.L., Fadok, V.A., Henson, P.M. 2002. Phosphatidylserine-dependent ingestion of apoptotic cells promotes TGF-beta1 secretion and the resolution of inflammation. J. Clin. Invest. 109, 41.

Ignotz, R.A., Massague, J. 1986. Transforming growth factor-beta stimulates the expression of fibronectin and collagen and their incorporation into the extracellular matrix. J. Biol. Chem. 261, 4337.

Julkunen, H., Kurki, P., Kaaja, R., et al. 1993. Isolated congenital heart block. Long-term outcome of mothers and characterization of the immune response to SS-A/Ro and to SS-B/La. Arthritis Rheum. 36, 1588.

Kalush, F., Rimon, E., Keller, A., et al. 1994. Neonatal lupus erythematosus with cardiac involvement in offspring of mothers with experimental systemic lupus erythematosus. J. Clin. Immunol. 14, 314.

Kim, S.J., Glick, A., Sporn, M.B., et al. 1989. Characterization of the promoter region of the human transforming growth factor-beta 1 gene. J. Biol. Chem. 264, 402.

Kolonin, M.G., Pasqualini, R., Arap, W. 2002. Teratogenicity induced by targeting a placental immunoglobulin transporter. Proc. Natl Acad. Sci. USA 99, 13055.

Korb, L.C., Ahearn, J.M. 1997. C1q binds directly and specifically to surface blebs of apoptotic human keratinocytes: complement deficiency and systemic lupus erythematosus revisited. J. Immunol. 158, 4525.

Lee, L.A. 1993. Neonatal lupus erythematosus. J. Invest Dermatol. 100, 9S.

Lee, L.A., Coulter, S., Erner, S., et al. 1987. Cardiac immunoglobulin deposition in congenital heart block associated with maternal anti-Ro autoantibodies. Am. J. Med. 83, 793.

Litsey, S.E., Noonan, J.A., O'Connor, W.N., et al. 1985. Maternal connective tissue disease and congenital heart block. Demonstration of immunoglobulin in cardiac tissue. N. Engl. J. Med. 312, 98.

Lyden, T.W., Robinson, J.M., Tridandapani, S., et al. 2001. The Fc receptor for IgG expressed in the villus endothelium of human placenta is Fc gamma RIIb2. J. Immunol. 166, 3882.

Manfredi, A.A., Rovere, P., Galati, G., et al. 1998. Apoptotic cell clearance in systemic lupus erythematosus. I. Opsonization by antiphospholipid antibodies. Arthritis Rheum. 41, 205.

Miranda-Carus, M.E., Boutjdir, M., Tseng, C.E., et al. 1998. Induction of antibodies reactive with SSA/Ro-SSB/La and development of congenital heart block in a murine model. J. Immunol. 161, 5886.

In this study, a murine model of CHB was established. The study shows that anti-Ro/anti-La antibodies are necessary but not sufficient for disease.

Miranda-Carus, M.E., Askanase, A.D., Clancy, R.M., et al. 2000. Anti-SSA/Ro and anti-SSB/La autoantibodies bind the surface of apoptotic fetal cardiocytes and promote secretion of TNF-alpha by macrophages. J. Immunol. 165, 5345.

Misra, U.K., Gawdi, G., Pizzo, S.V. 1999. Ligation of low-density lipoprotein receptor-related protein with antibodies elevates intracellular calcium and inositol 1,4,5-trisphosphate in macrophages. Arch. Biochem. Biophys. 372, 238.

Miyagawa, S., Fukumoto, T., Hashimoto, K., et al. 1997a. Neonatal lupus erythematosus: haplotypic analysis of HLA class II alleles in child/mother pairs. Arthritis Rheum. 40, 982.

Miyagawa, S., Shinohara, K., Kidoguchi, K., et al. 1997b. Neonatal lupus erythematosus: HLA-DR and -DQ distributions are different among the groups of anti-Ro/SSA-positive mothers with different neonatal outcomes. J. Invest Dermatol. 108, 881.

Moffatt, O.D., Devitt, A., Bell, E.D., et al. 1999. Macrophage recognition of ICAM-3 on apoptotic leukocytes. J. Immunol. 162, 6800.

Moulin, V., Tam, B.Y., Castilloux, G., et al. 2001. Fetal and adult human skin fibroblasts display intrinsic differences in contractile capacity. J. Cell Physiol. 188, 211.

Nakamura, Y., Tate, L., Ertl, R.F., et al. 1995. Bronchial epithelial cells regulate fibroblast proliferation. Am. J. Physiol. 269, L377.

Nakano, T., Ishimoto, Y., Kishino, J., et al. 1997. Cell adhesion to phosphatidylserine mediated by a product of growth arrest-specific gene 6. J. Biol. Chem. 272, 29411.

Nelson, D.P., Setser, E., Hall, D.G., et al. 2000. Proinflammatory consequences of transgenic fas ligand expression in the heart. J. Clin. Invest. 105, 1199.

Ogden, C.A., deCathelineau, A., Hoffmann, P.R., et al. 2001. C1q and mannose binding lectin engagement of cell surface calreticulin and CD91 initiates macropinocytosis and uptake of apoptotic cells. J. Exp. Med. 194, 781.

Phan, S.H., Kunkel, S.L. 1992. Lung cytokine production in bleomycin-induced pulmonary fibrosis. Exp. Lung Res. 18, 29.

Piecyk, M., Wax, S., Beck, A.R., et al. 2000. TIA-1 is a translational silencer that selectively regulates the expression of TNF-alpha. Embo. J. 19, 4154.

Platt, N., Suzuki, H., Kurihara, Y., et al. 1996. Role for the class A macrophage scavenger receptor in the phagocytosis of apoptotic thymocytes in vitro. Proc. Natl Acad. Sci. USA 93, 12456.

Platt, N., da Silva, R.P., Gordon, S. 1998. Recognizing death: the phagocytosis of apoptotic cells. Trends Cell Biol. 8, 365.

Pociot, F., Briant, L., Jongeneel, C.V., et al. 1993. Association of tumor necrosis factor (TNF) and class II major histocompatibility complex alleles with the secretion of TNF-alpha and TNF-beta by human mononuclear cells: a possible link to insulin-dependent diabetes mellitus. Eur. J. Immunol. 23, 224.

Polizzi, A., Huson, S.M., Vincent, A. 2000. Teratogen update: maternal myasthenia gravis as a cause of congenital arthrogryposis. Teratology 62, 332.

Riemersma, S., Vincent, A., Beeson, D., et al. 1996. Association of arthrogryposis multiplex congenita with maternal antibodies inhibiting fetal acetylcholine receptor function. J. Clin. Invest. 98, 2358.

Rigotti, A., Acton, S.L., Krieger, M. 1995. The class B scavenger receptors SR-BI and CD36 are receptors for anionic phospholipids. J. Biol. Chem. 270, 16221.

Sah, V.P., Minamisawa, S., Tam, S.P., et al. 1999. Cardiac-specific overexpression of RhoA results in sinus and atrioventricular nodal dysfunction and contractile failure. J. Clin. Invest. 103, 1627.

Savill, J. 1997. Recognition and phagocytosis of cells undergoing apoptosis. Br. Med. Bull. 53, 491.

Savill, J., Fadok, V. 2000. Corpse clearance defines the meaning of cell death. Nature 407, 784.

Scott, R.S., McMahon, E.J., Pop, S.M., et al. 2001. Phagocytosis and clearance of apoptotic cells is mediated by MER. Nature 411, 207.

Shiratsuchi, A., Kawasaki, Y., Ikemoto, M., et al. 1999. Role of class B scavenger receptor type I in phagocytosis of apoptotic rat spermatogenic cells by Sertoli cells. J. Biol. Chem. 274, 5901.

Siren, M.K., Julkunen, H., Kaaja, R., et al. 1999a. Role of HLA in congenital heart block: susceptibility alleles in children. Lupus 8, 60.

Siren, M.K., Julkunen, H., Kaaja, R., et al. 1999b. Role of HLA in congenital heart block: susceptibility alleles in mothers. Lupus 8, 52.

Sporn, M.B., Roberts, A.B., Wakefield, L.M., et al. 1986. Transforming growth factor-beta: biological function and chemical structure. Science 233, 532.

Svensson, P.A., Johnson, M.S., Ling, C., et al. 1999. Scavenger receptor class B type I in the rat ovary: possible role in high density lipoprotein cholesterol uptake and in the recognition of apoptotic granulosa cells. Endocrinology 140, 2494.

Tait, J.F., Smith, C. 1999. Phosphatidylserine receptors: role of CD36 in binding of anionic phospholipid vesicles to monocytic cells. J. Biol. Chem. 274, 3048.

Takeda, K., Yu, Z.X., Nishikawa, T., et al. 1996. Apoptosis and DNA fragmentation in the bulbus cordis of the developing rat heart. J. Mol. Cell Cardiol. 28, 209.

Tintut, Y., Patel, J., Territo, M., et al. 2002. Monocyte/macrophage regulation of vascular calcification in vitro. Circulation 105, 650.

Tran, H.B., Macardle, P.J., Hiscock, J., et al. 2002a. Anti-La/SSB antibodies transported across the placenta bind apoptotic cells in fetal organs targeted in neonatal lupus. Arthritis Rheum. 46, 1572.

This study shows that a consequence physiological apoptosis is the translocation of SSB/La and binding of anti-SSB/La antibodies in the developing murine heart.

Tran, H.B., Ohlsson, M., Beroukas, D., et al. 2002b. Subcellular redistribution of la/SSB autoantigen during physiologic apoptosis in the fetal mouse heart and conduction system: a clue to the pathogenesis of congenital heart block. Arthritis Rheum. 46, 202.

Ucker, D.S. 1991. Death by suicide: one way to go in mammalian cellular development? New Biol. 3, 103.

Werth, V.P., Zhang, W., Dortzbach, K., et al. 2000. Association of a promoter polymorphism of tumor necrosis factor-alpha with subacute cutaneous lupus erythematosus and distinct photoregulation of transcription. J. Invest Dermatol. 115, 726.

Wiener, E., Mawas, F., Coates, P., et al. 2000. HPA-1a-mediated platelet interaction with monocytes in vitro: involvement of Fcgamma receptor (FcgammaR) classes and inhibition by humanised monoclonal anti-FcgammaRI H22. Eur. J. Haematol. 65, 399.

Wilson, A.G., de Vries, N., Pociot, F., et al. 1993. An allelic polymorphism within the human tumor necrosis factor alpha promoter region is strongly associated with HLA A1, B8, and DR3 alleles. J. Exp. Med. 177, 557.

Yehualaeshet, T., O'Connor, R., Green-Johnson, J., et al. 1999. Activation of rat alveolar macrophage-derived latent transforming growth factor beta-1 by plasmin requires interaction with thrombospondin-1 and its cell surface receptor, CD36. Am. J. Pathol. 155, 841.

TGFbeta is produced as a latent molecule. This study demonstrated local activation of TGFbeta via a Thrombospondin-1 dependent pathway.

PART II

Immune Mechanisms Involved in Atherosclerosis

Handbook of Systemic Autoimmune Diseases, Volume 1
The Heart in Systemic Autoimmune Diseases
A. Doria and P. Pauletto, editors

CHAPTER 5

Innate Immunity, Inflammation, and Atherogenesis

Marcello Rattazzi[a], Yehuda Shoenfeld[b], Paolo Pauletto[*,a]

[a]*Dipartimento di Medicina Clinica e Sperimentale, Università di Padova and Medicina Interna I^ - Ospedale Ca'Foncello, Via Ospedale, 1, 31100 Treviso, Italy*
[b]*Department of Medicine 'B' and Center of Autoimmune Diseases, Sheba Medical Center, Tel-Hashomer, and Sackler Faculty of Medicine, Tel-Aviv University, Tel-Aviv, Israel*

1. Introduction

Atherosclerosis is recognized as the pathological basis of cardiovascular disease (CVD). To date, many risk factors for atherosclerosis development, progression and complication have been identified in clinical, experimental, and population-based studies (such as hypertension, hypercholesterolemia, diabetes, obesity, cigarette smoking, etc.). These are known as 'traditional risk factors', and are currently used to assess the cardiovascular global risk carried by each individual. As a matter of fact, despite the strong relationship linking traditional risk factors, atherosclerosis development, and cardiovascular events, a number of subjects still face an 'unexplained atherosclerosis' (Spence et al., 1999).

Recent advances in basic science have shown that atherosclerosis should be considered as a chronic inflammatory process and that a pivotal role of inflammation is evident from initiation through progression and complication of atherosclerosis (Ross, 1999; Libby, 2002). Based on this emerging evidence, many studies have demonstrated the potentiality for biochemical markers of inflammation to act as predictors of CVD risk in a variety of clinical settings. Specific subsets of subjects with chronic inflammatory diseases, such as patients with periodontitis (DeStefano et al., 1993), end-stage renal disease (Foley et al., 1998), or autoimmune disorders (Gordon, 2002; Goodson, 2002), are at increased risk of developing CVD compared to the general population. Many studies have demonstrated that all these clinical conditions are characterized by a significant elevation in systemic markers of inflammation (Loos et al., 2000; Gordon et al., 2001). Moreover, some epidemiological studies showed that a systemic chronic inflammatory state could promote atherosclerosis progression independently from traditional risk factors (Kiechl et al., 2001). This evidence raises the question whether or not an increase in circulating inflammatory molecules from an inflammatory remote source could per se promote the progression of the atherosclerotic process in different vascular districts. Many of these molecules (such as acute phase proteins or cytokines) belong to the innate immunity and act as the first-line response of the immune system against injurious elements, mainly infectious agents. It is still debated whether or not some of these inflammatory mediators could actively contribute to atherosclerotic lesion formation and instability. If so, in the near future, these molecules could be useful to complement traditional risk factors, to identify new categories of subjects prone to atherosclerosis development, and could become another potential target for therapeutic strategies.

* Corresponding author.
E-mail address: ppauletto@ulss.tv.it (P. Pauletto).

DOI: 10.1016/S1571-5078(03)01005-5

2. Inflammation and atherogenesis

During the last decade, an impressive body of evidence has grown showing that atheroma development represents an inflammatory process. Recent reviews on this topic have described in detail the mechanisms involved in the different phases of atherogenesis (Libby, 2002). Great attention has been paid to the network of inflammatory mediators (cytokines, chemokines, and growth factors) and cellular receptors that drive the cellular communication and activation inside the arterial wall. Atherogenesis is characterized by many interconnected phases that could be summarized as: (i) lipids accumulation and modification (such as oxidation, aggregation, proteolysis) inside the arterial wall which, in turn, can promote endothelial inflammatory activation; (ii) recruitment of inflammatory elements into the vascular intima, driven by the expression on endothelial surface of adhesion molecules such as vascular cell adhesion molecule-1 (VCAM-1) and P- and E-selectins; (iii) activation of macrophages and lymphocytes secreting many kinds of cytokines and growth factors and leading to foam cell accumulation; (iv) smooth muscle cells (SMC) dedifferentiation, proliferation, and migration from the media into the intima layer (Sartore et al., 1997). Many of the mechanisms involved in atherogenesis are not so different from those observed in other chronic inflammatory diseases (Ross, 1999). The onset of a chronic inflammatory process is usually characterized by the development of an aggressive immune response against an injurious element, together with the parallel activation of systems deputed to tissue reparation. If the initial trigger is not eliminated in a short time, inflammation will progress and the inherently protective response could shift to a harmful process. These concepts apply to almost all the steps of atherosclerosis development and may have a special relevance for plaque rupture. It has been shown that vulnerable atherosclerotic lesions have an increased number of activated inflammatory elements with relatively scarce SMC content (Pauletto et al., 2000). In this phase, the integrity of the atherosclerotic plaque depends on a dynamic balance of extracellular matrix production (mainly due to SMC) and enzymatic degradation. The latter is influenced by inflammatory elements secreting proteolytic enzymes that increase the risk of thrombotic complications by weakening the protective fibrous cap and eventually inducing its rupture (Libby, 2002).

The view that the atherosclerotic process is essentially a chronic inflammatory disease highlights the pivotal role played by the immune system. The latter is endowed with two different types of response against infection: the innate immunity and the adaptive immunity (Medzhitov and Janeway, 2000). The former represents the first-line defence against injurious elements and relies on inflammatory cells (macrophages, monocytes, neutrophils, basophils, mast cells, eosinophils, natural killer cells), complement, acute phase proteins, and different kinds of cytokines. The adaptive response is mainly based on the development of the antigen-specific immunological memory characterized by proliferation of B and T lymphocytes together with secretion of immunoglobulins, activation of macrophages, and killing of infected cells. Elements of the innate immunity system recognize a broad range of non-self molecular patterns present on pathogens (such as LPS, peptidoglycan, lipoteichoic acid, etc.) mainly through scavenger receptors (SR) and toll-like receptors (TLRs). Given their crucial role in the first identification of these highly conserved pathogen antigens, these structures are also called pattern-recognition receptors. They are expressed on the surface of many effector cells of the innate system (such as macrophages, dendritic cells, etc.) and trigger the initial activation of the immune response. The innate immunity response is also characterized by secretion of cytokines (such as IL-1, IL-6, TNFα), chemokines, such as monocyte chemoattractant protein-1 (MCP-1), and presentation by MHC of pathogen-derived proteins to the T cells with subsequent triggering of the adaptive immunity. Recent evidence suggests that the innate immune system could play a pivotal role during the development of autoimmune disorders (Carroll, 2001). This system is, in fact, deputed to the first contact with non-self antigens and plays a crucial role for the clearance of necrotic and apoptotic cells, thereby preventing the exposure to potential autologous antigens (such as nuclear antigens). Deregulations of the elements of this system could be actively involved in the start and progression of the autoimmune process. This aspect applies especially to the receptor elements (such as SR and TLRs), the acute phase proteins (especially those belonging to the pentraxin family), and the cellular elements deputed to the first-line response (such as NK). Cells and inflammatory molecules belonging to both the innate and adaptive immunities are also involved in the atherosclerotic process (Hansson et al., 2002). Once activated, both the innate and adaptive immune system elements could participate in all the stages of atherogenesis. Antigen-specific response of the adaptive immunity can develop against oxidized low-density lipoproteins (oxLDL), heat shock proteins (HSP), and β_2-glycoprotein I (these aspects are described in detail in chapter 6 of this book). The active role played by the cellular inflammatory elements during atherosclerosis development has been widely investigated and many of the pathophysiological mechanisms that drive the inflammatory cell activation (i.e. foam cells formation, T lymphocytes activation) are now well defined. Conversely, the potential involvement in atherogenesis of other molecules or receptors belonging to the innate immunity represents an emerging field of investigation. Until now, these latter components have been mainly considered in the light of their role in the onset of inflammatory response to pathogens. In this chapter, we will overview the emerging evidence of the pro-atherogenic potential displayed by molecules belonging to the innate immunity system.

3. Innate immunity and atherogenesis

3.1. *Pentraxins*

Pentraxins are a group of several proteins highly conserved among vertebrates, which are deputed to the innate resistance against pathogens. Based on their size, these proteins are now divided into two subfamilies: the classical 'short' proteins (25 kDa), whose C-reactive protein (CRP) is the main component, and the new, recently described 'long' (40–50 kDa) proteins, which are twice the size of the classical ones.

3.1.1. *C-reactive protein*

CRP is considered the major acute phase reactant in humans, and its plasma levels rapidly increase in response to inflammatory stimuli. This protein was discovered in 1930 in the blood of patients with acute pneumococcal pneumonia and named because of its reactivity with the C-polysaccharide of the pneumococcal cell wall. CRP is synthesized mainly by the liver in response to different pro-inflammatory cytokines. IL-6 acts as the principal inducer of the CRP gene while a minor role is attributed to other cytokines, such as IL-1 and TNFα, or to complement activation products and glucocorticoids (Volanakis, 2001; Du Clos, 2000). Moreover, an extrahepatic expression of this protein has also been documented in human neurons (Yasojima et al., 2000), alveolar macrophages (Dong and Wright, 1996), inside atherosclerotic lesions (Yasojima et al., 2001), in the kidney (Jabs et al., 2003), and in the adipose tissue (Ouchi et al., 2003). CRP has a Ca^{2+}-dependent binding specificity for phosphocholine (PC). The latter is an important constituent of many bacterial and fungal polysaccharides and is also present in the outer leaflet of most biological membranes. CRP also binds in a Ca^{2+}-dependent way to membrane and nuclear constituents such as histones, chromatine, and small nuclear ribonucleoproteins of necrotic cells. The 'effector' face of CRP contains the binding site for C1q and can initiate the classical complement pathway activation. CRP promotes the opsonic clearance of cellular debris or infectious elements without determining an inflammatory lytic damage of the host membranes. CRP completes its defensive properties by directly mediating the phagocytosis of its ligands through the FcγRIIa that is expressed on both macrophages and neutrophils (Volanakis, 2001; Du Clos, 2000). Thus, CRP is an important first-line host defence molecule, which is able to recognize pathogens and damaged cells and promote their elimination by activating the complement system and mediating their phagocytic clearance as well.

To date, several large prospective epidemiological studies have consistently shown that CRP plasma level is a strong, independent predictor of risk of future CVD events in patients with unstable angina (UA) or history of myocardial infarction (MI) (Liuzzo et al., 1994; Zebrack et al., 2002). Even in subjects without known CVD, high levels of CRP are independent determinants of the risk of coronary heart disease, stroke, and peripheral arterial disease (Kuller et al., 1996; Ridker et al., 2002).

The more obvious interpretation of the above results is that CRP can be considered just as a sensitive marker of the inflammatory process that characterizes progression and complication of atherosclerosis. However, reports seem to support the hypothesis that CRP could be directly involved in the pathogenesis of atherosclerotic lesions.

Several studies demonstrated the presence of CRP inside atherosclerotic lesions (see Fig. 1) from different vascular districts (Yasojima et al., 2001; Torzewski et al., 1998). Some recent reports raise the hypothesis that CRP plasma levels could be related with its content inside atherosclerotic lesions (Burke et al., 2002), and that a high content of this protein inside vascular lesions is also related with a decreased plaque stability (Ishikawa et al., 2003). Many in vivo and in vitro studies showed that CRP could interact with lipoproteins undergoing the enzymatic or oxidative modifications often occurring during their trapping inside arterial intima (Taskinen et al., 2002; Chang et al., 2002). The binding of CRP to lipoproteins is accompanied by augmentation of complement-activating capacity (Bhakdi et al., 1999), and enhanced uptake of lipoproteins by macrophages (Zwaka et al., 2001). Moreover, it has been shown that CRP could promote activation of monocytes by increasing the secretion of IL-1 and TNFα (Galve-de Rochemonteix et al., 1993) and by augmenting the expression of tissue factor (TF) (Cermak et al., 1993) and CD40 (Garlichs et al., 2001). CRP could also induce adhesion molecule expression (ICAM-1, VCAM-1, E-selectin) and increase the secretion rate of endothelin-1 (ET-1), IL-6, MCP-1, and plasminogen activator inhibitor-1 (PAI-1) by endothelial cells (EC) (Pasceri et al., 2000, 2001; Devaraj et al., 2003). In addition, recent studies reported that CRP could play an active role in modulating endothelial nitric oxide synthase (eNOS) bioactivity. In fact, EC incubated with CRP decreased eNOS expression and nitric oxide (NO) release as well (Venugopal et al., 2002). Two recent reports suggest that CRP could also promote activation of SMC. It has been shown that SMC incubated with CRP secrete MCP-1, IL-6 and express angiotensin-1 receptor (ATR). Moreover, the stimulation with CRP promotes SMC proliferation and migration in vitro and in vivo as well (Hattori et al., 2003; Wang et al., 2003).

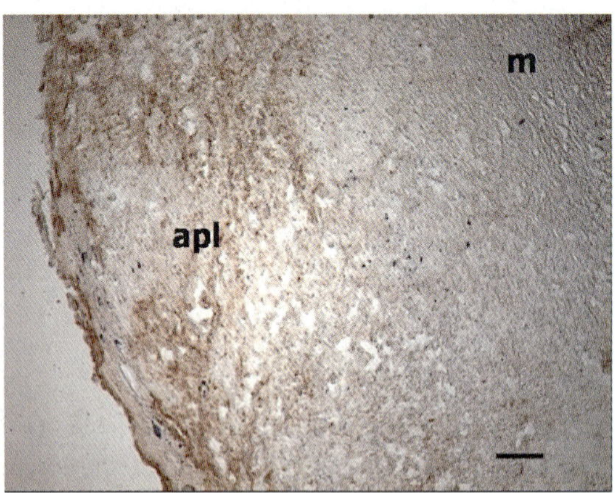

Figure 1. Representative testing for tissue CRP. Immunocytochemical analysis of CRP distribution in atherosclerotic lesion of human thoracic aorta. Areas of brown staining indicate the presence of CRP. Bar = 100 μm. Apl, atherosclerotic plaque; m, tunica media.

In summary, all the potential pro-atherogenic actions described above may contribute both to growth of the atherosclerotic plaque from the very beginning and to the onset of the atherothrombotic complications. A direct pathogenic role of CRP in the atherosclerosis progression cannot be ruled out. However, further studies are needed to upgrade this protein from the role of passive epiphenomenon to hard atherosclerotic risk factor.

3.1.2. PTX3

PTX3 was the first long pentraxin to be discovered and is now one of the most tracked molecules for a possible involvement in CVD. Different from CRP, PTX3 is not synthesized by hepatocytes. This protein is in fact produced by different cell types (such as monocytes/macrophages, fibroblasts, and EC) under stimulation of primary cytokines (IL-1 and TNFα) or LPS (Goodman et al., 1996). Some authors showed that after injection of LPS in mice, the PTX3 plasma levels were increased. Expression of the protein was mainly observed in the vascular EC of the heart and skeletal muscle. Probably this protein is mainly produced at the site of inflammation and could exert a sort of local amplification of the inflammatory response. Like CRP, PTX3 is able to interact with dying or apoptotic cells by mediating the clearance of cellular debris and, probably, also by promoting the complement activation (Rovere et al., 2000; Nauta et al., 2003). The first demonstration that PTX3 could be actively involved in human inflammatory disease was obtained in patients with autoimmune disease. Specifically, some authors observed an increase in the expression of PTX3 in the synovial fluid from patients with rheumatoid arthritis (RA). Beyond monocytes/macrophages and EC, synoviocytes could also be the potential source of PTX3, and through complement activation this protein could amplify the inflammatory tissue damage in RA (Luchetti et al., 2000). Increased PTX3 plasma level was also observed in patients suffering from acute MI, and its peak preceded that of CRP. The protein localized in intact cardiomyocytes and was probably released by dying or necrotic cells suggesting a potential for amplification of myocardial damage (Peri et al., 2000). Recently, the PTX3 expression has been documented inside advanced human carotid atherosclerotic lesions. This protein was mainly produced by macrophages and EC and, to a lesser extent, also by SMC (Rolph et al., 2002). Actually, little is known about the role played by this molecule during atherogenesis. In a recent report, it has been shown that PTX3 could increase the TF expression by EC (Napoleone et al., 2002). Thus, in analogy to other inflammation processes, PTX3 could participate in the inflammatory and pro-thrombotic activities inside atherosclerotic plaques with a potential detrimental effect on the plaque stability.

3.2. Pattern-recognition receptors

3.2.1. Toll-like receptors

TLRs are mainly expressed on macrophage surface and are able to recognize some molecular patterns commonly found on pathogens. At variance with the SR, which lead to endocytosis of their ligands, activation of the TLRs is accompanied by the activation of the NF-κB and MAPK pathways with subsequent synthesis of a number of pro-inflammatory mediators (Muzio et al., 1998; Faure et al., 2000). These mediators, in turn, modulate the activation of the different phases of the inflammatory process (such as leukocyte recruitment, production of reactive oxygen species, and phagocytosis). Recent studies suggest that these receptors may actively participate in promoting autoimmune disorders through the induction of autoantibodies to nuclear antigens such as self-DNA (Leadbetter et al., 2002). Moreover, TLRs are also expressed on the surface of cellular elements usually involved in the atherosclerotic process (such as EC and macrophages) (Faure et al., 2001; Medzhitov et al., 1997). Some authors observed that inside atherosclerotic lesions, both EC and macrophages expressed TLRs, and the receptor expression could be upregulated by oxLDL (Edfeldt et al., 2002; Xu et al., 2001). The activation of TLR elements by bacterial products is accompanied by the endothelial production of cytokines (such as IL-1), adhesion molecules, ET-1, chemokines, and reactive oxygen species (Hansson et al., 2002). Moreover, it has been recently shown that interaction of TLR4 with LPS (its main ligand) is accompanied in vivo by the inflammatory activation of the vascular adventitia, with secretion of different kinds of cytokines (IL-10, IL-1, IL-6, IL-8) and the development of intimal lesions (Vink et al., 2002). The HSP60 (which can be either autologous or derived from pathogens) can also activate TLR4 in a manner similar to LPS (Ohashi et al., 2000). As it has been widely demonstrated that both LPS and HSP60 could participate in accelerating the progression of atherosclerotic lesions (Xu, 2002; Ostos et al., 2002), it is plausible that the TLRs may offer a potential link between bacterial infection, activation of the inflammatory response inside the atherosclerotic plaque, and atherosclerosis progression that is observed in patients suffering from chronic inflammatory disease. According to this hypothesis, it has been recently demonstrated that a polymorphism of the TLR4 (Asp299Gly), which is related with a reduced inflammatory response to gram-negative pathogens, is also associated with a decreased risk of atherosclerosis progression (Kiechl et al., 2002).

3.2.2. Scavenger receptors

The SR are another group of molecules deputed to the identification of molecular patterns commonly found on pathogens. These receptors are expressed by myeloid cells (especially macrophages and dendritic cells) and are involved in phagocytosis of bacteria and clearance of necrotic and apoptotic cells. Their ligation is characterized by endocytosis and lysosomial degradation of the recognized particle. The latter is then presented to the T cells with the triggering of the adaptive immune response (Peiser et al., 2002). During the last few years, a large number of different SR sharing related functions, such as SR-AI and AII, MARCO, CD36, SR-PSOX, and macrosialin, have been described. A large amount of information about the SR structure and functions has been obtained through basic research studies investigating their potential involvement in the atherogenesis. Several studies showed that these receptors recognized altered molecular patterns on the surface of lipoproteins undergoing enzymatic and oxidative modification after their trapping inside the arterial wall. The SR, such as SR-A and CD36, can in fact mediate phagocytosis by macrophages of modified lipoproteins, oxLDL in particular (Kita et al., 2001). This phenomenon, promotes the intracellular accumulation of lipids and represents a crucial event for foam cell formation (Li and Glass, 2002). The pivotal role played by these receptors during atherogenesis is suggested by studies showing that hyperlipidemic mice lacking some of these receptors did develop less atherosclerotic lesions (Babaev et al., 2000; Febbraio et al., 2000).

3.3. Cytokines

3.3.1. IL-1 and TNFα

IL-1 and TNFα are primary pro-inflammatory cytokines, which are mainly produced by monocytes and macrophages, and play a crucial role in the initial amplification of the inflammatory response. They can promote endothelial activation, induce secretion of chemokines, and through the induction of IL-6 promote the synthesis of the acute phase proteins by the liver. It is widely known that these cytokines exert a crucial role during autoimmune disease. While IL-1 is more involved in determining the inflammatory damage of cartilage and bone at the local level, TNFα seems to play a prominent role in promoting the systemic inflammatory state. In this view, both cytokines have become an important therapeutic target. In the last few years, it has been shown that many other cell types (such as EC, SMC, and T lymphocytes) can express these molecules and, hence, it is not surprising that both cytokines are expressed inside atherosclerotic lesions (Young et al., 2002). In vivo and in vitro basic research has highlighted their potential pro-atherogenic action. In particular, it has been shown that both TNFα and IL-1 could induce the expression of adhesion molecules by EC (Myers et al., 1992), promote the secretion of different cytokines and chemokines by monocytes (Sica et al., 1990), and may enhance the SMC proliferation and migration even through the induction of PDGF secretion by EC (Hajjar et al., 1987). They can also induce the expression of CD40 and CD40L (Karmann et al., 1995) and actively participate in the process of foam cell formation mainly through the induction of growth factors (such as M-CSF and GM-CSF) by SMC, EC, and macrophages (Clinton and Libby, 1992). These cytokines could also play a crucial role in the later stage of atheroma development by hampering plaque stability. In fact, both IL-1 and TNFα stimulate the expression of metalloproteinases in EC, SMC as well as in macrophages (Galis et al., 1994) and they can induce TF in both monocytes and differentiated macrophages (Young et al., 2002). Thus, these molecules mediate inflammatory processes that drive not only the initiation of the atherosclerotic process but also modulate later events that eventually promote the atherosclerotic plaque rupture with the onset of clinical cardiovascular events.

3.3.2. IL-6

IL-6 is a secondary inflammatory cytokine of 26 kDa produced by different kinds of cellular elements such as activated macrophages, lymphocytes, fibroblasts, EC, and vascular SMC under stimulation by IL-1 and TNFα. During the acute phase response, IL-6 exerts its main inflammatory functions by acting on hepatocytes and lymphocytes in several ways as it promotes: (i) the synthesis by hepatocytes of the acute phase response proteins such as CRP and fibrinogen; (ii) the B lymphocyte terminal differentiation; (iii) the co-stimulation of T lymphocytes and thymocytes; (iv) the proliferation of haematopoietic progenitors; and (v) some anti-viral effects.

Some studies demonstrated that both cellular and extracellular IL-6 deposits were present inside human atherosclerotic lesions in different vascular districts (Seino et al., 1994). IL-6 is particularly expressed within the shoulder region of human coronary plaques and inside this region, IL-6 co-localizes with angiotensin II. The latter enhances the IL-6 in vitro expression by monocytes and SMC (Schieffer et al., 2000; Funakoshi et al., 1999). Previous studies on mice models of atherosclerosis showed that IL-6 was synthesized in the atherosclerotic plaque (Sukovich et al., 1998) and the exogenous cytokine administration accelerated fatty lesion development (Huber et al., 1999).

IL-6 could act in a pro-inflammatory and procoagulant way with implications on atherosclerosis progression and thrombotic complications. In fact, it has been shown that IL-6 stimulates macrophages to secrete MCP-1 (Biswas et al., 1998), promotes expression of adhesion molecules and secretion of other cytokines by EC (Romano et al., 1997), augments fibrinogen production by hepatocytes, promotes the transcription of the factor VIII gene, increases the TF surface expression on cultured monocytes, augments the von Willebrand factor circulating levels, and reduces the synthesis of protein S and anti-thrombin, which act as inhibitors of coagulation. Furthermore, IL-6 enhances platelet production and aggregation, probably by acting on both megakaryocyte maturation and their thrombin-induced activation (Kerr et al., 2001). Many in vitro studies demonstrated that SMC are able to produce IL-6. The cytokine expression was promoted by different kinds of stimuli, such as endotoxin (Detmer et al., 2001), thrombin (Tokunou et al., 2001), ET-1 (Browatzki et al., 2000), MCP-1 (Viedt et al., 2002). Even angiotensin II is able to increase the IL-6 release by SMC in a dose-dependent way. Some other studies demonstrated that stimulation of cultured SMC with IL-6 promoted their proliferation and migration (Kranzhofer et al., 1999).

In analogy to observations related to plasma levels of CRP in the last few years, some large population-based studies showed that IL-6 plasma level could also be used as a prognostic marker of CVD outcome, both in patients with UA and in healthy subjects (Biasucci et al., 1996; Ridker et al., 2000).

Taken together, IL-6 may exert an important direct pathogenic role in atherosclerosis development and progression, especially through inflammatory elements recruitment and SMC activation. Moreover, circulating or locally produced IL-6 may favour the onset of a pro-thrombotic state, which could increase the risk of atherosclerotic complications especially at the later stage of the atheroma development, when an increased inflammatory burden renders remarkably unsteady the balance between the pro-coagulant and the fibrinolytic systems.

4. Clinical and diagnostic value of inflammatory markers

The predictive cardiovascular power of many of the inflammatory molecules described would imply some usefulness of routine measurement of their plasma level to improve the cardiovascular risk stratification of patients with known or unknown risk for CVD. A recent report sponsored by the Center for Disease Control and Prevention and the American Heart Association was published concerning the application of markers of inflammation to clinical and public health practice (Pearson et al., 2003). Among the various markers considered for potential clinical use (adhesion molecules, cytokines included IL-6, acute phase reactants, and white blood count), high-sensitivity CRP (hs-CRP) emerged as more clinically sound in terms of predictive CVD value, assay availability, and standardization. Compared to routine automated methods for CRP quantification, the hs-CRP methods are characterized by a lower detection limit, which allows a better analysis of CRP distribution within the normal range in the general population. Even using different hs-CRP methods, the protein values appear to be relatively stable over time as a consequence of its long half-life (Macy et al., 1997) with baseline concentrations in healthy humans that are subject to neither diurnal nor seasonal variation (Meier-Ewert et al., 2001; Frohlich et al., 2002). However, the recommendations for clinical and public health practice limit the optional hs-CRP use to relatively few conditions. The assessment of hs-CRP in fact could be useful in primary prevention to identify patients who may be at higher absolute risk than estimated by traditional risk factors. Within this category, the hs-CRP value may stimulate the physician to promote further diagnostic evaluation (imaging, exercise testing, etc.) or initiate specific therapies (aspirin, statins, etc.), particularly in subjects judged at intermediate risk. In addition, hs-CRP assessment could be useful in the secondary prevention setting (stable angina, UA, and patients undergoing percutaneous coronary intervention) to estimate the risk of future CVD. This information could be used to promote an aggressive application of the secondary prevention care, although these interventions should not depend on hs-CRP levels. This report advises against the widespread screening of the general population for hs-CRP or the protein level measurement as a guide to establish measures of secondary prevention, different from those described by the current guideline for the management of acute coronary syndrome. Moreover, levels of hs-CRP should not influence pharmacological options nor be used to monitor the effects of the treatment. According to the joint statement, hs-CRP measurement should be done twice, two weeks apart in metabolic stable patients. In the case of hs-CRP higher than 10 mg/l, the test should be repeated and patients screened for a potential source of inflammation. The relative risk of CVD based on hs-CRP level should be stratified as follows: low for hs-CRP level < 1 mg/l, average for hs-CRP level between 1.0 and 3.0 mg/l, high for hs-CRP level higher than 3.0 mg/l.

5. Potential treatment strategies

The progressive elucidation of the pivotal role played by inflammation during atherogenesis raises the question whether anti-inflammatory treatments could reduce the risk of CVD disease. Except for aspirin, pharmacological intervention studies specifically designed to clarify this issue using different anti-inflammatory strategies are still lacking. However, many preclinical and clinical researches demonstrated that some categories of drugs used for management of high blood pressure, hyperlipemia, or insulin resistance could exert a series of additive anti-inflammatory activities. In the clinical ground, these effects have been documented by the reduction of plasma levels of some pro-inflammatory cytokines. Many studies demonstrated that statins may exert a direct anti-atherosclerotic and anti-inflammatory effect on the arterial wall by acting on SMC, EC, and macrophages (Takemoto and Liao, 2001; Shovman et al., 2002). These effects could explain the reduction observed in circulating levels of many pro-inflammatory cytokines after treatment. In this context, plenty of data has been obtained mainly for CRP, even though similar results were observed for other cytokines such as IL-6 (Wiklund et al., 2002). Unfortunately, data in the literature are not compelling enough to support the view that the lowering of these inflammatory molecules leads to a risk reduction. Moreover, a recent study showed that statin therapy can also suppress the SR expression in differentiating monocytes (Fuhrman et al., 2002). PPAR agonists represent another drug class able to reduce the circulating level of these molecules (Staels et al., 1998), whereas ACE inhibitors/ATR antagonists induced a reduction in plasma MCP-1, TNFα, IL-6, and some other adhesion molecules (Brasier et al., 2002; Tsutamoto et al., 2000) without affecting CRP levels. Specific intervention studies should be conducted to establish whether or not these reductions of inflammatory molecules are accompanied by a decrease of risk of CVD. Finally, it should be noted that natural antibodies and anti-idiotypic antibodies within intravenous immunoglobulin (IVIg) could affect the atherosclerosis progression (Sherer and Shoenfeld, 2002). The treatment of mice prone to the development of atherosclerosis with IVIg was able to reduce the progression of both fatty streak and fibrofatty lesions. Recently it has also been shown that IVIg could attenuate the expression of metalloproteinase-9 in monocytes (Shapiro et al., 2002). These results display a potential usefulness of this treatment in reducing the atherosclerotic plaque instability.

6. Conclusion

During the last decade, a growing body of evidence yielded to a progressive overcoming of the formulation that atherosclerosis merely represents a process of lipids accumulation inside the arterial wall. Inflammatory cellular elements as well as cytokines, chemokines, or growth factors have emerged as key active elements in all phases of atherosclerosis progression. The atherosclerosis process, per se, might be considered as a chronic effort to eradicate a local inflammatory trigger. In a time span of years, this initially protective reaction could turn into a harmful, self-perpetuated process inside the arterial wall. This process could also be exacerbated by inflammatory systemic conditions and some inflammatory molecules could be involved in atherogenesis independent from their original source. Many molecules belonging to the innate immune system and closely linked together have emerged as potential active perpetrators of the atherogenic process. Indeed, many of the mechanisms described above (such as EC and macrophage activation with subsequent induction of cytokines secretion and receptor expression) are compatible with the physiological activity with which these molecules are deputed to during the inflammatory process. We do not clearly know whether these actions could shift into a harmful process, which may favour atherosclerosis progression. If so, they could become the another potential target for therapeutic intervention.

Key points

- Some categories of patients affected by chronic inflammatory disease (including patients with autoimmune disorders) are at increased risk of developing CVD compared to the general population and often experience an accelerated atherosclerosis.
- The innate immune system elements (including cellular receptors, cytokines, and acute phase response proteins) could be directly involved in the atherosclerotic process.
- Among the different inflammatory markers, hs-CRP assessment emerged as the main tool for stratifying cardiovascular risk in patients with either known or unknown cardiovascular disease.
- Some categories of drugs (statins in particular) exert a series of additional anti-inflammatory effects, which could contribute to their efficacy in preventing cardiovascular events.

References

Babaev, V.R., Gleaves, L.A., Carter, K.J., et al. 2000. Reduced atherosclerotic lesions in mice deficient for total or macrophage-specific expression of scavenger receptor-A. Arterioscler. Thromb. Vasc. Biol. 20, 2593.

Bhakdi, S., Torzewski, M., Klouche, M., et al. 1999. Complement and atherogenesis: binding of CRP to degraded, nonoxidized LDL enhances complement activation. Arterioscler. Thromb. Vasc. Biol. 19, 2348.

Biasucci, L.M., Vitelli, A., Liuzzo, G., et al. 1996. Elevated levels of interleukin-6 in unstable angina. Circulation 94, 874.

Biswas, P., Delfanti, F., Bernasconi, S., et al. 1998. Interleukin-6 induces monocyte chemotactic protein-1 in peripheral blood mononuclear cells and in the U937 cell line. Blood 91, 258.

Brasier, A.R., Recinos, A. III, Eledrisi, M.S. 2002. Vascular inflammation and the renin–angiotensin system. Arterioscler. Thromb. Vasc. Biol. 22, 1257.

Browatzki, M., Schmidt, J., Kubler, W., et al. 2000. Endothelin-1 induces interleukin-6 release via activation of the transcription factor NF-kappaB in human vascular smooth muscle cells. Basic Res. Cardiol. 95, 98.

Burke, A.P., Tracy, R.P., Kolodgie, F., et al. 2002. Elevated C-reactive protein values and atherosclerosis in sudden coronary death: association with different pathologies. Circulation 105, 2019.

Carroll, M. 2001. Innate immunity in the etiopathology of autoimmunity. Nat. Immunol. 2, 1089.

Cermak, J., Key, N.S., Bach, R.R., et al. 1993. C-reactive protein induces human peripheral blood monocytes to synthesize tissue factor. Blood 82, 513.

Chang, M.K., Binder, C.J., Torzewski, M., et al. 2002. C-reactive protein binds to both oxidized LDL and apoptotic cells through recognition of a common ligand: phosphorylcholine of oxidized phospholipids. Proc. Natl Acad. Sci. USA 99, 13043.

Clinton, S.K., Libby, P. 1992. Cytokines and growth factors in atherogenesis. Arch. Pathol. Lab. Med. 116, 1292.

DeStefano, F., Anda, R.F., Kahn, H.S., et al. 1993. Dental disease and risk of coronary heart disease and mortality. BMJ 306, 688.

Detmer, K., Wang, Z., Warejcka, D., et al. 2001. Endotoxin stimulated cytokine production in rat vascular smooth muscle cells. Am. J. Physiol. Heart Circ. Physiol. 281, H661.

Devaraj, S., Xu, D.Y., Jialal, I. 2003. C-reactive protein increases plasminogen activator inhibitor-1 expression and activity in human aortic endothelial cells: implications for the metabolic syndrome and atherothrombosis. Circulation 107, 398.

Dong, Q., Wright, J.R. 1996. Expression of C-reactive protein by alveolar macrophages. J. Immunol. 156, 4815.

Du Clos, T.W. 2000. Function of C-reactive protein. Ann. Med. 32, 274.

Edfeldt, K., Swedenborg, J., Hansson, G.K., et al. 2002. Expression of toll-like receptors in human atherosclerotic lesions: a possible pathway for plaque activation. Circulation 105, 1158.

Faure, E., Equils, O., Sieling, P.A., et al. 2000. Bacterial lipopolysaccharide activates NF-kappaB through toll-like receptor 4 (TLR-4) in cultured human dermal endothelial cells. Differential expression of TLR-4 and TLR-2 in endothelial cells. J. Biol. Chem. 275, 11058.

Faure, E., Thomas, L., Xu, H., et al. 2001. Bacterial lipopolysaccharide and IFN-gamma induce toll-like receptor 2 and toll-like receptor 4 expression in human endothelial cells: role of NF-kappa B activation. J. Immunol. 166, 2018.

Febbraio, M., Podrez, E.A., Smith, J.D., Hajjar, D.P., Hazen, S.L., Hoff, H.F., Sharma, K., Silverstein, R.L. 2000. Targeted disruption of the class B scavenger receptor CD36 protects against atherosclerotic lesion development in mice. J. Clin. Invest. 105, 1049.

Foley, R.N., Parfrey, P.S., Sarnak, M.J. 1998. Epidemiology of cardiovascular disease in chronic renal disease. J. Am. Soc. Nephrol. 9, S16.

Frohlich, M., Sund, M., Thorand, B., et al. 2002. Lack of seasonal variation in C-reactive protein. Clin. Chem. 48, 575.

Fuhrman, B., Koren, L., Volkova, N., et al. 2002. Atorvastatin therapy in hypercholesterolemic patients suppresses cellular uptake of oxidized-LDL by differentiating monocytes. Atherosclerosis 164, 179.

Funakoshi, Y., Ichiki, T., Ito, K., et al. 1999. Induction of interleukin-6 expression by angiotensin II in rat vascular smooth muscle cells. Hypertension 34, 118.

Galis, Z.S., Sukhova, G.K., Lark, M.W., et al. 1994. Increased expression of matrix metalloproteinases and matrix degrading activity in vulnerable regions of human atherosclerotic plaques. J. Clin. Invest. 94, 2493.

Galve-de Rochemonteix, B., Wiktorowicz, K., Kushner, I., et al. 1993. C-reactive protein increases production of IL-1 alpha, IL-1 beta, and TNF-alpha, and expression of mRNA by human alveolar macrophages. J. Leukoc. Biol. 53, 439.

Garlichs, C.D., John, S., Schmeisser, A., et al. 2001. Upregulation of CD40 and CD40 ligand (CD154) in patients with moderate hypercholesterolemia. Circulation 104, 2395.

Goodman, A.R., Cardozo, T., Abagyan, R., et al. 1996. Long pentraxins: an emerging group of proteins with diverse functions. Cytokine Growth Factor Rev. 7, 191.

Goodson, N. 2002. Coronary artery disease and rheumatoid arthritis. Curr. Opin. Rheumatol. 14, 115.

Gordon, C. 2002. Long-term complications of systemic lupus erythematosus. Rheumatology 41, 1095.

Gordon, P.A., George, J., Khamashta, M.A., et al. 2001. Atherosclerosis and autoimmunity. Lupus 10, 249.

Hajjar, K.A., Hajjar, D.P., Silverstein, R.L., et al. 1987. Tumor necrosis factor-mediated release of platelet-derived growth factor from cultured endothelial cells. J. Exp. Med. 166, 235.

Hansson, G.K., Libby, P., Schonbeck, U., et al. 2002. Innate and adaptive immunity in the pathogenesis of atherosclerosis. Circ. Res. 23, 281.

In this recent review, the evidence for the involvement of mediators of innate and acquired immunity during atherogenesis is discussed in detail. In particular, the authors focused on the role played by the pattern-recognition receptors and on the mobilization of the adaptive immune response as well.

Hattori, Y., Matsumura, M., Kasai, K. 2003. Vascular smooth muscle cell activation by C-reactive protein. Cardiovasc. Res. 58, 186.

Huber, S.A., Sakkinen, P., Conze, D., et al. 1999. Interleukin-6 exacerbates early atherosclerosis in mice. Arterioscler. Thromb. Vasc. Biol. 19, 2364.

Introna, M., Alles, V.V., Castellano, M., et al. 1996. Cloning of mouse ptx3, a new member of the pentraxin gene family expressed at extrahepatic sites. Blood 87, 1862.

Ishikawa, T., Hatakeyama, K., Imamura, T., et al. 2003. Involvement of C-reactive protein obtained by directional coronary atherectomy in plaque instability and developing restenosis in patients with stable or unstable angina pectoris. Am. J. Cardiol. 91, 287.

Jabs, W.J., Logering, B.A., Gerke, P., et al. 2003. The kidney as a second site of human C-reactive protein formation in vivo. Eur. J. Immunol. 33, 152.

Karmann, K., Hughes, C.C., Schechner, J., et al. 1995. CD40 on human endothelial cells: inducibility by cytokines and functional regulation of adhesion molecule expression. Proc. Natl Acad. Sci. USA 92, 4342.

Kerr, R., Stirling, D., Ludlam, C.A. 2001. Interleukin 6 and haemostasis. Br. J. Haematol. 115, 3.

Kiechl, S., Egger, G., Mayr, M., et al. 2001. Chronic infections and the risk of carotid atherosclerosis: prospective results from a large population study. Circulation 103, 1064.

Kiechl, S., Lorenz, E., Reindl, M., et al. 2002. Toll-like receptor 4 polymorphisms and atherogenesis. N. Engl. J. Med. 347, 185.

Kita, T., Kume, N., Minami, M., et al. 2001. Scavenger receptors, oxidized LDL, and atherosclerosis. Ann. NY Acad. Sci. 947, 214.

Kranzhofer, R., Schmidt, J., Pfeiffer, C.A., et al. 1999. Angiotensin induces inflammatory activation of human vascular smooth muscle cells. Arterioscler. Thromb. Vasc. Biol. 19, 1623.

Kuller, L.H., Tracy, R.P., Shaten, J., et al. 1996. Relation of C-reactive protein and coronary heart disease in the MRFIT nested case-control study. Multiple Risk Factor Intervention Trial. Am. J. Epidemiol. 144, 537.

Leadbetter, E.A., Rifkin, I.R., Hohlbaum, A.M., et al. 2002. Chromatin–IgG complexes activate B cells by dual engagement of IgM and toll-like receptors. Nature 416, 603.

Li, A.C., Glass, C.K. 2002. The macrophage foam cell as a target for therapeutic intervention. Nat. Med. 8, 1235.

Libby, P. 2002. Inflammation in atherosclerosis. Nature 420, 868.

This is an extensive overview on the pathophysiological mechanisms involved in the atherosclerotic process. In particular, the author described in detail the pivotal role played by cellular and humoral inflammatory elements from initiation through progression and complication of atherosclerosis.

Liuzzo, G., Biasucci, L.M., Gallimore, J.R., et al. 1994. The prognostic value of C-reactive protein and serum amyloid a protein in severe unstable angina. N. Engl. J. Med. 331, 417.

Loos, B.G., Craandijk, J., Hoek, F.J., et al. 2000. Elevation of systemic markers related to cardiovascular diseases in the peripheral blood of periodontitis patients. J. Periodontol. 71, 1528.

Luchetti, M.M., Piccinini, G., Mantovani, A., et al. 2000. Expression and production of the long pentraxin PTX3 in rheumatoid arthritis (RA). Clin. Exp. Immunol. 119, 196.

Macy, E.M., Hayes, T.E., Tracy, R.P. 1997. Variability in the measurement of C-reactive protein in healthy subjects: implications for reference intervals and epidemiological applications. Clin. Chem. 43, 52.

Medzhitov, R., Janeway, C. 2000. Innate immunity. N. Engl. J. Med. 343, 338.

Medzhitov, R., Preston-Hurlburt, P., Janeway, C.A. 1997. A human homologue of the Drosophila toll protein signals activation of adaptive immunity. Nature 388, 394.

Meier-Ewert, H.K., Ridker, P.M., Rifai, N., et al. 2001. Absence of diurnal variation of C-reactive protein concentrations in healthy human subjects. Clin. Chem. 47, 426.

Muzio, M., Natoli, G., Saccani, S., et al. 1998. The human toll signaling pathway: divergence of nuclear factor kappaB and JNK/SAPK activation upstream of tumor necrosis factor receptor-associated factor 6 (TRAF6). J. Exp. Med. 187, 2097.

Myers, C.L., Wertheimer, S.J., Schembri-King, J., et al. 1992. Induction of ICAM-1 by TNF-alpha, IL-1 beta, and LPS in human endothelial cells after downregulation of PKC. Am. J. Physiol. 263, C767.

Napoleone, E., Di Santo, A., Bastone, A., et al. 2002. Long pentraxin PTX3 upregulates tissue factor expression in human endothelial cells: a novel link between vascular inflammation and clotting activation. Arterioscler. Thromb. Vasc. Biol. 22, 782.

Nauta, A.J., Bottazzi, B., Mantovani, A., et al. 2003. A biochemical and functional characterization of the interaction between pentraxin 3 and C1q. Eur. J. Immunol. 33, 465.

Ohashi, K., Burkart, V., Flohe, S., et al. 2000. Cutting edge: heat shock protein 60 is a putative endogenous ligand of the toll-like receptor-4 complex. J. Immunol. 164, 558.

Ostos, M.A., Recalde, D., Zakin, M.M., et al. 2002. Implication of natural killer T cells in atherosclerosis development during a LPS-induced chronic inflammation. FEBS Lett. 519, 23.

Ouchi, N., Kihara, S., Funahashi, T., et al. 2003. Reciprocal association of C-reactive protein with adiponectin in blood stream and adipose tissue. Circulation 107, 671.

Pasceri, V., Willerson, J.T., Yeh, E.T. 2000. Direct proinflammatory effect of C-reactive protein on human endothelial cells. Circulation 102, 2165.

Pasceri, V., Cheng, J.S., Willerson, J.T., et al. 2001. Modulation of C-reactive protein-mediated monocyte chemoattractant protein-1 induction in human endothelial cells by anti-atherosclerosis drugs. Circulation 103, 2531.

Pauletto, P., Puato, M., Faggin, E., et al. 2000. Specific cellular features of atheroma associated with development of neointima after carotid endarterectomy: the carotid atherosclerosis and restenosis study. Circulation 102, 771.

Pearson, T.A., Mensah, G.A., Alexander, R.W., Centers for Disease Control and Prevention, American Heart Association, et al. 2003. Markers of inflammation and cardiovascular disease: application to clinical and public health practice: a statement for healthcare professionals from the Centers for Disease Control and Prevention and the American Heart Association. Circulation 107, 499.

This report was recently published by the AHA to focus on the suitability of markers of inflammation for clinical and public health practice. Among the various markers considered for potential clinical use (adhesion molecules, cytokines, acute phase reactants, and white blood count) hs-CRP emerged as the more clinically sound in terms of predictive cardiovascular disease value, assay availability, and standardization. This report represents an useful guide for the correct assessment and interpretation of the hs-CRP in the clinical ground.

Peiser, L., Mukhopadhyay, S., Gordon, S. 2002. Scavenger receptors in innate immunity. Curr. Opin. Immunol. 14, 123.

Peri, G., Introna, M., Corradi, D., et al. 2000. PTX3, a prototypical long pentraxin, is an early indicator of acute myocardial infarction in humans. Circulation 102, 636.

Ridker, P.M., Rifai, N., Stampfer, M.J., et al. 2000. Plasma concentration of interleukin-6 and the risk of future myocardial infarction among apparently healthy men. Circulation 101, 1767.

Ridker, P.M., Rifai, N., Rose, L., et al. 2002. Comparison of C-reactive protein and low-density lipoprotein cholesterol levels in the prediction of first cardiovascular events. N. Engl. J. Med. 347, 1557.

Many population based studies have suggested that hs-CRP assessment could predict the risk of future cardiovascular events among healthy subjects. This is the largest study (nearly 28,000 healthy women) on this topic. C-reactive protein level predicted the risk of subsequent cardiovascular events after a mean follow up of 8 years, and emerged as a stronger predictor than the LDL cholesterol level.

Rolph, M.S., Zimmer, S., Bottazzi, B., Garlanda, C., Mantovani, A., Hansson, G.K. 2002. Production of the long pentraxin PTX3 in advanced atherosclerotic plaques. Arterioscler. Thromb. Vasc. Biol. 22, e10.

Romano, M., Sironi, M., Toniatti, C., et al. 1997. Role of IL-6 and its soluble receptor in induction of chemokines and leukocyte recruitment. Immunity 6, 315.

Ross, R. 1999. Atherosclerosis—an inflammatory disease. N. Engl. J. Med. 340, 115.

Rovere, P., Peri, G., Fazzini, F., et al. 2000. The long pentraxin PTX3 binds to apoptotic cells and regulates their clearance by antigen-presenting dendritic cells. Blood 96, 4300.

Sartore, S., Chiavegato, A., Franch, R., et al. 1997. Myosin gene expression and cell phenotypes in vascular smooth muscle during development, in experimental models, and in vascular disease. Arterioscler. Thromb. Vasc. Biol. 17, 1210.

Schieffer, B., Schieffer, E., Hilfiker-Kleiner, D., et al. 2000. Expression of angiotensin II and interleukin 6 in human coronary atherosclerotic plaques: potential implications for inflammation and plaque instability. Circulation 101, 1372.

Seino, Y., Ikeda, U., Ikeda, M., et al. 1994. Interleukin 6 gene transcripts are expressed in human atherosclerotic lesions. Cytokine 6, 87.

Shapiro, S., Shoenfeld, Y., Gilburd, B., et al. 2002. Intravenous gamma globulin inhibits the production of matrix metalloproteinase-9 in macrophages. Cancer 95, 2032.

Sherer, Y., Shoenfeld, Y. 2002. Immunomodulation for treatment and prevention of atherosclerosis. Autoimmun. Rev. 1, 21.

Shovman, O., Levy, Y., Gilburd, B., et al. 2002. Antiinflammatory and immunomodulatory properties of statins. Immunol. Res. 25, 271.

Sica, A., Wang, J.M., Colotta, F., et al. 1990. Monocyte chemotactic and activating factor gene expression induced in endothelial cells by IL-1 and tumor necrosis factor. J. Immunol. 144, 3034.

Spence, J.D., Barnett, P.A., Bulman, D.E., et al. 1999. An approach to ascertain probands with a non-traditional risk factor for carotid atherosclerosis. Atherosclerosis 144, 429.

Staels, B., Koenig, W., Habib, A., et al. 1998. Activation of human aortic smooth-muscle cells is inhibited by PPARalpha but not by PPARgamma activators. Nature 393, 790.

Sukovich, D.A., Kauser, K., Shirley, F.D., et al. 1998. Expression of interleukin-6 in atherosclerotic lesions of male ApoE-knockout mice: inhibition by 17beta-estradiol. Arterioscler. Thromb. Vasc. Biol. 18, 1498.

Takemoto, M., Liao, J.K. 2001. Pleiotropic effects of 3-hydroxy-3-methylglutaryl coenzyme a reductase inhibitors. Arterioscler. Thromb. Vasc. Biol. 21, 1712.

Taskinen, S., Kovanen, P.T., Jarva, H., et al. 2002. Binding of C-reactive protein to modified low-density-lipoprotein particles: identification of cholesterol as a novel ligand for C-reactive protein. Biochem. J. 367, 403.

Tokunou, T., Ichiki, T., Takeda, K., et al. 2001. Thrombin induces interleukin-6 expression through the cAMP response element in vascular smooth muscle cells. Arterioscler. Thromb. Vasc. Biol. 21, 1759.

Torzewski, J., Torzewski, M., Bowyer, D.E., et al. 1998. C-reactive protein frequently colocalizes with the terminal complement complex in the intima of early atherosclerotic lesions of human coronary arteries. Arterioscler. Thromb. Vasc. Biol. 18, 1386.

Tsutamoto, T., Wada, A., Maeda, K., et al. 2000. Angiotensin II type 1 receptor antagonist decreases plasma levels of tumor necrosis factor alpha, interleukin-6 and soluble adhesion molecules in patients with chronic heart failure. J. Am. Coll. Cardiol. 35, 714.

Venugopal, S.K., Devaraj, S., Yuhanna, I., et al. 2002. Demonstration that C-reactive protein decreases eNOS expression and bioactivity in human aortic endothelial cells. Circulation 106, 1439.

Viedt, C., Vogel, J., Athanasiou, T., et al. 2002. Monocyte chemoattractant protein-1 induces proliferation and interleukin-6 production in human smooth muscle cells by differential activation of nuclear factor-kappaB and activator protein-1. Arterioscler. Thromb. Vasc. Biol. 22, 914.

Vink, A., Schoneveld, A.H., van der Meer, J.J., et al. 2002. In vivo evidence for a role of toll-like receptor 4 in the development of intimal lesions. Circulation 106, 1985.

Volanakis, J.E. 2001. Human C-reactive protein: expression, structure, and function. Mol. Immunol. 38, 189.

Wang, C.H., Li, S.H., Weisel, R.D., et al. 2003. C-reactive protein upregulates angiotensin type 1 receptors in vascular smooth muscle. Circulation. 107, 1783.

Wiklund, O., Mattsson-Hulten, L., Hurt-Camejo, E., et al. 2002. Effects of simvastatin and atorvastatin on inflammation markers in plasma. J. Intern. Med. 251, 338.

Xu, Q. 2002. Role of heat shock proteins in atherosclerosis. Arterioscler. Thromb. Vasc. Biol. 22, 1547.

Xu, X.H., Shah, P.K., Faure, E., et al. 2001. Toll-like receptor-4 is expressed by macrophages in murine and human lipid-rich atherosclerotic plaques and upregulated by oxidized LDL. Circulation 104, 3103.

Yasojima, K., Schwab, C., McGeer, E.G., et al. 2000. Human neurons generate C-reactive protein and amyloid P: upregulation in Alzheimer's disease. Brain. Res. 887, 80.

Yasojima, K., Schwab, C., McGeer, E.G., et al. 2001. Generation of C-reactive protein and complement components in atherosclerotic plaques. Am. J. Pathol. 158, 1039.

Young, J.L., Libby, P., Schonbeck, U. 2002. Cytokines in the pathogenesis of atherosclerosis. Thromb. Haemost. 88, 554.

Zebrack, J.S., Anderson, J.L., Maycock, C.A., et al. 2002. Usefulness of high-sensitivity C-reactive protein in predicting long-term risk of death or acute myocardial infarction in patients with unstable or stable angina pectoris or acute myocardial infarction. Am. J. Cardiol. 89, 145.

Zwaka, T.P., Hombach, V., Torzewski, J. 2001. C-reactive protein-mediated low density lipoprotein uptake by macrophages: implications for atherosclerosis. Circulation 103, 1194.

Handbook of Systemic Autoimmune Diseases, Volume 1
The Heart in Systemic Autoimmune Diseases
A. Doria and P. Pauletto, editors

CHAPTER 6

Atherosclerosis and Autoimmunity

Yaniv Sherer[a], Paolo Pauletto[b], Yehuda Shoenfeld[*,a]

[a]*Department of Medicine 'B', Center of Autoimmune Diseases, Sheba Medical Center, Tel-Hashomer, Sackler Faculty of Medicine, Tel-Aviv University, Tel-Aviv, Israel*[1]

[b]*Dipartimento di Medicina Clinica e Sperimentale, Università di Padova, Padova, Italy*

1. Introduction

Cardiovascular diseases are the leading cause of death in the Western world. Atherosclerosis (AS) is by far the most common underlying pathologic process leading to cardiovascular-related morbidity and mortality. Several factors, termed 'traditional' risk factors for cardiovascular disease, are associated with AS, and include smoking, hypertension, diabetes mellitus, hypercholesterolemia, and family history. The presence of these risk factors cannot always explain cardiovascular diseases (Braunwald, 1997). Other 'novel' factors are now considered to be associated with AS and its complications, including infectious agents, inflammatory processes and autoimmunity (Shoenfeld et al., 2001a,b). In this chapter we describe the contribution of autoimmunity to AS development in the general population and in patients affected with autoimmune diseases.

2. Etiology/pathogenesis

The etiology of AS is multi-factorial (which is also true for autoimmune diseases) and includes involvement of classical risk factors, infectious agents, inflammation and autoimmunity. Wick et al. (2001) summarized the classical concepts for the development of AS as including the 'respone to injury', 'altered-lipoprotein' and 'monoclonal smooth muscle cells proliferation' hypotheses. The first related to endothelial dysfunction in the basis of AS, whilst the 'altered-lipoprotein' hypothesis relates to oxidized LDL (oxLDL) as responsible for foam cells formation. These and other theories which were not mentioned are beyond the scope of this chapter. These authors also reviewed findings that support the role of inflammatory-immune processes in the development of AS. These include, for example, T cells infiltrating the intima at sites of development of AS lesions, and production of various mediators (such as interleukin-1, tumor necrosis factor alpha and various other cytokines) by leukocytes and endothelial cells in the AS plaque. Moreover, several of the cytokines are considered pro-atherogenic while others have anti-atherogenic effects (Sherer and Shoenfeld, 2002a).

2.1. *Autoantigens and autoantibodies in atherosclerosis*

Autoimmune diseases are characterized by pathological immune reactions against the self. Autoantigens and autoantibodies usually involved have been recognized, even though in the case of the latter, their pathogenic role is not always established. Similarly, several autoantigens and autoantibodies are also

Abbreviations: AS, Atherosclerosis; β2GPI, β2-glycoprotein-I; HSP, Heat-shock protein; oxLDL, oxidized LDL.

[1] Incumbent of the chair of autoimmunity, Laura Schwartz-Kipp, Tel Aviv University.

*Corresponding author.
E-mail address: shoenfel@post.tau.ac.il (Y. Shoenfeld).

DOI: 10.1016/S1571-5078(03)01006-7

implicated in AS pathogenesis (Shoenfeld et al., 2000). Most are considered pro-atherogenic, whereas some might even have a protective role against AS.

2.1.1. β2-glycoprotein-I as an autoantigen in atherosclerosis

Human β2GPI is a 50-kDa plasma glycoprotein that binds negatively charged surfaces and substances, and it is formed from four complement control protein modules and a fifth C-terminal domain that forms an elongated J-shaped molecule (Schwarzenbacher et al., 1999). β2GPI is considered the real autoantigen in the antiphospholipid syndrome, which is characterized by variety of clinical manifestations (most characteristics are thrombosis and obstetrical complications) and antiphospholipid antibodies (Sherer and Shoenfeld, 1999). β2GPI is also found in human AS lesions obtained from carotid endarterectomies, is abundantly expressed within the sub-endothelial regions and the intimal-medial border of human AS plaques, and co-localizes with CD4 + lymphocytes (George et al., 1999b).

Anti-β2GPI antibodies exert a pro-coagulant activity and they are also pro-atherogenic. Whereas β2GPI inhibited the in vitro uptake of oxLDL by murine macrophages, the binding of oxLDL to macrophages was significantly increased by simultaneous addition of anti-β2GPI antibodies (Hasunuma et al., 1997). The role of these antibodies *in vivo* was studied (as were other autoantibodies) in animal models of AS. The apo-E knockout mice developed spontaneous hypercholesterolemia and AS lesions, while the LDL-receptor-deficient mice developed AS plaques only when fed a high-fat diet. These models have morphological characteristics similar to human AS, and the AS in these mice develops from the proximal to distal aorta. A representative figure of an AS lesion obtained from the aortic sinus (the most proximal part of the aorta) of a mouse is shown in Fig. 1. Immunization of these mouse strains with β2GPI resulted in pronounced cellular and humoral response to β2GPI with high titers of anti-β2GPI antibodies concomitant with larger AS lesions which contained abundant CD4 + cells (Afek et al., 1999; George et al., 1998b). Upon transfer of lymphocytes obtained from β2GPI-immunized LDL-receptor deficient mice into syngeneic mice, the recipients exhibited larger fatty streaks compared with mice that received lymphocytes from control mice. T cell depletion of lymphocytes failed to induce this effect (George et al., 2000). Therefore, T cells specific to β2GPI are capable of increasing AS, suggesting that β2GPI is a target autoantigen in AS.

2.1.2. Anti-cardiolipin antibodies

Anti-cardiolipin antibodies are the hallmark of the antiphospholipid syndrome and are also used for its diagnosis. Immunization of LDL-receptor deficient mice with anti-cardiolipin antibodies resulted in development of high titers of mouse anti-cardiolipin and increased AS compared with controls (George et al., 1997). The presence of high levels of anti-cardiolipin antibodies was found as an independent risk factor for myocardial infarction or cardiac death in middle-aged men (Vaarala et al., 1995), and we found elevated levels of anti-cardiolipin, anti-β2GPI, and anti-oxLDL antibodies in patients having coronary artery disease compared with control subjects (Sherer et al., 2001a).

2.1.3. Oxidized low-density lipoprotein as an autoantigen in atherosclerosis

LDL is the ultimate source of cholesterol which accumulates in foam cells. LDL particles contain hundreds of molecules of phospholipids, free cholesterol, cholesterol esters and triglycerides (Steinberg, 1997). OxLDL as opposed to native LDL, contains large amounts of lysophosphatidylcholine and can increase adherence and penetration of monocytes. While enhanced oxidation of LDL is considered a pro-atherogenic step, the nature of the immune reaction against oxLDL regarding its effects on AS is less clear. Elevated levels of anti-oxLDL antibodies usually signify enhanced AS and presence of its manifestations. Hence, anti-oxLDL are elevated in patients with early-onset peripheral vascular disease, severe carotid atherosclerosis, angiographically verified coronary artery disease, and are predictive of carotid atherosclerosis progression, myocardial infarction occurrence and mortality (Bergmark et al., 1995; Maggi et al., 1994; Lehtimaki et al., 1999; Bui et al., 1996; Salonen et al., 1992; Wu et al., 1997). In addition, patients who underwent PTCA and were positive for the presence of anti-oxLDL antibodies

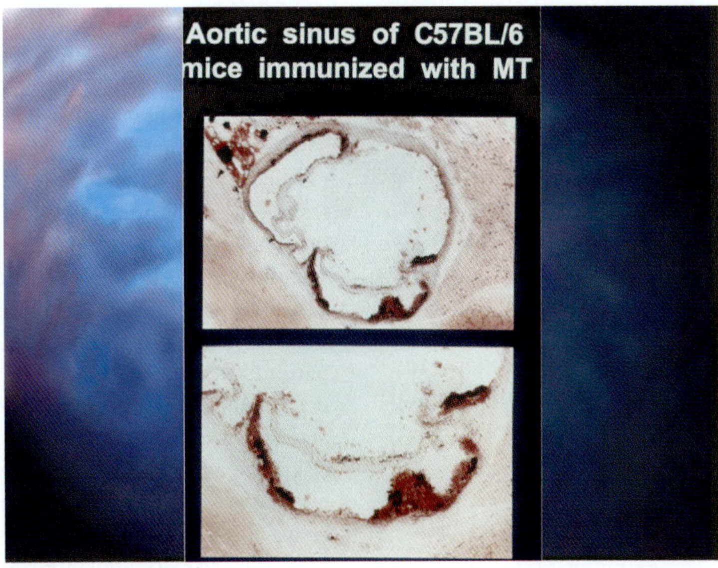

Figure 1. Atherosclerosis induced experimentally in C57BL/6 mice following immunization with *Mycobacteria* which are rich in HSP65 (George et al., 1999c).

were more likely to develop restenosis within 6 months compared with patients with no subsequent restenosis (George et al., 1999a).

As opposed to the above-mentioned studies, in animal models AS immunization with oxLDL resulted in induction of anti-oxLDL antibodies but suppression rather than aggravation of early atherogenesis (George et al., 1998a; Ameli et al., 1996). These results support the presence of different types of anti-oxLDL antibodies. As oxLDL is a particle rather than an antigen, different autoantibodies against it might have opposite effects. We have recently (Wu et al., 2003) found autoantibodies against oxLDL and also anti-idiotypes directed towards these antibodies (namely anti-anti-oxLDL) within commercial preparations of intravenous immunoglobulins. Of note is that treatment of animals with intravenous immunoglobulins could decrease AS extent. We speculated that the repertoire of anti-oxLDL in humans include both 'protective' and 'pathogenic' autoantibodies. Under normal circumstances, anti-oxLDL might help clear oxLDL by immune complexes. However, upon enhanced oxidation of LDL (which can occur due to smoking, lack of anti-oxidants, etc.), anti-oxLDL with higher affinity or different target epitopes are generated and can enhance AS. In this latter scenario, the anti-idiotypes to anti-oxLDL can have their beneficial effect, similar to their effect in various autoimmune diseases (Sherer and Shoenfeld, 2000).

2.1.4. Heat shock proteins as autoantigens in atherosclerosis

HSPs have important functions in conjugation with the folding and intracellular transport of proteins. They are phylogenetically highly conserved, and thus human HSP60 and mycobacterial HSP65 have 55% homology (Jones et al., 1993). As HSPs are antigenic components of infectious agents, almost all human subjects have immune reactivity against them. Hence, immune cross-reactivity against human HSP60 might arise. Indeed, using sonographic assessment of carotid lesions, subjects with AS lesions had significantly elevated levels of anti-HSP65 antibodies compared with controls (Xu et al., 1993). This difference was found only in 60–79 year old patients, but not in younger subjects. Follow-up of these patients disclosed that these antibodies were also associated with increased mortality (Xu et al., 1999).

The association between HSPs and AS is also demonstrated in animal models. Rabbits that were immunized with material containing HSP65, either in the form of mycobacteria or recombinant HSP65 alone developed AS lesions (Xu et al., 1992). In another study, C57BL/6 mice were injected with either HSP65, HSP65-rich *Mycobacterium tuberculosis*, or PBS. Early AS was significantly enhanced in high-cholesterol diet fed mice that were immunized with HSP65 or *M. tuberculosis*, compared with the PBS-injected mice, and the lesions found in the former two groups were associated with extensive deposits of immunoglobulins and infiltration of CD4 lymphocytes (George et al., 1999c). In a similar study, LDL receptor deficient mice that were immunized with HSP65 developed significantly larger fatty streaks compared with the BSA immunized group (Afek et al., 2000).

2.2. Cellular or humoral-mediated autoimmunity?

The above-mentioned studies are mainly dealing with the association of the humoral immune system, namely autoantibodies, with AS. However, the cellular immune system is also involved in AS development and progression (Sherer and Shoenfeld, 2002b). The importance of T cells in AS is emphasized in the a study in which CD4 + and CD8 + T cell depletion reduced fatty streak formation in C57BL/6 mice, indicating that T cells aggravate fatty streak formation (Emeson et al., 1996). Immunosuppression could be more specific. Cells within AS plaques express CD40 and CD40 ligand. Treatment with antibody against mouse CD40 ligand limited AS in LDL receptor deficient mice (Mach et al., 1998). AS probably includes both cellular and humoral components in its underlying pathophysiology, as occurring in many autoimmune diseases. A study in which lymph node cells, splenocytes and IgG were obtained from LDL-receptor-deficient mice immunized with HSP65 emphasizes this point. Adaptive transfer of HSP65-reactive1 lymph node cells increased fatty-streak formation in comparison with mice treated with BSA-primed cells, and in addition repeated intraperitoneal administration of IgG from serum of HSP65-immunized mice enhanced fatty-streak formation in mice in comparison with controls (George et al., 2001). This study supports a pro-atherogenic role for both cellular and humoral immune systems.

3. Clinical manifestations

The clinical manifestations of AS include various aspects of cardiovascular morbidity and mortality. These include angina pectoris, myocardial infarction, cardiac arrest, limb claudication, heart failure, transient ischemic attack, stroke, multi-infarct dementia, renal failure, and actually all the clinical manifestations associated with AS, decreased perfusion to target organs or arterial thrombosis. This is true in general population, but is evident also in patients having autoimmune diseases, who are occasionally characterized by enhanced AS (Sherer and Shoenfeld, 2001). One example for the increased risk of cardiovascular diseases in systemic lupus erythematosus, the disease most commonly associated with secondary antiphospholipid syndrome, is that the risk of hospitalization for myocardial infarction, cerebrovascular accidents and congestive heart failure was 2.27, 2.03 and 3.01 times, respectively, greater for patients between 18 and 44 years compared with controls (Ward, 1999). In a study where 22 patients with systemic lupus erythematosus and/or antiphospholipid syndrome were matched with controls, and underwent carotid ultrasonography and echocardiography, there was a 4.5-fold increase in the presence of carotid AS in the patient group versus controls, and similarly a 6-fold increase in the prevalence of left ventricular hypertrophy (Roman et al., 2001). In a recent study by Doria et al. (2003, in press), the predictors of AS in systemic lupus erythematosus were not only traditional including age and hypertension, but also 'non-traditional' including cumulative prednisone uptake, renal involvement, and the levels of anti-oxidized palmitoyl arachidonoyl phosphocholine antibodies.

4. Diagnostic investigations

Diagnosis of significant AS state is based on patients' symptoms, and objective signs detected in the physical examination. All of the above-mentioned manifestations of AS have more or less characteristic clinical presentation. Regarding imaging studies, the gold standard for coronary artery disease is still the coronary angiography which can best demonstrate the state of the coronary vessels. Similarly, ultrasound studies can evaluate narrowing and intimal plaques in the carotid arteries, and Doppler studies can aid in the evaluation of renal artery stenosis, for example.

Nonetheless, in the setting of autoimmunity-associated AS, other less conventional methods can be used for estimation of AS risk or extent, even though their efficacy has not yet been proven. Regarding serologic evaluation of patients, the presence of higher levels of antiphospholipid antibodies might indicate an increased risk or presence of enhanced AS. We failed to identify any difference in the level of anti-oxLDL antibodies between coronary artery disease patients regarding the status of their risk factors (Sherer et al., 2001a), whereas a comparison of anti-β2GPI antibody levels in these patients disclosed that the non-smokers had higher anti-β2GPI levels than smokers with coronary artery disease. Eleven patients in this cohort who were not smokers, and did not have hypercholesterolemia or hypertension had higher levels of anti-β2GPI antibodies than 11 patients who had all of these three risk factors (Sherer et al., 2002). All of these patients had coronary artery disease, but those who almost did not have any classical risk factor for AS had higher levels of autoantibody suggesting that this antibody might be a non-classical risk factor for AS. It is early to determine, however, whether this assumption is true.

An alternative way to estimate the burden of AS is by non-invasive techniques, such as the dual-helical computerized tomography. This method can assess calcific coronary deposits, which are closely associated with AS. It has been proved as a non-invasive test with a good sensitivity for the detection of coronary wall AS (Budoff et al., 1996). We measured the levels of anti-oxLDL, anti-cardiolipin and anti-β2GPI antibodies in patients having coronary artery disease, and failed to find a positive correlation between autoantibody levels and extent of coronary calcium as determined by spiral CT (Sherer et al., 2001a). Moreover, patients without any coronary calcification had elevated levels of anti-oxLDL antibodies compared with patients who had any degree of coronary calcification. As the role of anti-oxLDL antibodies is not clearly understood, this finding supports a negative association between higher levels of oxLDL antibodies and calcified AS lesions. We did identify higher levels of both coronary calcium and anti-cardiolipin antibodies in patients having typical chest pain for angina pectoris, compared with patients with atypical or no chest pain (Sherer et al., 2001b). Moreover, elevated levels of both anti-cardiolipin and coronary calcium score could differentiate better than any of those independently between patients with typical and atypical chest pain.

5. Treatment

Treatment of overt cardiovascular disease should be according to the clinical presentation. Many patients at risk for thrombosis, such as systemic lupus erythematosus/antiphospholipid syndrome patients are given aspirin which can decrease the chance of arterial thrombosis, regardless of the underlying mechanism (the pro-coagulant activity of autoantibodies, or the enhanced AS state characterizing these diseases). However, one should remember that the best treatment is prevention. Patients having autoimmune diseases are at increased risk for cardiovascular diseases and enhanced AS not only due to the autoimmune process, but also due to drugs such as steroids, or disease complications such as nephritis leading to hypertension, and nephrotic syndrome. Additionally, other classical risk factors might be found in autoimmune diseases. In systemic lupus erythematosus, there are elevated triglycerides and VLDL cholesterol, decreased HDL cholesterol and apolipoprotein A-1 (Borba and Bonfa, 1997), and also elevated levels of homocysteine (Petri et al., 1996). Therefore, patients should receive preventive therapy with education for regular exercise, blood pressure control, and when appropriate use of statins and/or folic acid. Immunomodulation of AS is also an option, even though it is only in the experimental stages now (Sherer and Shoenfeld, 2002a). It includes use of intravenous immunoglobulins, immunosuppression, oral tolerance with autoantigens such as oxLDL, bone-marrow transplantation, cytokine inhibitors, and gene therapy.

Key points

- AS is a pathological process which is associated with inflammation, infections and autoimmunity. These components contribute to AS in the general population as well as in patients having autoimmune diseases.
- Several autoantigens and autoantibodies are associated with AS including anti-cardiolipin, oxLDL, HSPs and β2GPI.
- Both the cellular and humoral immune systems are involved in autoimmune AS.
- Patients having certain autoimmune diseases (e.g. systemic lupus erythematosus, vasculitis, rheumatoid arthritis) are prone to enhanced AS and its complications.
- Aggressive preventive measures are necessary in order to minimize the risk of cardiovascular diseases in patients with autoimmune diseases.
- AS can be immunomodulated.

References

Afek, A., George, J., Shoenfeld, Y., et al. 1999. Enhancement of atherosclerosis in beta-2-glycoprotein I-immunized apolipoprotein E-deficient mice. Pathobiology 67, 19.

Afek, A., George, J., Gilburd, B., et al. 2000. Immunization of low-density lipoprotein receptor deficient (LDL-RD) mice with heat shock protein 65 (HSP-65) promotes early atherosclerosis. J. Autoimmun. 14, 115.

Ameli, S., Hultgardh-Nilsson, A., Regnstrom, J., et al. 1996. Effect of immunization with homologous LDL and oxidized LDL on early atherosclerosis in hypercholesterolemic rabbits. Arterioscler. Thromb. Vasc. Biol. 16, 1074.

Bergmark, C., Wu, R., de Faire, U., et al. 1995. Patients with early-onset peripheral vascular disease have increased levels of autoantibodies against oxidized LDL. Arterioscler. Thromb. Vasc. Biol. 15, 441.

Borba, E.F., Bonfa, E. 1997. Dyslipoproteinemias in systemic lupus erythematosus: influence of disease, activity and anticardiolipin antibodies. Lupus 6, 533.

Braunwald, E. 1997. Shattuck lecture—cardiovascular medicine at the turn of the millennium: triumphs, concerns and opportunities. N. Engl. J. Med. 337, 1360.

Budoff, M.J., Georgiou, D., Brody, A., et al. 1996. Ultrafast computed tomography as a diagnostic modality in the detection of coronary artery disease. Circulation 93, 898.

Bui, M.N., Sack, M.N., Moutsatsos, G., et al. 1996. Autoantibody titers to oxidized low-density lipoprotein in patients with coronary atherosclerosis. Am. Heart. J. 131, 663.

Doria, A., Shoenfeld, Y., Wu, R., et al. 2003. A five-year prospective study on risk factors for subclinical atherosclerosis in patients with systemic lupus erythematosus. Ann. Rheuamt. Dis. 62, 1071–1077.

Emeson, E.E., Shen, M.L., Bell, C.G., Qureshi, A. 1996. Inhibition of atherosclerosis in CD4 T-cell-depleted and nude (nu/nu) C57BL/6 hyperlipidemic mice. Am. J. Pathol. 149, 675.

George, J., Afek, A., Gilburd, B., Levy, Y., Blank, M., Kopolovic, J., et al. 1997. Atherosclerosis in LDL-receptor knockout mice is accelerated by immunization with anticardiolipin antibodies Lupus 6, 723.
One of the first studies demonstrating the pro-atherogenic role of antiphospholipid antibodies.

George, J., Afek, A., Gilburd, B., et al. 1998a. Hyperimmunization of apo-E mice with homologous malondialdehyde low-density lipoprotein suppresses early atherogenesis. Atherosclerosis 138, 147.

George, J., Afek, A., Gilburd, B., et al. 1998b. Induction of early atherosclerosis in LDL-receptor-deficient mice immunized with beta2-glycoprotein I. Circulation 98, 1108.

George, J., Harats, D., Bakshi, E., et al. 1999a. Anti-oxidized low density lipoprotein antibody determination as a predictor of restenosis following percutaneous transluminal coronary angioplasty. Immunol. Lett. 68, 263.

George, J., Harats, D., Gilburd, B., et al. 1999b. Immunolocalization of β2-glycoprotein I (apolipoprotein H) to human atherosclerotic plaques: potential implications for lesion progression. Circulation 99, 2227.

George, J., Shoenfeld, Y., Afek, A., et al. 1999c. Enhanced fatty streak formation in C57BL/6J mice by immunization with heat shock protein-65. Arterioscler. Thromb. Vasc. Biol. 19, 505.

George, J., Harats, D., Gilburd, B., et al. 2000. Adoptive transfer of beta-2-glycoprotein-I-reactive lymphocytes enhances early atherosclerosis in LDL receptor-deficient mice. Circulation 102, 1822.
A study which best emphasizes the importance of T cells in promotion of atherosclerosis.

George, J., Afek, A., Gilburd, B., et al. 2001. Cellular and humoral immune responses to heat shock protein 65 are both involved in promoting fatty-streak formation in LDL-receptor deficient mice. J. Am. Coll. Cardiol. 38, 900.

Hasunuma, Y., Matsuura, E., Makita, Z., et al. 1997. Involvement of beta 2-glycoprotein I and anticardiolipin antibodies in oxidatively modified low-density lipoprotein uptake by macrophages. Clin. Exp. Immunol. 107, 569.

Jones, D.B., Coulson, A.F., Duff, G.W. 1993. Sequence homology between hsp60 and autoantigens. Immunol. Today 14, 115.

Lehtimaki, T., Lehtinen, S., Solakivi, T., et al. 1999. Autoantibodies against oxidized low density lipoprotein in patients with angiographically verified coronary artery disease. Arterioscler. Thromb. Vasc. Biol. 19, 23.

Mach, F., Schonbeck, U., Sukhova, G.K., et al. 1998. Reduction of atherosclerosis in mice by inhibition of CD40 signaling. Nature 394, 200.

Maggi, E., Chiesa, R., Melissano, G., et al. 1994. LDL oxidation in patients with severe carotid atherosclerosis: a study in vitro and in vivo oxidation markers. Arterioscler. Thromb. 14, 1892.

Petri, M., Roubenoff, R., Dallal, G.E., et al. 1996. Plasma homocysteine as a risk factor for atherosclerotic events in systemic lupus erythematosus. Lancet 348, 1120.

Roman, M.J., Salmon, J.E., Sobel, R., et al. 2001. Prevalence and relation to risk factors of carotid atherosclerosis and left ventricular hypertrophy in systemic lupus erythematosus and antiphospholipid antibody syndrome. Am. J. Cardiol. 87, 663.

Salonen, J.T., Yla-Herttuala, S., Yamamoto, R., et al. 1992. Autoantibodies against oxidized LDL and progression of carotid atherosclerosis. Lancet 339, 883.

Schwarzenbacher, R., Zeth, K., Diederichs, K., et al. 1999. Crystal structure of human beta 2-glycoprotein I: implications for phospholipid binding and the antiphospholipid syndrome. EMBO J. 18, 6228.

Sherer, Y., Shoenfeld, Y. 1999. The antiphospholipid (Hughes') syndrome—an entity to be expanded. Am. J. Reprod. Immunol. 41, 113.

Sherer, Y., Shoenfeld, Y. 2000. The idiotypic network in antinuclear-antibody-associated diseases. Int. Arch. Allergy Immunol. 123, 10.

Sherer, Y., Shoenfeld, Y. 2001. Antiphospholipid syndrome, antiphospholipid antibodies, and atherosclerosis. Curr. Atheroscler. Rep. 3, 328.

Sherer, Y., Shoenfeld, Y. 2002a. Immunomodulation for treatment and prevention of atherosclerosis. Autoimmun. Rev. 1, 21.

A thorough review of the options to immunomodulate atherosclerosis.

Sherer, Y., Shoenfeld, Y. 2002b. Is atherosclerosis a cellular or humoral mediated autoimmune disease? Ann. Rheum. Dis. 61, 97.

Sherer, Y., Shemesh, J., Tenenbaum, A., et al. 2000. Coronary calcium and anti-cardiolipin antibody are elevated in patients with typical chest pain. Am. J. Cardiol. 86, 1306.

Sherer, Y., Tenenbaum, A., Blank, M., et al. 2001a. Coronary artery disease but not coronary calcification is associated with elevated levels of cardiolipin, β-2-glycoprotein-I, and oxidized-LDL antibodies. Cardiology 95, 20.

Sherer, Y., Tenenbaum, A., Blank, M., et al. 2001b. Autoantibodies to oxidized low-density lipoprotein in coronary artery disease. Am. J. Hypertens. 14, 149.

Sherer, Y., Tenenbaum, A., Praprotnik, S., et al. 2002. Autoantibodies to cardiolipin and beta-2-glycoprotein-I in coronary artery disease patients with and without hypertension. Cardiology 97, 2.

Shoenfeld, Y., Sherer, Y., George, J., et al. 2000. Autoantibodies associated with atherosclerosis. Ann. Med. 32 (Suppl. 1), 37.

Shoenfeld, Y., Harats, D., Wick, G. 2001a. Atherosclerosis and Autoimmunity. Elsevier, Amsterdam.

Shoenfeld, Y., Sherer, Y., Harats, D. 2001b. Atherosclerosis as an infectious, inflammatory and autoimmune disease. Trends Immunol. 22, 293.

Steinberg, D. 1997. Low density lipoprotein oxidation and its pathophysiological significance. J. Biol. Chem. 272, 20963.

Vaarala, O., Manttari, M., Manninen, V., et al. 1995. Anticardiolipin antibodies and risk of myocardial infarction in a prospective cohort of middle-aged men. Circulation 91, 23.

Ward, M.M. 1999. Premature morbidity from cardiovascular and cerebrovascular diseases in women with systemic lupus erythematosus. Arthritis Rheum. 42, 338.

Wick, G., Millonig, G., Xu, Q. 2001. The autoimmune pathogenesis of atherosclerosis—an evolutionary-Darwinian concept. In: Y. Shoenfeld, D. Harats, G. Wick (Eds.), Atherosclerosis and Autoimmunity. Elsevier, Amsterdam, p. 5.

Wu, R., Nityanand, S., Berglund, L., et al. 1997. Antibodies against cardiolipin and oxidatively modified LDL in 50-year-old men predict myocardial infarction. Arterioscler. Thromb. Vasc. Biol. 17, 3159.

Wu, R., Shoenfeld, Y., Sherer, Y., et al. 2003. Anti-idiotypes against oxidized LDL antibodies in intravenous immunoglobulin preparations—possible immunomodulation of atherosclerosis. Autoimmunity 36, 91.

Xu, Q., Dietrich, H., Steiner, H.J., et al. 1992. Induction of arteriosclerosis in normocholesterolemic rabbits by immunization with heat shock protein 65. Arterioscler. Thromb. 12, 789.

Xu, Q., Willeit, J., Marosi, M., et al. 1993. Association of serum antibodies to heat-shock protein 65 with carotid atherosclerosis. Lancet 341, 255.

Xu, Q., Kiechl, S., Mayr, M., et al. 1999. Association of serum antibodies to heat-shock protein 65 with carotid atherosclerosis: clinical significance determined in a follow-up study. Circulation 100, 1169.

Handbook of Systemic Autoimmune Diseases, Volume 1
The Heart in Systemic Autoimmune Diseases
A. Doria and P. Pauletto, editors

Chapter 7

Statins and Autoimmunity

Victor S. Gurevich

Mechnicov's State Medical Academy, The Center of Atherosclerosis and Lipid Disorders, 194291 pr.Kultury 4, CMSD-122 St Petersburg, Russia

1. Introduction

Statins (HMG-CoA reductase inhibitors) have been used broadly for the treatment of hypercholesterolemia over the last two decades. However, current understanding of the pharmacological effects of statins is progressing toward the insight that these agents do more than simply lower cholesterol. Their role as lipid lowering agents is now surpassed by their effects on endothelial, immune and smooth muscle cells. Statins may provide benefits both by decreasing cholesterol and by use of lipid-independent mechanisms. Extensive research carried out recently suggests that the clinical benefits of these drugs could be related to an improvement in endothelial dysfunction, a reduction in blood thrombogenicity, anti-inflammatory properties, and, finally, immunomodulatory actions. It is thought that they will become valuable tools for controlling inflammatory and immune responses. Below, the positive role of statins in the treatment of autoimmune reactions is presented.

2. Statin drug family

Lovastatin, pravastatin, and simvastatin are derived from fungal fermentation. Fluvastatin and atorvastatin are entirely synthetic. Lovastatin, simvastatin and atorvastatin exploit the cytochrome P 450 (CYP) 3A4 pathway for metabolism or biotransformation (Lennernas and Fager, 1997). Fluvastatin metabolism occurs via CYP2C9, but pravastatin does not use the CYP pathway significantly. Pravastatin is extremely hydrophilic compared with other statins except for fluvastatin, which has intermediate physicochemical properties. This difference in hydrophilicity has not been demonstrated to have clinical significance (Maron et al., 2000). Two more drugs of this class have been developed recently—rosuvastatin and pitavastatin (Gotto, 2003). Despite having a lipid lowering effect comparable with atorvastatin and simvastatin, further investigation of their effectiveness in prevention of coronary events is warranted.

3. Molecular mechanisms of statins action

All statins are competitive inhibitors of HMG-CoA reductase because of their structural similarity to hydroxymethylglutaryl-coenzyme A(HMG-CoA), a precursor of cholesterol. This enzyme regulates an important step in cholesterol synthesis. The resulting decrease in intracellular cholesterol level leads to transcriptional upregulation of LDL-receptor synthesis, increases the LDL entry into the hepatic cells and thus reduces LDL levels in the circulation.

Statins also inhibit the synthesis of important isoprenoid intermediates in the cholesterol biosynthesis pathway: farnesylpyrophosphate (FPP) and geranylgeranylpyrophosphate (GGPP) (Goldstein and Brown, 1990). These intermediates operate as

E-mail address: gur@cards.lanck.net (V.S. Gurevich).

DOI: 10.1016/S1571-5078(03)01007-9

lipid attachments for the posttranslational modification of an assortment of proteins, in particular, the small GTP-binding Ras-protein and Ras-like proteins, such as Rho, Rab, Rac, Ral, and Rap. Protein isoprenylation sanctions the covalent attachment, subcellular localization, and intracellular translocation of membrane-associated proteins. Members of the Ras and Rho GTPase family are major substrates for posttranslational modification by prenylation (Van Aelst and D' Souza-Schorey, 1997; Hall, 1998). Ras and Rho are small GTP-binding proteins that rotate between the inactive and active GTP-bound states. Ras translocation from the cytoplasm to the plasma membrane is dependent on farnesylation, whereas Rho translocation is dependent on geranylgeranylation (Laufs and Liao, 1998). Statins inhibit Ras and Rho isoprenylation, leading to the accumulation of inactive Ras and Rho in the cytoplasm.

4. Hypolipidemic and pleiotropic effects of statins

The hypolipidemic action of statins remains the important beneficial characteristic of this drug class in the treatment and the prevention of clinical complications of atherosclerosis because serum cholesterol levels are strongly associated with coronary atherosclerotic disease (Shepherd et al., 1995). For a long time it has been generally assumed that cholesterol reduction by statins is the only mechanism underlying their positive effects in cardiovascular diseases (Downs et al., 1998). However, subgroup analyses of large clinical trials have disputed this point of view. It has been suggested that the beneficial effects of statins may also be explained by mechanisms beyond cholesterol reduction. For instance, subgroup analysis of WOSCOP and CARE studies have indicated that statin-treated individuals have a significantly lower risk of coronary heart disease than do age-matched placebo-controlled individuals, despite comparable serum cholesterol levels (Sacks et al., 1996; Packard, 1998). Furthermore, meta-analyses of cholesterol-lowering trials suggest that the risk of myocardial infarction in individuals treated with statins is significantly lower than that in individuals treated with other cholesterol-lowering agents or modalities despite comparable reductions in serum cholesterol levels in both groups (Brown et al., 1993). An additional important observation regarding the effectiveness of statins has suggested that their positive effect on clinical outcomes considerably exceed the influence on regression of coronary stenosis and volume of lipid core in atherosclerotic plague (Fuster and Badimon, 1995; Gotto, 1997). These findings suggest that statins may have beneficial effects further than cholesterol lowering (Takemoto and Liao, 2001). According to the generally accepted viewpoint, the pleiotropic effects of statins influence on atherogenesis are selected as antiatherosclerotic and antithrombotic. The spectrum of direct antiatherogenic properties integrates the maintenance of endothelial function, tissue antioxidant capacity, inhibition of smooth muscle cell proliferation and inflammation. Following plaque disruption, statins may influence thrombosis through variable inhibitory actions on platelet function, coagulation factors, reology and fibrinolysis (Shovman et al., 2002). All these parameters, as well as immune cells reactions, could become unbalanced in a number of specific autoimmune and inflammation conditions including those taking place in atherosclerosis, type 1 diabetes, thyroid autoimmunity, antiphospholipid syndrome and multiple sclerosis. This is the reason why interest in the pleiotropic effects of statins has grown recently.

5. Atherosclerosis, lipid disorders and autoimmunity

The classical cholesterol concept of atherogenesis was upgraded principally by Brown and Goldstein (1983) when the idea was put forward that circulating LDL must undergo some kind of structural modification before it becomes completely atherogenic. They found out that the macrophages, the precursors of the cholesterol-loaded foam cells, took up native LDL at a rate that was not enough to provide the cell with cholesterol. They also called attention to the fact that patients who fully lack the native LDL receptor nevertheless accumulate sufficient amounts of cholesterol in their macrophages. It has been suggested that modifications of LDL must occur, leading to uptake of the modified forms through receptors other than the classic LDL receptors. Soon afterwards, these so-called 'scavenger receptors' were discovered and identified (Kodama et al., 1988; Krieger and Herz, 1994). The fundamental correctness of this conception of LDL modification is now supported by many lines of evidence (Steinberg and Witztum, 1990). Later studies showed that autoantibodies are generated against oxidized LDL and that the titers are correlated with the extent of atherosclerosis (Salonen et al., 1992).

It is also well known that atherosclerotic lesions are filled with immune cells that can orchestrate and affect inflammatory responses (Hansson et al., 1989; Van der Wal et al., 1989). The first lesions of atherosclerosis consist of macrophages and T cells. Unstable plaques are rich in activated immune cells, suggesting that they may initiate plaque destabilization. There is a remarkable increase in the understanding of the mechanisms that manage the recruitment, differentiation, and activation of immune cells in atherosclerosis (Hansson, 2001).

Experimental and clinical studies have identified several candidate lipid antigens and autoantibodies suggested to play important role in cardiovascular disorders. Anticardiolipin (aCL) antibodies and lupus anticoagulant are the main antibodies associated with the antiphospholipid syndrome, which manifests clinically as vascular thrombosis and pregnancy morbidity. It is known that aCL antibodies require a serum cofactor, β_2-glycoprotein I (β_2GPI) or apolipoprotein H, for binding to cardiolipin in vitro. Antibodies to β_2GPI can be measured directly and were shown to be more specific than aCL antibodies for the clinical manifestations of antiphospholipid syndrome (Tsutsumi et al., 1996). The enhanced risk of cardiovascular disease (CVD) in a major autoimmune disease, systemic lupus erythematosus, is therefore, highly relevant, and in addition to being an important clinical problem, SLE-related CVD could give insights into the nature of autoimmunity in atherosclerosis and CVD in general. Frostegard (2002) recently defined traditional and non-traditional risk factors for CVD in SLE. These include increased atherosclerosis (as determined by intima-media thickness of carotid artery); raised oxidized low density lipoprotein (OxLDL) and autoantibodies to OxLDL; dyslipidemia with raised triglycerides and Lp(a) and decreased HDL-cholesterol concentrations; raised systemic inflammation; presence of anti-phospholipid antibodies including lupus anticoagulant, homocysteine-levels and more frequent osteoporosis. Taken together, immune reactions are highly relevant in atherosclerosis, and patients with autoimmune disease like SLE are at high risk of CVD. It was suggested that if prospectively confirmed, non-traditional risk factors like OxLDL in the circulation, autoantibodies against OxLDL and phospholipids and inflammation could lead to new therapeutic strategies and insights into disease mechanisms.

Subclinical hypothyroidism and thyroid autoimmunity may also result in accelerated atherosclerosis and premature coronary heart disease, more often in middle-aged women presumably because of the associated hypercholesterolemia, hypertriglyceridemia, elevated total cholesterol/HDL-cholesterol ratio and hypertension (Luboshitzky et al., 2002). Lotz and Salabe (1997) have demonstrated in males and postmenopausal females an association between thyroid autoimmunity and increased levels of lipoprotein(a). However, it should be emphasized that the relation between the development of CVD in these patients and autoimmunity remains to be confirmed (Miura et al., 1996).

The role of infectious agents in the pathogenesis of atherosclerosis has long been suggested (Danesh et al., 1997). On the one hand the pathogens initiate the development of an inflammatory reaction, the first step in the atherogenesis. On the other hand bacterial and viral infections can induce autoimmune reactivity against host lipoproteins, phospholipids and other autoantigens, for example, heat shock proteins, which may serve as a target for autoimmune reactions (Wick et al., 1995).

Since organ-specific autoimmune diseases are sometimes accompanied by broad alterations of serum autoreactive antibody repertoires, Caligiuri et al. (2003) investigated antibody repertoires at a global level, using a technique of immunoblotting that allows for the quantitative screening of antibody reactivities in complex antibody mixtures toward a large panel of antigens derived from homologous tissue extracts. The autoreactive IgG repertoire in 20 patients with documented coronary atherosclerosis and in 20 matched healthy controls has been analyzed. Total proteins from atherosclerotic carotid specimens, normal arterial tissues (target organs) and from kidney, liver, and stomach (non-target control organs) were used as panels of antigens. Patients had a significantly perturbed antibody repertoire and an enhanced autoreactivity of IgG to target and non-target organs, as compared with controls. Reactivity of purified IgG to plaque and normal artery proteins was greater in patients, but reactivity of IgG in the whole serum toward normal arterial tissue was lower than in controls. It has been suggested that, in patients, autoreactivity toward normal arteries is regulated by serum factors. These data indicate that atherosclerotic patients develop a perturbed humoral immune response directed toward arterial proteins, which impacts on the overall autoreactive repertoire. These findings further substantiate that autoimmune processes take place in atherosclerosis and most likely influence disease progression.

HDL, unlike LDL, are not capable of becoming antigenic. However, HDL can intensively influence, atherogenic autoimmune reactivity because normal HDL contains at least four enzymes as well as apolipoproteins that can prevent the formation of the LDL-derived oxidized phospholipids or inactivate them after they are formed (Klimov et al., 1993; Watson et al., 1995). Under some conditions, for example, due to viral infection, HDL can lose its protective potential. Therefore, it has been proposed recently that LDL-derived oxidized phospholipids and HDL may be part of a system of non-specific innate immunity. Any disbalance in this system increases the susceptibility to atherosclerosis (Navab et al., 2001).

6. Cellular and molecular targets for immunomodulatory effects of statins

6.1. Effects of statins on macrophages

Macrophages are involved in all the phases of atherosclerosis from initiation through progression and finally plaque rupture and thrombosis. Several works have demonstrated that macrophages proliferate in human and hypercholesterolemic rabbit atheroma (Gordon et al., 1990; Rosenfeld and Ross, 1990; Rekhter and Gordon, 1995). Survival factors such as macrophages-colony stimulating factor (M-CSF) and granulocyte macrophage-colony stimulating factor (GM-CSF) induce macrophage proliferation in vitro (Becker et al., 1987; Metcalf, 1989) and ox-LDL enhances their action (Sakai et al., 1996; Hamilton et al., 1999). Macrophage proliferation may contribute to the formation of macrophage-rich vulnerable atheroma. Additional problems from macrophages in the pathogenesis of atherosclerosis are associated with over-expression by them of matrix metalloproteinases (MMPs) such as MMP-1 (collagenase-1), MMP-3 (stromelysin-1), and MMP-9 (gelatinase-B) (Henney et al., 1991; Galis et al., 1994; Nikkari et al., 1995) as well as tissue factor (TF), a strong activator of blood coagulation (Wilcox et al., 1989; Mach et al., 1997). Regarding the context of this chapter, the initiation by macrophages adaptive immune responses through the presentation of foreign antigens to T cells is most important. Nevertheless all these activities may be significant in atherogenesis.

Several studies provide new evidence for an effect of HMG-CoA reductase inhibitors on macrophage function beyond lipid lowering. Interestingly, Shiomi and Ito (1999) have demonstrated that statin treatment retarded enlargement of plaque size and reduced accumulation of macrophages in Watanabe heritable hyperlipidemic (WHHL) rabbits, which have endogenous hypercholesterolemia due to LDL-receptor deficiency. Moreover, Pauletto et al. (2000) observed, using a panel of monoclonal antibodies specific to macrophages, that statin treatment at doses comparable with those used in humans radically reduced macrophage accumulation in the intima of the thoracic aorta in heterozygous WHHL rabbits, who developed mild hypercholesterolemia along with focal atherosclerotic lesions in the thoracic aorta.

These data were reinforced by Aikawa et al. (2001) who reported that, additionally, statins reduced growth of macrophages both in vivo and in vitro as well as decreasing cell proliferation. Reduced macrophage function in terms of expression of MMPs and TF were also observed in atheroma of WHHL rabbits. Similar results regarding the proteolytic activity ascribable to MMP-9 and TF expression after coincubation with statin were determined in vitro (Aikawa et al., 2001). The last finding is compatible with previous data entailing reduction of MMP-9 expression by human macrophage in vitro with fluvastatin treatment (Bellosta et al., 1998) and decreased TF expression with fluvastatin and simvastatin (Colli et al., 1997). Significant reduction of MMPs expression but not macrophage number in vivo by pravastatin or simvastatin compared with placebo was demonstrated by Fukumoto et al. (2001). This fact reflects a direct effect of statins on macrophage function.

6.2. The effect of statins on different T cell function

T cells are prominent components of both early and late atherosclerotic lesions and the role of Th1/Th2 cell subsets in the evolution and rupture of the plaque is currently under investigation. Suppression of lymphoid cell function in vitro such as proliferation or natural killer cell activity by lovastatin (Cutts and Bankhurst, 1989) and simvastatin (Kurakata et al., 1996) have been reported. Identification of the mechanism by which statins may modulate immune function was found by Kwak et al. (2000). Indeed, it has been demonstrated that statins inhibited the interferon-gamma induced expression of class II major histocompatibility complexes (MHCII) on antigen-presenting cells. This effect of statins resulted from the reduced activation of the inducible promoter IV on the transactivator CIITA (Steimle et al., 1994) and was observed in several cell types, including primary human macrophages (Kwak et al., 2000). The MHCII are required for antigen presentation and T cell activation through the T cell receptor. This T cell receptor (following activation) may trigger proliferation of other T cells, their differentiation into two distinct effector cell populations (Th1 and Th2), and effector functions such as cytokine release. Th1 cells secrete proinflammatory cytokines: interferon-gamma and tissue necrosis factor alpha (TNF-alfa). Th2 cells produce antiinflammatory cytokines interleukin-4 (IL-4), IL-10, IL-13, and transforming growth-factor-beta. The ability of the statins to down-regulate the expression of MHCII may lead to decreased Th1 activation in vivo and inhibition of proinflammatory cytokine release. However, statins may induce an opposite effect via a similar impact on Th2 proliferation and effector functions or shift toward a Th1 immune response (Palinski, 2000). These results may provide an explanation for several previous works, which have studied the impact of statins on cytokine production. Thus, inhibition of important proinflammatory cytokines TNF-alfa by pravastatin (Rosenson et al., 1999; Grip et al., 2000), simvastatin (Musial et al., 2001), or lovastatin (Pahan et al., 1997), and IL-6 by lovastatin (Pahan et al., 1997) were examples of the alteration of the Th1 function. IL-8 secretion by *Chlamidia pneumoniae*-infected human macrophages was also attenuated by statins (Kothe et al., 2000). Complementary properties of statins, which are unrelated to HMG-CoA reductase inhibition and, at the same time, may explain their antiinflammatory and immunomodulatory effects, were reported by Weitz-Schmidt et al. (2001). It has been indicated that statins, generally lovastatin and mevastatin, selectively block lymphocyte function associated antigen-1 (LFA-1), which is a glycoprotein belonging to the β2-integrin family. LFA-1 is involved in adhesion of leukocytes to ICAM-1 and also in lymphocyte recirculation and effective T cell activation by antigen-presenting cells. Inhibition of LFA-1 by compounds of the statin class resulted in a decrease of lymphocyte adhesion to ICAM-1 and impaired T cell costimulation. It has been proved that this effect occurred via binding to the novel allosteric site within LFA-1 (Weitz-Schmidt et al., 2001).

7. The clinical relevance of immunomodulatory activity of statins

Clinical trials with statins have demonstrated a marked reduction of cardiovascular mortality (Sacks et al., 1996; Downs et al., 1998). Now it is generally accepted that these clinical benefits stem not only from powerful cholesterol-lowering effects of statins but are due in part to their cholesterol-independent effects on vascular function, plaque growth, plaque rupture, or thrombosis (Bellosta et al., 2000). The identification of several mechanisms through which statins decrease the recruitment of macrophages and T cells into the arterial wall and inhibit T cell activation and proliferation in vitro have confirmed speculations that immunomodulatory effects of statins may also be beneficial in prevention of cardiovascular events (Kwak et al., 2000).

Many of these effects are related to the inhibition of isoprenoid synthesis mentioned above, which serves as a lipid attachment for a variety of proteins implicated in intracellular signaling (Van Aelst and D'Souza-Schorey, 1997; Hall, 1998). It should be also noted that all statins remarkably increase serum HDL levels. Such an effect can be considered by some means as a pleiotropic because statins increase HDL by preventing the geranylgeranylation of Rho A and phosphorylation of peroxisome proliferation activator receptor-alfa, which mediates apo AI transcriptional regulation (Martin et al., 2001). This mechanism may also mediate many of the effects of statins not related to a reduction in LDL levels. It should be taken into consideration that HDL is not only involved in reverse cholesterol transport, prevents endothelial dysfunction and platelet hyperactivation, but also inhibits the homing of monocytes and has antioxidant properties preventing LDL from antigenic modification (Navab et al., 2000).

The first clinical observations suggesting a beneficial effect of statin on decreasing the incidence of severe acute rejection episodes, and therefore, a significant improvement in 1 year survival in heart transplant recipients was reported by Katznelson and Kobashigawa (1995). These data were obtained by these authors in a prospective randomized study of kidney transplant recipients, which demonstrated a reduction in the incidence of acute rejection episodes under pravastatin treatment. The finding of the immunomodulatory and immunosuppressory effects of statins provided a rationale for their clinical employment not only in organ transplantations but also for cancer and several autoimmune diseases. The antitumor impact of statin compounds has been demonstrated in several experimental animal studies (Rao et al., 1999; Wheeler, 1998), but these results were inconsistent with the concerns raised by a review of the carcinogenisity of lipid lowering drugs (Newman and Hulley, 1996). According to this review, statins are not mutagenic but they may increase the frequency of several cancers in rodents. Metaanalysis of several large randomized trials of statins (Shepherd et al., 1995; Sacks et al., 1996; Downs et al., 1998) concluded that neither cancer incidence nor total mortality were increased in patients taking statins compared with those taking placebos (Bjerre and LeLorier, 2001).

Publication from cholesterol and recurrent events (CARE) (Ridker et al., 1999) has shown a reduction in stroke incidence in patients treated with statins. Because of the controversy over the role of LDL cholesterol as a risk factor for stroke, it is possible that non-lipid mechanisms may be important, especially antiinflammatory effects. For example, statins resulted in a reduction of the CRP level in a LDL-independent manner (Ridker et al., 1999) and were effective in decreasing events associated with elevated CRP levels (Ridker et al., 1998). The high CRP levels are a potential risk factor for thromboembolic stroke, whereas total and LDL cholesterol levels are not. Thus, the above-listed data invite further clinical investigation to stroke treatment and prevention, and also decipher the pathogenic mechanisms of statin in stroke.

Meroni et al. (2001) have shown that endothelial thrombogenic activation mediated by anti-beta2GPI antibody can be inhibited by statins. Because of the suggested role of endothelial cell activation in the pathogenesis of antiphospholipid syndrome (APS), these data provide a basis for using statins as an additional therapeutic tool in APS. Fluvastatin in this study reduced, in a concentration-dependent manner, the expression of E-selectin and ICAM-1 induced by anti-beta2GPI antibodies as well as by cytokines or LPS. Another lipophilic statin, simvastatin, displayed similar effects but to a lesser extent than fluvastatin. Mevalonate greatly prevented the inhibitory effect of statins.

Leung et al. (2003) explored the activities of simvastatin in a Th1-driven model of murine inflammatory arthritis. It was shown in this study that simvastatin markedly inhibited not only developing but also clinically evident collagen-induced arthritis in doses that were unable to significantly alter cholesterol concentrations in vivo. Ex vivo analysis demonstrated significant suppression of collagen-specific Th1 humoral and cellular immune responses. Moreover, simvastatin reduced anti-CD3/anti-CD28 proliferation and IFN-gamma release from mononuclear cells derived from peripheral blood and synovial fluid. Proinflammatory cytokine production in vitro by T cell contact-activated macrophages was suppressed by simvastatin, suggesting that such observations have direct clinical relevance.

Finally, recent exciting findings indicate that statins may also be beneficial in the treatment of multiple sclerosis and neurodegenerative diseases (Stuve et al., 2003). Multiple sclerosis is a central nervous system (CNS) inflammatory demyelinating disease that is thought to have an autoimmune pathogenesis. Youssef et al. (2002) have shown that oral atorvastatin prevented or reversed chronic and relapsing paralysis. Atorvastatin induced secretion of Th2 antiinflamatory cytokines (IL-4, IL-5 and IL-10) and transforming growth factor (TGF)-beta. Conversely, secretion of Th1 proinflamatory cytokines (IL-2, IL-12), interferon (IFN)-gamma and tumour necrosis factor alfa (TNF-alpha) were suppressed. Atorvastatin promoted differentiation of Th0 cells into Th2 cells and reduced CNS infiltration and major histocompatibility complex (MHC) class II expression. Mevalonate, the product of HMG-CoA reductase, reversed atorvastatin's effects. Additionally, Aktas et al. (2003) have demonstrated that both subcutaneous and oral administration of atorvastatin inhibits the development of actively induced chronic experimental autoimmune encephalomyelitis in SJL/J mice and significantly reduce the inflammatory infiltration into the CNS. When treatment was started after disease onset, atorvastatin reduced the incidence of relapses and protected from the development of further disability. Both the reduced autoreactive T cell response measured by proliferation toward the encephalitogenic peptide PLP139-151 and the cytokine profile indicate a potent blockade of Th1 immune response. In in vitro assays, atorvastatin not only inhibited antigen-specific responses, but also decreased T cell proliferation independently of MHC class II and LFA-1. Inhibition of proliferation was not due to apoptosis induction, but linked to a negative regulation on cell cycle progression. However, early T cell activation was unaffected, as reflected by unaltered calcium fluxes. Thus, these results also provide promising evidence for a beneficial role of statins in the treatment of autoimmune attack on the CNS.

Key points

- The reality of the mechanisms that manage the recruitment, differentiation, and activation of immune cells in atherosclerosis is now generally admitted.
- Concurrently, understanding of the pharmacological effects of HMG-CoA reductase inhibitors—statins is progressing toward the insight that these agents do more than simply lower cholesterol.
- The identification of mechanisms through which these drugs decrease the enrollment of macrophages and T-cells into the arterial wall and inhibit T-cell activation and proliferation has confirmed the concept that immunomodulatory effects of statins may be effective not only in the prevention of cardiovascular events.
- The finding of the immunomodulatory and immunosuppressory effects of statins provided a rationale for their clinical employment in antiphospholipid syndrome, organ transplantations, thyroid autoimmunity, multiple sclerosis, neurodegenerative diseases and cancer.

References

Aikawa, M., Rabkin, E., Sugiyama, S., et al. 2001. An HMG-CoA reductase inhibitor, cerivastatin, suppresses growth of macrophages expressing matrix metalloproteinases and tissue factor in vivo and in vitro. Circulation 103, 276.

Aktas, O., Waiczies, S., Smorodchenko, et al. 2003. Treatment of relapsing paralysis in experimental encephalomyelitis by targeting Th1 cells through atorvastatin. J. Exp. Med. 197, 725.

Becker, S., Warren, M.K., Haskill, S. 1987. Colony-stimulating factor-induced monocyte survival and differentiation into macrophages in serumfree cultures. J. Immunol. 139, 3703.

Bellosta, S., Via, D., Canavesi, M. 1998. HMG-CoA reductase inhibitors reduce MMP-9 secretion by macrophages. Arterioscler. Thromb. Vasc. Biol. 18, 1671.

Bellosta, S., Ferri, N., Arnaboldi, L., et al. 2000. Pleiotropic effects of statins in atherosclerosis and diabetes. Diabetes Care 23 (Suppl. 2), B72.

Bjerre, L.M., LeLorier, J. 2001. Do statins cause cancer? A metaanalysis of large randomized clinical trials. Am. J. Med. 110, 716.

It was concluded that neither cancer incidence nor total mortality were increased in patients taking statins compared with those taking placebo.

Brown, M.S., Goldstein, J.L. 1983. Lipoprotein metabolism in the macrophage: implications for cholesterol deposition in atherosclerosis. Annu. Rev. Biochem. 52, 223.

Brown, B.G., Zhao, X.Q., Sacco, D.E., et al. 1993. Lipid lowering and plaque regression: new insights into prevention of plaque disruption and clinical events in coronary disease. Circulation 87, 1781.

Caligiuri, G., Stahl, D., Kaveri, S., et al. 2003. Autoreactive antibody repertoire is perturbed in atherosclerotic patients. Lab. Invest. 83, 939.

These data indicate that atherosclerotic patients develop a perturbed humoral immune response directed toward arterial proteins, which impacts on the overall autoreactive repertoire.

Colli, S., Eligini, S., Lalli, M., et al. 1997. Vastatins inhibit tissue factor in cultured human macrophages. A novel mechanism of protection against atherothrombosis. Arterioscler. Thromb. Vasc. Biol. 17, 265.

Cutts, J.L., Bankhurst, A.D. 1989. Suppression of lymphoid cell function in vitro by inhibition of 3-hydroxy-3-methylglutaryl coenzyme A reductase by lovastatin. Int. J. Immunopharmacol. 11, 863.

Danesh, J., Collins, R., Peto, R. 1997. Chronic infections and coronary heart disease: is there a link? Lancet 350, 430.

Downs, J.R., Clearfield, M., Weis, S., et al. 1998. Primary prevention of acute coronary events with lovastatin in men and women with average cholesterol levels: results of AFCAPS/TexCAPS: Air Force/Texas Coronary Atherosclerosis Prevention Study. JAMA 279, 1615.

Frostegard, J. 2002. Autoimmunity, oxidized LDL and cardiovascular disease. Autoimmun. Rev. 4, 233.

Fukumoto, Y., Libby, P., Rabkin, E., et al. 2001. Statins alter smooth muscle cell accumulation and collagen content in established atheroma of watanabe heritable hyperlipidemic rabbits. Circulation 103, 993.

Fuster, V., Badimon, J.J. 1995. Regression or stabilization of atherosclerosis means regression or stabilization of we don't see in the arteriogram. Eur. Heart J. 16 (Suppl. E), 6.

Galis, Z.S., Sukhova, G.K., Lark, et al. 1994. Increased expression of matrix metalloproteinases and matrix degrading activity in vulnerable regions of human atherosclerotic plaques. J. Clin. Invest. 94, 2493.

Goldstein, J.L., Brown, M.S. 1990. Regulation of the mevalonate pathway. Nature 343, 425.

Statins inhibit the synthesis of isoprenoid intermediates operating as lipid attachments of a assortment of proteins which are important in cell signalling.

Gordon, D., Reidy, M.A., Benditt, et al. 1990. Cell proliferation in human coronary arteries. Proc. Natl Acad. Sci. USA 87, 4600.

Gotto, A.M. Jr 1997. Cholesterol management in theory and practice. Circulation 96, 4424.

Gotto, A.M. Jr 2003. reating hypercholesterolemia: looking forward. Clin. Cardiol. 26 (Suppl. 1), I21.

Grip, O., Janciauskiene, S., Lindgren, S. 2000. Pravastatin downregulates inflammatory mediators in human monocytes in vitro. Eur. J. Pharmacol. 410, 83.

Hall, A. 1998. Rho GTPases and the actin cytoskeleton. Science 279, 509.

Hamilton, J.A., Myers, D., Jessup, W., et al. 1999. Oxidized LDL can induce macrophage survival, DNA synthesis, and enhanced proliferative response to CSF-1 and GM-CSF. Arterioscler. Thromb. Vasc. Biol. 19, 98.

Hansson, G.K. 2001. Immune mechanisms in atherosclerosis. Arterioscler. Thromb. Vasc. Biol. 21, 1876.

Hansson, G.K., Holm, J., Jonasson, L. 1989. Detection of activated T lymphocytes in the human atherosclerotic plaque. Am. J. Pathol. 135, 169.

Henney, A.M., Wakeley, P.R., Davies, M.J. 1991. Localization of stromelysin gene expression in atherosclerotic plaques by in situ hybridization. Proc. Natl Acad. Sci. USA 88, 8154.

Katznelson, S., Kobashigawa, J.A. 1995. Dual roles of HMG-CoA reductase inhibitors in solid organ transplantation: lipid lowering and immunosuppression. Kidney Int. Suppl. 52, S112.

Klimov, A.N., Gurevich, V.S., Nikiforova, A.A., et al. 1993. Antioxidative activity of high density lipoproteins in vivo. Atherosclerosis 100, 13.

Normal HDL can prevent the formation of the oxidized LDL in patients with coronary heart disease or inactivate them after they are formed.

Kodama, T., Reddy, P., Kishimoto, C., et al. 1988. Purification and characterization of a bovine acetyl low density lipoprotein receptor. Proc. Natl Acad. Sci. USA 85, 9238.

Kothe, H., Dalhoff, K., Rupp, J., et al. 2000. Hydroxymethylglutaryl coenzyme A reductase inhibitors modify the inflammatory response of human macrophages and endothelial cells infected with Chlamydia pneumoniae. Circulation 101, 1760.

Krieger, M., Herz, J. 1994. Structures and functions of multiligand lipoprotein receptors: macrophage scavenger receptors and LDL receptor-related protein (LRP). Annu. Rev. Biochem. 63, 601.

Kurakata, S., Kada, M., Shimada, Y., et al. 1996. Effects of different inhibitors of 3-hydroxy-3-methylglutaryl coenzyme A (HMG-CoA) reductase, pravastatin sodium and simvastatin, on sterol synthesis and immunological functions in human lymphocytes in vitro. Immunopharmacology 34, 51.

Kwak, B., Mulhaupt, F., Myit, S., et al. 2000. Statins as a newly recognized type of immunomodulator. Nat. Med. 6, 1399.

Statins inhibit the expression of class II major histocompatibility complexes. This effect was observed in several cell types including primary human macrophages.

Laufs, U., Liao, J.K. 1998. Post-transcriptional regulation of endothelial nitric oxide synthase mRNA stability by Rho GTPase. J. Biol. Chem. 273, 24266.

Lennernas, H., Fager, G. 1997. Pharmacodynamics and pharmacokinetics of the HMG-CoA reductase inhibitors: similarities and differences. Clin. Pharmacokinet. 32, 403.

Lovastatin, simvastatin, atorvastatin, fluvastatin and pravastatin exploit the different pathways for metabolism or biotransformation.

Leung, B.P., Sattar, N., Crilly, A., et al. 2003. A novel anti-inflammatory role for simvastatin in inflammatory arthritis. J. Immunol. 170, 1524.

LIPID Study Group, 1998. Prevention of cardiovascular events and death with pravastatin in patients with coronary heart disease and a broad range of initial cholesterol levels. The long-term intervention with pravastatin in ischaemic disease. N. Engl. J. Med. 339, 1349.

Lotz, H., Salabe, G.B. 1997. Lipoprotein(a) increase associated with thyroid autoimmunity. Eur. J. Endocrinol. 136, 87.

Luboshitzky, R., Aviv, A., Herer, P., et al. 2002. Risk factors for cardiovascular disease in women with subclinical hypothyroidism. Thyroid 12, 421.

Mach, F., Schonbeck, U., Bonnefoy, J.Y., et al. 1997. Activation of monocyte/macrophage functions related to acute atheroma complication by ligation of CD40: induction of collagenase, stromelysin, and tissue factor. Circulation 96, 396.

Maron, D.J., Fazio, S., Linton, M.F. 2000. Current perspectives on statins. Circulation 101, 207.

Martin, G., Duez, H., Blanquart, C., et al. 2001. Statin-induced inhibition of the Rho-signaling pathway activates PPAR alpha and induces HDL apo AI. J. Clin. Invest. 107, 1423.

Meroni, P.L., Raschi, E., Testoni, C., et al. 2001. Statins prevent endothelial cell activation induced by antiphospholipid (anti-beta2-glycoprotein I) antibodies: effect on the proadhesive and proinflammatory phenotype. Arthritis Rheum. 44, 2870.

The data obtained provide a basis for using statins as an additional therapeutic tool in APS.

Metcalf, D. 1989. The molecular control of cell division, differentiation commitment and maturation in haemopoietic cells. Nature 339, 27.

Miura, S., Iitaka, M., Suzuki, S., et al. 1996. Decrease in serum levels of thyroid hormone in patients with coronary heart disease. Endocr. J. 43, 657.

Musial, J., Undas, A., Gajewski, P., et al. 2001. Anti-inflammatory effects of simvastatin in subjects with hypercholesterolemia. Int. J. Cardiol. 77, 247.

Navab, M., Hama, S.Y., Anantharamaiah, G.M., et al. 2000. Normal high density lipoprotein inhibits three steps in the formation of mildly oxidized low density lipoprotein: steps 2 and 3. J. Lipid Res. 41, 1495.

Navab, M., Berliner, J.A., Subbanagounder, G., et al. 2001. HDL and the inflammatory response induced by LDL-derived oxidized phospholipids. Arterioscler. Thromb. Vasc. Biol. 21, 481.

It has been proposed that oxidized LDL and HDL may be part of a system of nonspecific innate immunity.

Newman, T.B., Hulley, S.B. 1996. Carcinogenicity of lipid-lowering drugs. JAMA 275, 55.

Nikkari, S.T., O'Brien, K.D., Ferguson, M., et al. 1995. Interstitial collagenase (MMP-1) expression in human carotid atherosclerosis. Circulation 92, 1393.

Packard, C.J. 1998. Influence of pravastatin and plasma lipids on clinical events in the West of Scotland Coronary Prevention Study (WOSCOPS). Circulation 97, 1440.

Pahan, K., Sheikh, F.G., Namboodiri, A.M., et al. 1997. Lovastatin and phenylacetate inhibit the induction of nitric oxide synthase and cytokines in rat primary astrocytes, microglia, and macrophages. J. Clin. Invest. 100, 2671.

Palinski, W. 2000. Immunomodulation: a new role for statins? Nature Med. 12, 1311.

Pauletto, P., Puato, M., Faggin, E., et al. 2000. Low-dose cerivastatin inhibits spontaneous atherogenesis in heterozygous watanabe hyper lipidemic rabbits. J. Vasc. Res. 37, 189.

It has been firstly shown that statin treatment radically reduced macrophage accumulation in the intima of the thoracic aorta in heterozygous WHHL rabbits.

Rao, S., Porter, D.C., Chen, X., et al. 1999. Lovastatin-mediated G1 arrest is through inhibition of the proteasome, independent of hydroxymethyl glutaryl-CoA reductase. Proc. Natl Acad. Sci. USA 96, 7797.

Rekhter, M.D., Gordon, D. 1995. Active proliferation of different cell types, including lymphocytes, in human atherosclerotic plaques. Am. J. Pathol. 147, 668.

Ridker, P.M., Rifai, N., Pfeffer, M.A., et al. 1998. Inflammation, pravastatin, and the risk of coronary events after myocardial infarction in patients with average cholesterol levels. Cholesterol and Recurrent Events (CARE) Investigators. Circulation 98, 839.

Ridker, P.M., Rifai, N., Pfeffer, M.A., et al. 1999. Long-term effects of pravastatin on plasma concentration of C-reactive protein. The cholesterol and recurrent events (CARE) investigators. Circulation 100, 230.

Rosenfeld, M.E., Ross, R. 1990. Macrophage and smooth muscle cell proliferation in atherosclerotic lesions of WHHL and comparably hypercholesterolemic fat-fed rabbits. Arteriosclerosis 10, 680.

Rosenson, R.S., Tangney, C.C., Casey, L.C. 1999. Inhibition of proinflammatory cytokine production by pravastatin. Lancet 353, 983.

Sacks, F.M., Pfeffer, M.A., Moye, L.A., et al. 1996. The effect of pravastatin on coronary events after myocardial infarction in patients with average cholesterol levels. Cholesterol and Recurrent Events Trial investigators. N. Engl. J. Med. 335, 1001.

Sakai, M., Miyazaki, A., Hakamata, H., et al. 1996. Lysophosphatidylcholine potentiates the mitogenic activity of modified LDL for human monocyte-derived macrophages. Arterioscler. Thromb. Vasc. Biol. 16, 600.

Salonen, J.T., Yla-Herttuala, S., Yamamotto, R., et al. 1992. Autoantibody against oxidised LDL and progression of carotid atherosclerosis. Lancet 339, 883.

It has been shown that oxidised LDL are antigenic and the titers of autoantibodies against oxidized LDL are correlated with the extent of atherosclerosis.

Shepherd, J., Cobbe, S.M., Ford, I., et al. 1995. Prevention of coronary heart disease with pravastatin in men with hypercholesterolemia. West of Scotland Coronary Prevention Study Group. N. Engl. J. Med. 333, 1301.

Shiomi, M., Ito, T. 1999. Effect of cerivastatin sodium, a new inhibitor of HMG-CoA reductase, on plasma lipid levels, progression of atherosclerosis, and the lesional composition in the plaques of WHHL rabbits. Br. J. Pharmacol. 126, 961.

Shovman, O., Levy, Ya., Gilburd, B., et al. 2002. Antiinflamatory and immunomodulatory properties of statins. Immunol. Res. 25, 271.

Statins may influence thrombosis through variable inhibitory actions on platelet function, coagulation factors, reology and fibrinolysis.

Steimle, V., Siegrist, C.A., Mottet, A., et al. 1994. Regulation of MHC class II expression by interferon-gamma mediated by the transactivator gene CIITA. Science 265, 106.

Steinberg, D., Witztum, J.L. 1990. Lipoproteins and atherogenesis: current concepts. JAMA 264, 3047.

Stuve, O., Youssef, S., Steinman, L., et al. 2003. Statins as potential therapeutic agents in neuroinflammatory disorders. Curr. Opin. Neurol. 16, 393.

Takemoto, M., Liao, J.K. 2001. Pleiotropic effects of 3-hydroxy-3-methylglutaryl coenzyme a reductase inhibitors. Arterioscler. Thromb. Vasc. Biol. 21, 1712.

Tsutsumi, A., Matsuura, E., Ichikawa, K., et al. 1996. Antibodies to β_2-glycoprotein I and clinical manifestations in patients with systemic lupus erythematosus. Arthritis Rheum. 39, 1466.

Van Aelst, L., D' Souza-Schorey, C. 1997. Rho GTPases and signaling networks. Genes Dev. 11, 2295.

Van der Wal, A.C., Das, P.K., Van de Berg, D.B., et al. 1989. Atherosclerotic lesions in humans: in situ immunophenotypic analysis suggesting an immune mediated response. Lab. Invest. 61, 166.

Watson, A.D., Berliner, J.A., Hama, S.Y., et al. 1995. Protective effect of high density lipoprotein associated paraoxonase: inhibition of the biological activity of minimally oxidized low density lipoprotein. J. Clin. Invest. 96, 2882.

Weitz-Schmidt, G., Welzenbach, K., Brinkmann, V. 2001. Statins selectively inhibit leukocyte function antigen-1 by binding to a novel regulatory integrin site. Nat. Med. 7, 687.

Wheeler, D.C. 1998. Are there potential non-lipid-lowering uses of statins? Drugs 56, 517.

Wick, G., Schett, G., Amberger, A., et al. 1995. Is atherosclerosis an immunologically mediated disease? Immunol. Today 16, 27.

Wilcox, J.N., Smith, K.M., Schwartz, S.M., et al. 1989. Localization of tissue factor in the normal vessel wall and in the atherosclerotic plaque. Proc. Natl Acad. Sci. USA 86, 2839.

Youssef, S., Stuve, O., Patarroyo, J.C., et al. 2002. The HMG-CoA reductase inhibitor, atorvastatin, promotes a Th2 bias and reverses paralysis in central nervous system autoimmune disease. Nature 420, 78.

The article provides promising evidence for a beneficial role of statins in the treatment of autoimmune attack on the CNS.

PART III

Cardiac Involvement in Autoimmune Connective Tissue Diseases

Handbook of Systemic Autoimmune Diseases, Volume 1
The Heart in Systemic Autoimmune Diseases
A. Doria and P. Pauletto, editors

CHAPTER 8

Cardiac Imaging Techniques in Systemic Autoimmune Diseases

Maurizio Turiel[*,a], Piercarlo Sarzi-Puttini[b], Ricard Cervera[c]

[a]*Cardiology Unit, Istituto Ortopedico Galeazzi, University of Milan, Via Galeazzi 4, 20161 Milan, Italy*

[b]*Rheumatology Unit, L. Sacco University Hospital, Milan, Italy*

[c]*Department of Autoimmune Diseases, Hospital Clinic, Barcelona, Catalonia, Spain*

1. Introduction

Cardiac involvement in patients suffering from systemic autoimmune diseases is an important clinical problem because of its high incidence and potential severity. There are multiple tests and strategies for the evaluation of a suspected or known coronary artery disease (Table 1), heart valve lesion or cardiac arrhythmia (Lee and Boucher, 2001). Furthermore, there is a need for guidelines to diagnose and manage these patients in specialized and multidisciplinary centers. In such patients, an early and careful diagnosis may significantly improve the management and provide insights into the prognosis. Additionally, the choice of an imaging technique should take into consideration the test that is most trusted and available at a given institution.

Several authors reported the wide variety of cardiac manifestations in rheumatoid arthritis (RA) (Braunwald, 1997). In particular, the most common lesion is pericarditis, which occurs in 11–50% of the patients. Vasospasm, microvascular disease or thrombosis, with or without atherosclerosis, also present an even greater challenge.

The incidences of cardiac involvement in systemic lupus erythematosus (SLE) and antiphospholipid syndrome (APS) are also very high with a widespread range of manifestations (Cervera et al., 1992). By means of two-dimensional (2D) echocardiography, 57% of SLE patients show valvular, myocardial or pericardial abnormalities (Nihoyannopoulos et al., 1990; Omdal et al., 2001).

Additionally, it is well known that there is a significant association between several systemic autoimmune diseases, such as SLE, and early or accelerated atherosclerosis. Cerebrovascular, coronary and peripheral vascular thromboembolic events are major causes of morbidity and mortality in SLE patients. Factors implicated in early atherosclerosis and occlusive arteritis include immune-mediated endothelial injury, hypertension, hyperlipidemia, morbid obesity, corticosteroid therapy, coronary artery spasm, hypercoagulability related to antiphospholipid antibodies (aPL) and elevated plasma levels of homocysteine (Ghaffary, 1999; Manzi et al., 2000; Jiménez et al., 2001).

Prognostic information, obtained by imaging techniques, can help in the management of these disorders and, therefore, improve the outcome in patients with these diseases. In this chapter, we will review the role and choice of several cardiac techniques that are commonly used in patients with systemic autoimmune diseases.

* Corresponding author.
E-mail address: maurizio.turiel@unimi.it (M. Turiel).

DOI: 10.1016/S1571-5078(03)01008-0

Table 1
Algorithm for diagnostic work-up in patients suspected of having coronary artery disease (CAD)

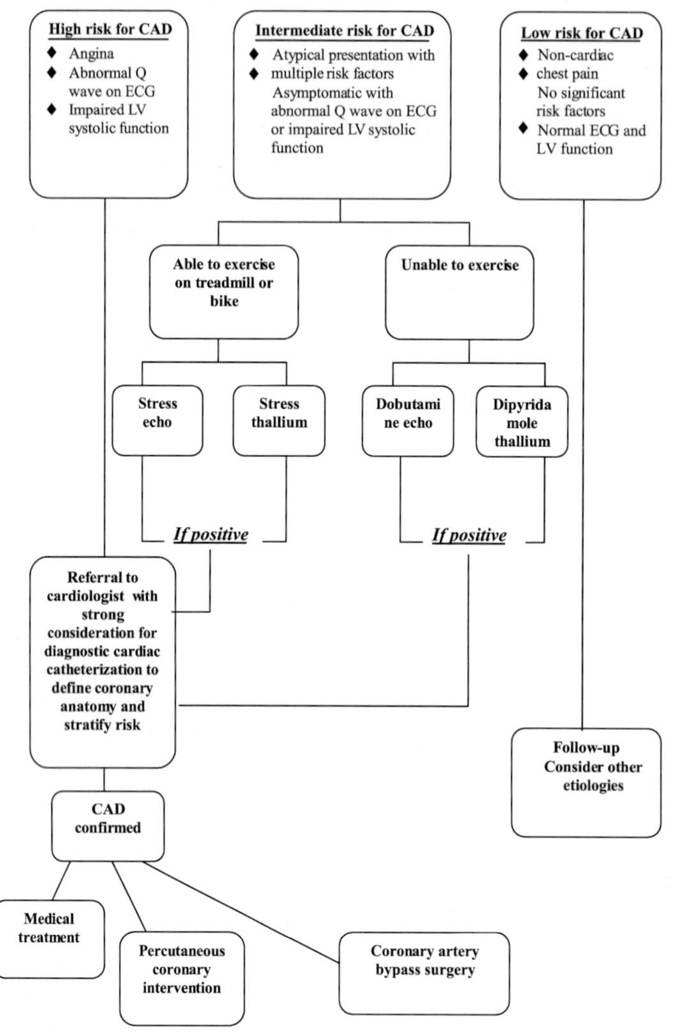

Cardiac imaging techniques can be divided into: (1) non-invasive imaging techniques, including electrocardiography (ECG), echocardiography and radionuclide perfusion imaging; (2) semi-invasive techniques, such as transesophageal echocardiography (TEE); and (3) invasive techniques, such as angiography.

2. Electrocardiography

2.1. Holter ECG monitoring

An increased prevalence of arrhythmias and conduction system abnormalities is present in patients with connective tissue diseases. If 24 h ambulatory (Holter) ECG monitoring is used, the frequency of conduction system abnormalities and arrhythmias increases (Deswall and Follansbee, 1996). Some authors (Bijl et al., 2000) showed that an impaired left ventricular diastolic function in SLE patients with an overall decrease of ejection fraction of 10% can result in cardiac arrhythmias, ST-T wave changes and congestive heart failure.

Furthermore, it has been reported (Ferri et al., 1985) that 48 of 53 patients with systemic sclerosis (SSc) had, using Holter ECG monitoring, ventricular arrhythmias, with multiform ventricular premature beats in 21 (40%), pairs of runs of ventricular tachycardia in 15 (28%) and one or more runs of ventricular tachycardia in 7 (15%). Multiform and/or repetitive ventricular premature beats occurred more frequently in patients with echocardiographic abnormalities but were also present in patients who had normal findings on echocardiographic examination. According to these authors, Holter ECG monitoring and echocardiography study should be included in the routine work-up of patients who had SSc.

2.2. Signal-averaged ECG

The value of signal-averaged ECG in predicting high-risk arrhythmias and sudden death in patients with SSc was studied (Moser et al., 1991).They found that 60% of the SSc subjects with abnormalities on the signal-averaged ECG had complex or frequent ventricular ectopy and 78% of patients with complex or frequent ectopy had no evidence of ventricular late potentials. Thus, the signal-averaged ECG did not appear to be a good predictor of high-risk patients.

2.3. Exercise ECG (stress test)

Exercise ECG is the least expensive non-invasive test for myocardial ischemia (Legrand et al., 1997): the costs of stress echocardiography and stress single-photon-emission computed tomography (SPECT) are at least two and five times as high, respectively.

The rate of acute myocardial infarction or death is about 1 per 2500 tests and can safely be performed in outpatient settings by trained personnel who are under the supervision of a physician. During this test, the physician should be nearby and available in case of emergency.

Several drugs can influence the results of exercise ECG, including digoxin, beta-adrenergic-blocking agents, vasodilators and other antihypertensive agents that alter hemodynamic responses. Whenever possible, beta-blockers and other anti-ischemic drugs should be stopped four or five half-lives (usually about 2 days) before exercise testing is performed as part of the diagnostic work-up and initial risk stratification for patients with suspected coronary disease. Withdrawal of these medications is often not feasible. Nevertheless, even when medications are not withdrawn, the results of stress testing are usually abnormal in patients at highest risk for complications.

The major value of this test is in predicting prognosis, especially in patients with established coronary artery disease. Parameters associated with poor prognosis include (1) duration of less than 6.5 METS (metabolic equivalent, oxygen consumption at 3.5 mL O_2/kg/min); (2) exercise heart rate of less than 120 per min (off beta-blockers); (3) ischemic ST segment change at a heart rate of less than 120 per min or less than 6.5 METS; (4) ST segment depression greater than 2 mm, especially in multiple leads; (5) ST segment depression for more than 6 min in recovery; and (6) a decrease in blood pressure during exercise. Therefore, exercise treadmill testing can be used in active low-risk patients with non-anginal symptoms to provide assurance and verify the patient's conditioning level. In addition, efficacy of antianginal therapy can be assessed in patients with chronic stable angina pectoris and normal ventricular function.

Exercise-induced atrial and ventricular arrhythmias were reported in 35% of SSc patients (Follansbee et al., 1985). An association was noted between ventricular ectopy, an abnormal LVEF response to exercise and perfusion defects on thallium scintigraphy implying more advanced myocardial disease as the substrate for the ectopy.

3. Echocardiography

3.1. Transthoracic echocardiography

2D and Doppler echocardiography are able to detect myocardial abnormalities including valvular abnormalities, pericardial diseases and regional or global left ventricular defects (Cheitlin et al., 1997).

Echocardiographic screening of SSc patients has found a high prevalence of asymptomatic cardiac abnormalities with a high prevalence of pericardial effusion (Candell-Riera et al., 1996). Valvular abnormalities (predominantly of the mitral and aortic valves) were revealed in 61% of SLE patients (Roldan et al., 1996). Valvular thickening was the most common abnormality and valvular lesions frequently changed over time.

Interestingly, most studies have related valvulopathy to the presence of aPL (Khamashta et al., 1990; Brenner et al., 1991; Cervera et al., 1991; Galve et al., 1992). Cardiac involvement is also frequently present in patients with primary APS, as reported by several studies with transthoracic echocardiography (Giunta et al., 1993; Metz et al., 1994).

A 32–38% prevalence of valvular lesions, most frequently involving left-sided valves, valvular rings, cordae tendineae or any other location of ventricular or atrial endocardium was reported (Hojnik et al., 1996). Valvular lesions are characterized by diffuse leaflet thickening, sometimes, as far as valvular stenosis; these lesions are often associated with valvular regurgitation.

Intracardiac thrombosis is among the unusual manifestations of the APS (Cervera, 2000). This entity is usually seen in the clinical setting of left ventricular dysfunction. The thrombus can be found in all the chambers of the heart. This manifestation can occur in both the primary and the secondary APS. Rarely, this can present as intracardiac mass simulating myxoma, and diagnosis can only be made by histology.

Non-infective endocarditis has been reported in many patients with SLE and primary APS (Cervera, 2000). These patients can present with fever, cardiac murmurs, vegetations on the valves, negative blood cultures and elevated aPL. It is difficult to exclude infective endocarditis in these patients. The C reactive protein, white blood cell count and echocardiography findings may be helpful in differentiating these two conditions.

LV diastolic filling can be determined reliably by Doppler-derived mitral and pulmonary venous flow velocities. Diastolic filling abnormalities are broadly classified at their extremes to impaired relaxation and restrictive physiology with many patterns in-between. Based on 2D and Doppler echocardiographic evaluation, the following grading system for diastolic dysfunction is proposed: grade 1, impaired relaxation pattern; grade 2, pseudonormalized pattern; grade 3, reversible restrictive pattern; and grade 4, irreversible restrictive pattern.

An impaired relaxation pattern (grade 1 diastolic dysfunction) identifies patients with early stages of heart disease, and appropriate therapy may avert progression and functional disability. A pseudonormalized pattern (grade 2) is a transitional phase between abnormal relaxation and restrictive physiology and signifies increased filling pressures and decreased compliance. In this phase, reducing preload, optimizing afterload and treating the underlying disease, if possible, are clinically helpful. A restrictive physiology pattern (grade 3–4) identifies advanced, usually symptomatic disease with a poor prognosis. Therapeutic intervention is directed toward normalizing loading conditions and improving the restrictive filling pattern (grade 3 when reversible), although this may not be feasible in certain heart diseases (grade 4 when irreversible).

Many patients have LV filling patterns that appear indeterminate or mixed. In these cases, clinical information, LA and LV size, pulmonary venous flow velocity and alteration of preload with the Valsalva maneuver help assess diastolic function and estimate diastolic filling pressure measures.

Patients with APS can have isolated diastolic dysfunction too. Some authors performed Doppler echocardiography in 10 consecutive patients with APS (Hasnie et al., 1995). They found a decrease in peak early filling velocity, peak early to atrial filling velocity ratio and mean deceleration time of early filling velocity in this group in comparison to the control group. The left ventricular mass, systolic function and ejection fractions were normal in these patients. These findings may represent subclinical myocardial damage.

Finally, clinically apparent pericardial effusion is a rare cardiac manifestation in the APS. The prevalence of echocardiographic evidence of pericardial effusion is about 15–20%. The mechanism, prognosis and sequelae of this manifestation are not yet known.

3.2. Transesophageal echocardiography

The usefulness of TEE to identify not only minimal cardiac abnormalities or vegetations but also intracardiac embolic source is well known (Jafar et al., 1994; Asherson and Cervera, 1991; Espinola-Zavaleta et al., 1999) (Fig. 1). Our group (Turiel et al., 2000) found cardiac involvement (valvular thickening and/or regurgitation, vegetations or masses and potential embolic sources) in 33 out of 40 (82%) APS patients. Mitral valve thickening was the most common abnormality (63%) (Fig. 2). Our data demonstrated embolic sources in 10 out of 40 (25%) APS patients: 7 patients showed marked spontaneous echocontrast, 3 of whom had mitral stenosis. Furthermore, we found non-infective vegetations (Libman-Sacks endocarditis) in 3 patients (1 on aortic and 2 on tricuspid valve with severe tricuspid regurgitation). Indeed, our APS patients with anticardiolipin antibody titer higher than 40 GPL units showed a greater number of associated and/or recurrent thromboembolic events. Furthermore, APS patients with anticardiolipin antibody titer higher than 40 GPL units presented an increased number of potential embolic sources demonstrated by TEE in comparison with patients with anticardiolipin antibody titer lower than 40 GPL units ($\chi^2 = 10.03$, $p < 0.01$).

The use of TEE, therefore, should be recommended in APS patients with clinical findings and/or high anticardiolipin antibody titer in order to better define the cardiac abnormalities and detect embolic sources (Black et al., 1991) as well as to establish an appropriate antiplatelet and/or anticoagulant therapy.

Recently, 30 unselected RA patients, by means of TEE technique, showed an extremely common cardiac involvement, including echo-generating nodules on mitral or aortic valves, frequent atheroma of the aorta and mitral or aortic regurgitation (Guedes et al., 2001).

3.3. Stress echocardiography

Exercise echocardiography and exercise SPECT have similar sensitivities for the detection of coronary artery disease, but exercise echocardiography has better specificity and, therefore, higher overall discriminatory capabilities, as used in contemporary practice. Exercise echocardiography, thus, provides more clinical information at a lower cost without the

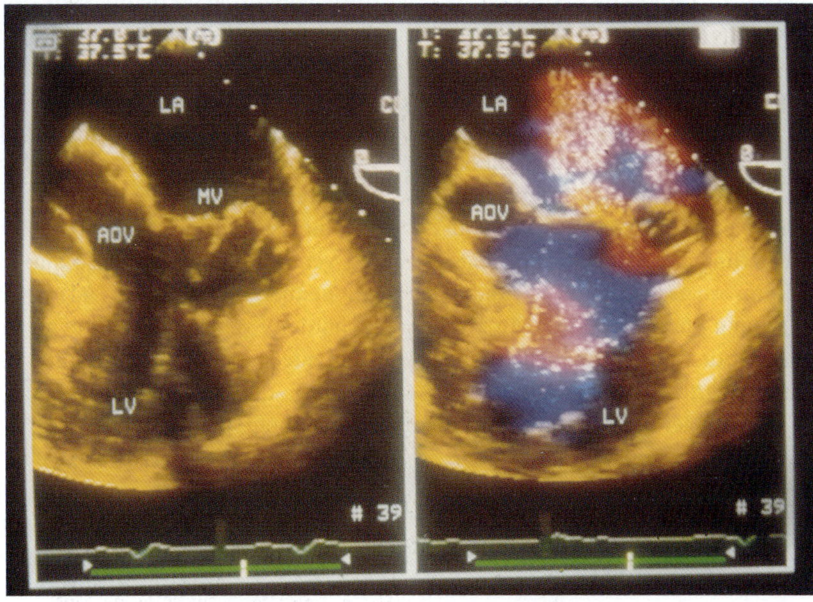

Figure 1. Floppy mitral valve prolapse (left) of posterior leaflets with moderate mitral regurgitation (right) (PAPS).

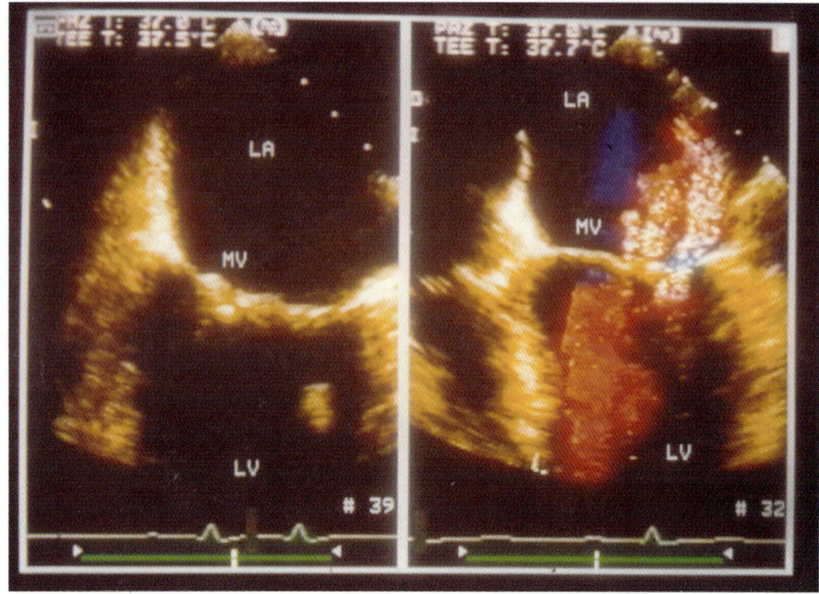

Figure 2. Marked mitral leaflet thickening (left) with moderate mitral regurgitation (right) (PAPS).

effect of ionizing radiation when compared with nuclear perfusion studies.

A pharmacological stress test is indicated for patients who are unable to adequately exercise because of rheumatologic, orthopedic, vascular or pulmonary conditions.

Dobutamine is a synthetic sympathomimetic amine that stimulates myocardial β receptors, resulting in an increase of left ventricular contractility and heart rate. Its half-life is 2 min; therefore, continuous infusion is necessary to sustain its effect. The protocol at our Institute is to use a continuous dobutamine infusion starting at 5 μg/kg/min, increasing the dose at 3 min stages to 10, 20 and a maximum of 40 μg/kg/min plus intravenous atropine 0.5–2.0 bolus administration to achieve minimum 85% (MPHR maximum heart rate). Heart rate, blood pressure, cardiac rhythm and left ventricular function are carefully monitored and recorded at each stage, including 6 min into recovery. Echocardiographic images are acquired from standard views at rest, during stress and in recovery. The images are recorded on videotape and digitized on optical disk. A single cardiac cycle at rest, intermediate and peak doses is looped and replayed, which allows side-by-side comparisons of left ventricular function at different phases of dobutamine infusions. The objective of this test is to detect new or worsening wall motion abnormalities or failure to increase contractility, which indicates myocardial ischemia. Dobutamine infusion is stopped and intravenous propranolol 1–5 mg is used if patients develop supra or ventricular tachyarrhythmias, uncontrolled hypertension or severe angina (Johns et al., 1995). This test offers an advantage over dipyridamole thallium since it allows online ‘live’ assessment of left ventricular function, also into the recovery phase (Eichenberger et al., 1994). Refined ultrasound technology and contrast echocardiography have eliminated to some extent the problem of poor image quality during dobutamine stress echocardiography.

If a patient is active and can do exercise, then treadmill or bike stress echocardiography is recommended. In addition to the assessment of valvular, pericardial and myocardial function at rest, stress echocardiography permits direct visualization of left ventricular cavity enlargement or wall motion

Table 2
Common indications for dobutamine stress echocardiography

Myocardial viability determination
Prognosis postmyocardial infarction
Emergency department chest pain evaluation
Aortic stenosis functional severity (especially with reduced systolic function)
Other valvular assessments
Cost effectiveness versus nuclear imaging or cardiac catheterization
Preoperative evaluation (risk stratification)
Typical and atypical cardiac symptom evaluation
Electrocardiographic baseline abnormalities

abnormalities, which imply significant myocardial ischemia. If the echocardiography laboratory does not have sufficient experience with this technique, thallium exercise is the next study of choice. If a patient is inactive or unable to exercise, dobutamine stress echocardiography is recommended (Table 2).

3.4. *Ultrasonic videodensitometry*

Quantitative analysis of 2D echocardiography pattern represents a novel approach for myocardial tissue characterization. Ultrasonic videodensitometric analysis may represent a non-invasive feasible method that can detect early myocardial changes in SSc patients, who could be related to both fibrosis and microcirculation abnormalities (Ferri et al., 1998). These authors demonstrated that myocardial tissue changes were detectable in the large majority of SSc patients (88%). These findings can be the expression of preclinical heart abnormalities in SSc patients with a normal left ventricular systolic function. Furthermore, tissue Doppler imaging technique (Plazak et al., 2002) has revealed a diastolic dysfunction in SSc patients only in the longitudinal myocardial fibers concentrated in the subendocardial left ventricular region.

3.5. *Tissue Doppler imaging*

Tissue Doppler imaging is a technique that allows recording of the low Doppler shift frequencies of high energy generated by the ventricular wall motion that are purposely filtered out in standard Doppler blood flow studies. Tissue Doppler imaging can be performed with the use of pulsed Doppler, color 2D Doppler and color M-mode Doppler. Pulsed Doppler tissue imaging offers a high temporal resolution and therefore can be appropriately used for analysis of temporal relation between myocardium systolic and diastolic velocity waves. Color 2D Doppler provides a good spatial resolution that permits differentiation of the velocity profiles between subendocardial and subepicardial layers but is limited by its poor temporal resolution. M-mode color-coded tissue imaging is characterized by a high spatial–temporal resolution, but sampling is only performed on a single line. Both 2D and M-mode color-coded tissue imaging require specific modification of the current ultrasound machines.

Since the early descriptions, extensive work has been published during the last few years demonstrating the potential of tissue Doppler imaging for assessing both systolic and diastolic functions. The use of tissue Doppler imaging combined with advanced analysis of left ventricular Doppler inflow as proposed recently will probably further expand the frontiers of Doppler echocardiography assessment of diastolic function.

3.6. *Myocardial contrast echocardiography*

Myocardial contrast echocardiography (MCE) is an emerging technique in which microbubble contrast agents are visualized in the coronary microvasculature. MCE is an ideal modality for the non-invasive evaluation of acute coronary syndromes because it provides portable, simultaneous assessment of regional wall motion and myocardial perfusion. Recent advances in microbubble contrast agents and ultrasound imaging technology have allowed new clinical applications of MCE in acute coronary syndromes. Studies suggest a promising role for MCE in the evaluation of chest pain, the diagnosis and prognosis in acute myocardial infarction, the assessment of the success of reperfusion and the differentiation of myocardial stunning from myocardial necrosis. Potential future applications of MCE in acute coronary syndromes include the detection of inflammation and ultrasound-induced thrombolysis.

3.7. Heart rate variability

Analysis of heart rate variability (HRV) has been proposed as a method for assessing autonomic cardiac function that provides specific information on changes in autonomic tone resulting from the interaction between the sympathetic and parasympathetic nervous activity. Fast Fourier transform was performed to separate RR interval fluctuations into their characteristic frequencies and to determine the square roots of areas under the power spectrum. From the 24 h HRV power spectra, the power within two frequency bands was calculated:

- 0.04–0.15 Hz, low-frequency (LF) power which reflects increased sympathetic or parasympathetic tone modulated by baroreflex activity;
- 0.15–0.40 Hz, high-frequency (HF) power, a specific measure of vagal tone, modulated primarily by breathing.

The HF component of HRV is synchronous with the respiratory cycle and is considered to be a reliable marker of parasympathetic activity in the supine position. The HF component is known to be almost completely mediated by the parasympathetic nervous system. Time-domain parameters are also related to vagal activity.

The analysis of HRV may be a reliable means of detecting severe coronary artery disease. Furthermore, the technique is relatively inexpensive, safe and non-invasive and the method merits further study on more patients. It would also be important to determine whether similar changes in HRV indices are present during the quiescent phases of coronary artery disease.

4. Radionuclide imaging

Most nuclear cardiology applications use SPECT to reconstruct anatomical slices of discrete thickness in standardized views. Positron-emission tomographic scanners include multiple rings of stationary detectors that detect emission from tracers, which can be used to determine regional myocardial blood flow and metabolic processes. However, these scanners are more costly than SPECT scanners and are not widely available for routine use.

The initial distribution of these tracers is proportional to myocardial blood flow, whereas the so-called redistribution images, which are obtained 3–4 h later, reflect myocardial viability and are unrelated to flow. A myocardial defect on an initial scan that subsequently resolves is an indicator of myocardium that is viable. A defect that is apparent on both scans suggests a region of myocardium that has died, presumably as a result of a myocardial infarction. However, additional injections of thallium after redistribution imaging may reveal viable myocardium within such areas (Table 3).

Ischemia can be provoked with physical exercise or pharmacologic agents. Dobutamine provokes ischemia by increasing myocardial work, whereas adenosine and dipyridamole are vasodilators that unmark coronary stenosis by causing relative increases in flow in coronary arteries that are not diseased. All three agents are useful in patients who are unable to perform physical exercise.

Radionuclide studies also provide prognostic information beyond that available from clinical evaluations and exercise ECG in both men and women. However, as is true of exercise ECG, radionuclide perfusion imaging is less accurate in women than in men. Some data suggest that the better imaging properties of technetium-99m sestamibi may make it a superior agent for the evaluation of obese patients or women with large breasts or breast implants.

Table 3
Indications for the use of radionuclide perfusion imaging rather than exercise ECG

Complete left bundle-branch block
Electronically paced ventricular rhythm
Preexcitation (Wolff—Parkinson—White) syndrome or other similar electrocardiographic conduction abnormalities
More than 1 mm of ST-segment depression at rest
Inability to exercise to a level high enough to give meaningful results on routine stress ECG
Angina and a history of revascularization

The guidelines were developed by the American College of Cardiology, the American Heart Association, the American College of Physicians and the American Society of Internal Medicine.

Tracers labeled with thallium-201 and technetium-99 are used to assess myocardial perfusion and viability. The uptake of these agents by myocardial cells depends on both the perfusion and viability of a specific region of myocardium. Although both tracers can be used to assess myocardial perfusion, thallium remains the most widely used agent for testing viability. While a few reports have described planar myocardial thallium scintigraphy in SSc and SLE patients, this method has limitation in the evaluation of patients with systemic autoimmune diseases because the myocardial lesions in such patients are usually patchy and focal.

Thallium perfusion abnormalities using SPECT have been noted in 100% of SSc patients and are able to predict mortality in these patients (Kahan et al., 1990).

Radionuclide perfusion studies using thallium-201 or positron-emission tomography have shown perfusion defects in SSc patients that, in the absence of coronary lesions, may be attributed to a local coronary spasm. These sustained or repeated episodes of vasospasm may be responsible for the myocardial fibrosis and contraction band necrosis that can be found in SSc patients.

Furthermore, using myocardial single photon emission tomography, a high incidence of abnormalities (82%) was reported in patients with systemic autoimmune diseases (Ishida et al., 2000).

5. Angiography

Coronary artery disease has a wide spectrum of presentations, from stable, predictable effort-related angina pectoris to sudden death from acute ventricular tachyarrhythmias. It causes significant morbidity and mortality in our society and is more common in patients with systemic autoimmune diseases, with a lower prevalence in women than in men. An ischemic response in a symptomatic patient requires, in most cases, further evaluation with cardiac catheterization.

Some authors reported that coronary disease is responsible for 40–50% of deaths in RA (Goodson, 2002); it is not clear why RA patients have higher rates of coronary disease not related to the duration of rheumatoid disease.

At the end, when a symptomatic patient demonstrates a positive functional test on dobutamine echocardiography or dipyridamole thallium imaging, he or she should be referred for consideration of cardiac catheterization, especially if a large ischemic territory is involved. For a minority of symptomatic patients with advanced coronary artery disease, who are not suitable candidates for either percutaneous coronary intervention or coronary artery bypass graft surgery, new experimental alternatives include gene therapy and angiogenesis using endothelial growth factor or transmyocardial laser revascularization.

Acknowledgements

I gratefully acknowledge Rossana Peretti MD for her assistance in the preparation of this manuscript.

Key points

- The heart and the vascular system are frequent and characteristic targets of several systemic autoimmune diseases (particularly SLE, RA and SSc).
- Coronary artery diseases, primarily due to atheromatosis, have a prevalence considerably in systemic autoimmune disease, presumably linked to increased survival time, long-term corticosteroid therapy and other associated factors.
- We pointed out guidelines for choosing among cardiac tests for myocardial ischemia or valvular abnormalities.
- A high prevalence of valvular abnormalities or masses has been detected by TEE superior to conventional transthoracic technique.
- Stress testing with radionuclide scintigraphy or echocardiography provide more information than exercise ECG alone.
- Uninterpretable electrocardiograms or unclear images need the employment of a pharmacologic agent able to provoke ischemia in patients with coronary artery disease.

References

Asherson, R.A., Cervera, R. 1991. Antiphospholipid antibodies and heart. Lessons and pitfalls for the cardiologist. Circulation 84, 920.

Bijl, M., Brouwer, J., Kallemberg, G.G.M. 2000. Grand rounds from international lupus centres. Cardiac abnormalities in SLE: pancarditis. Lupus 9, 236.

Black, I.W., Hopkins, A.P., Lee, L.C.L., et al. 1991. Left atrial spontaneous echo contrast: a clinical and echocardiographic analysis. J. Am. Coll. Cardiol. 18, 398.

Braunwald, E. 1997. Heart Disease: A Textbook of Cardiovascular Medicine, 5th ed., Saunders, London, p. 1776.

Brenner, B., Blumenfeld, Z., Markiewicz, W., et al. 1991. Cardiac involvement in patients with primary antiphospholipid syndrome. J. Am. Coll. Cardiol. 18, 931.

Candell-Riera, J., Armadans-Gil, L., Simeon, C.P., et al. 1996. Comprehensive noninvasive assessment of cardiac involvement in limited systemic sclerosis. Arthritis Rheum. 39, 1138.

Cervera, R. 2000. Recent advances in antiphospholipid antibody-related valvulopathies. J. Autoimmun. 15, 123.

Cervera, R., Khamashta, A., Font, J., et al. 1991. High prevalence of significant heart valve lesion in patients with the primary antiphospholipid syndrome. Lupus 1, 43.

Cervera, R., Font, J., Paré, C., et al. 1992. Cardiac disease in systemic lupus erythematosus. Prospective study of 70 patients. Ann. Rheum. Dis. 51, 156.

Cheitlin, M.S., Alpert, J.S., Armstrong, W.F., et al. 1997. ACC/AHA guidelines for the clinical application of echocardiography: executive summary. A report of the American College of Cardiology/American Heart Association Task Force on Practice Guidelines (Committee on Clinical Application of Echocardiography). J. Am. Coll. Cardiol. 29, 862.

Deswall, A., Follansbee, W.P. 1996. Cardiac involvement in scleroderma. Rheum. Dis. Clin. North Am. 22, 841.

Eichenberger, A.C., Schuiki, E., Kochli, D.V., et al. 1994. Ischaemic heart disease: assessment with gadolinium-enhanced ultrafast MR imaging and dipyridamole stress. J. Magn. Reson. Imag. 4, 425.

Espinola-Zavaleta, N., Vargas-Barracòn, J., Colmenares-Galvis, T., et al. 1999. Echocardiographic evaluation of patients with primary antiphospholipid syndrome. Am. Heart J. 137, 973.

Ferri, C., Bernini, L., Bongiorni, M.G., et al. 1985. Noninvasive evaluation of cardiac dysrhythmias, and their relationship with systemic symptoms, in progressive systemic sclerosis. Arthritis Rheum. 28, 1259.

Ferri, C., Di Bello, V., Martini, A., et al. 1998. Heart involvement in systemic sclerosis: an ultrasonic tissue characterisation study. Ann. Rheum. Dis. 57, 296.
This study evaluates SSc patients by ultrasonic videodensitometric analysis, a non-invasive method that can detect early myocardial changes related to both fibrosis and microcirculatory abnormalities.

Follansbee, W.P., Curtiss, E.I., Rahko, P.S., et al. 1985. The electrocardiogram in systemic sclerosis (scleroderma). Study of 102 consecutive cases with functional correlations and review of the literature. Am. J. Med. 79, 183.

Galve, E., Ordi, J., Barquinero, J., et al. 1992. Valvular heart disease in the primary antiphospholipid syndrome. Ann. Intern. Med. 116, 293.

Ghaffary, S. 1999. Detection and management of coronary artery disease in patients with rheumatological disorders. Rheum. Dis. Clin. North Am. 25, 657.

Giunta, A., Picillo, U., Maione, S., et al. 1993. Spectrum of cardiac involvement in systemic lupus erythematosus: echocardiographic, echo-Doppler observations and immunological investigation. Acta Cardiol. 2, 183.

Goodson, N. 2002. Coronary artery disease and rheumatoid arthritis. Curr. Opin. Rheumatol. 14, 115.

Guedes, C., Bianchi-Fior, P., Cormier, B., et al. 2001. Cardiac manifestations of rheumatoid arthritis: a case-control transesophageal echocardiography study in 30 patients. Arthritis Rheum. 45, 129.
This study analyzed 30 unselected rheumatoid arthritis patients by means of transesophageal echocardiography to evaluate the incidence and type of heart lesions. Cardiac involvement, particularly of the mitral valve, is extremely common in these patients.

Hasnie, A.M., Stoddard, M.F., Gleason C.B., et al. 1995. Diastolic dysfunction is a feature of the antiphospholipid syndrome. Am. Heart J. 129, 1009.

Hojnik, M., George, J., Ziporen, L., et al. 1996. Heart valve involvement (Libman-Sacks endocarditis) in the antiphospholipid syndrome. Circulation 93, 1579.

Ishida, R., Murata, Y., Sawada, Y., et al. 2000. Thallium-201 myocardial SPET in patients with collagen disease. Nucl. Med. Commun. 21, 729.

Jafar, M.Z., Morgan, M.C., Gorcsan, J. III 1994. Transesophageal echocardiographic detection of multiple mitral valve masses in primary antiphospholipid syndrome with stroke. Am. Heart J. 127, 445.

Jiménez, S., Ramos-Casals, M., Cervera, R., et al., 2001. Atherosclerosis in systemic lupus erythematosus: clinical relevance. In: Y. Shoenfeld, D. Harats, G. Wick (Eds.), Atherosclerosis and Autoimmunity. Elsevier, Amsterdam, p. 255.

Johns, J.P., Abraham, S.A., Eagle, K.A. 1995. Dipyridamol-thallium versus dobutamine echocardiographic stress testing: a clinician's view point. Am. Heart J. 130, 373.

Kahan, A., Devaux, J., Amor, B., et al. 1990. The effect of captopril on thallium 201 myocardial perfusion in systemic sclerosis. Clin. Pharmacol. Ter. 47, 483.

Khamashta, M.A., Cervera, R., Asherson, R.A., et al. 1990. Association of antibodies against phospholipids with heart valve disease in systemic lupus erythematosus. Lancet 335, 1541.

Lee, T.H., Boucher, C.A. 2001. Noninvasive tests in patients with stable coronary artery disease. N. Engl. J. Med. 344, 1840.
These authors review the indications of noninvasive tests in patients with known or suspected coronary heart disease. No single test or strategy has been proved to be superior to the others. The authors report their guidelines for these tests.

Legrand, V., Raskinet, B., Laarman, G., et al. 1997. Diagnostic value of exercise electrocardiography and angina after coronary artery stenting. Benestent Study Group. Am. Heart J. 133, 240.

Manzi, S., Kuller, L.H., Edmundowicz, D., et al. 2000. Vascular imaging: changing the face of cardiovascular research. Lupus 9, 176.

Metz, D., Jolly, D., Graciet-Richard, J., et al. 1994. Prevalence of valvular involvement in systemic lupus erythematosus and association with antiphospholipid syndrome: a matched echocardiographic study. Cardiology 85, 129.

Moser, D.K., Stevenson, W.G., Woo, M.A., et al. 1991. Frequency of late potentials in systemic sclerosis. Ann. Cardiol. 67, 541.

Nihoyannopoulos, P., Gomez, P.M., Joshi, J., et al. 1990. Cardiac abnormalities in systemic lupus erythematosus. Circulation 82, 369.

Omdal, R., Lunde, P., Rasmussen, K., et al. 2001. Transesophageal and transthoracic echocardiography and Doppler-examinations in systemic lupus erythematosus. Scand. J. Rheumatol. 30, 275.

This study examined 35 patients with SLE by 2D transthoracic and transesophageal echocardiography. Valve thickening and valve masses, often in combination, are the most frequent lesions in SLE patients (46%) and occur more often on the aortic than on the mitral valves.

Plazak, W., Zabinska-Plazak, E., Wojas-Pelc, A., et al. 2002. Heart structure and function in systemic sclerosis. Eur. J. Dermatol. 12, 257.

Roldan, C.A., Shively, B.K., Crawford, M.H. 1996. An echocardiographic study of valvular heart disease associated with systemic lupus erythematosus. N. Engl. J. Med. 335, 1424.

The authors studied 69 SLE patients by transesophageal echocardiography with a long-term follow-up of 57 months. Valvular heart diseases were common on the initial and the follow-up echocardiograms (61 and 53%, respectively). An important finding in this study is that over time valvular abnormalities frequently resolve or change and new ones often develop. The authors also demonstrated that most of the complications were related to valvular disease.

Turiel, M., Muzzupappa, S., Gottardi, B., et al. 2000. Evaluation of cardiac abnormalities and embolic sources in primary antiphospholipid syndrome by transesophageal echocardiography. Lupus 9, 406.

The authors performed a transesophageal echocardiographic study in a group of 40 patients with primary antiphospholipid syndrome (PAPS) to describe the prevalence of cardiac abnormalities or potential embolic sources. Cardiac involvement was present in 82% of these patients. PAPS patients with aCL titer >40 GPL-U represent a higher risk group for thromboembolic events.

Handbook of Systemic Autoimmune Diseases, Volume 1
The Heart in Systemic Autoimmune Diseases
A. Doria and P. Pauletto, editors

CHAPTER 9

Cardiac Involvement in Rheumatoid Arthritis

Nicola J. Goodson

ARC Epidemiology Unit, Stopford Building, University of Manchester, Oxford Road, Manchester M13 9PT, UK

1. Introduction

1.1. Rheumatoid arthritis

Rheumatoid arthritis (RA) is one of the more common systemic autoimmune disorders, affecting approximately 0.5–1% of the adult population, although its prevalence varies worldwide. The incidence of RA is 2–3 times higher in females than males and rises with increasing age. Over recent decades the incidence of RA appears to have reduced, particularly in women (Doran et al., 2002), and it is thought that this could be due to the use of oral contraceptive pill. RA also seems to have become less severe over recent years (Silman, 2002) and this may in part contribute to the falling disease prevalence. The exact aetiology of RA is not known but several genetic, host and environmental risk factors have been identified that influence susceptibility and progression of the disease (Symmons, 2002).

RA is characterised by chronic inflammation of synovial tissues in a characteristic joint distribution leading to joint damage and disability. However, although RA is primarily an inflammatory disease of joint tissues it also causes systemic symptoms, affects extra-articular tissues and can involve many organ systems including the cardiovascular system.

E-mail address: nicola.goodson@man.ac.uk (N.J. Goodson).

DOI: 10.1016/S1571-5078(03)01009-2

1.2. Mortality of rheumatoid arthritis

RA is not a benign disease. In addition to causing significant chronic morbidity it is associated with a substantial reduction in life expectancy. Many studies of mortality have been carried out using RA cohorts from around the world. Nearly all of these studies have reported increased mortality rates in RA patients compared to that in the general population (Table 1). The reported standardised mortality rates (SMR) from these RA cohorts range from 0.87 to 2.7. There has been a tendency, in recent studies, to report a more modest rise in RA mortality rates. However, different study designs, affecting patient selection, disease duration and follow-up duration, make comparison between studies difficult and may influence the magnitude of mortality excess reported (Ward, 2001). Also most SMRs are calculated using the indirect standardisation method, which is dependent on the study population's age and gender distribution, and this prevents direct comparison between studies (Hennekens and Buring, 1987). Three inception studies of RA patients with disease onset in the 1980s–1990s reported no increase in RA mortality (Kroot et al., 2000; Lindqvist and Eberhardt, 1999; Peltomaa et al., 2002). It has been suggested that these findings reflect either more effective drug therapy suppressing inflammatory disease (Bjornadal et al., 2002) or a reduction in the severity of RA over recent years (Silman, 1992). Conversely two population-based studies have failed to identify any recent

Table 1
Mortality studies in rheumatoid arthritis

Study design	Inclusion period	*n*	SMR	Increased cardiovascular mortality?
Inception cohort-population based				
Gabriel et al. (2003)	1955–1994	609	1.27	Not reported
Mikuls et al. (2002)	1986–1997	158	1.52[a]	Excess CVD deaths
Inception cohort-clinic based				
Reilly et al. (1990)	1957–1963	100	1.4	Excess CVD deaths
Lindqvist and Eberhardt (1999)	1985–1989	183	0.87	No excess CVD deaths
Kroot et al. (2000)	1985–1997	622	No increased mortality	No excess CVD deaths
Sokka et al. (1999)	1983–1989	135	1.28	No excess CVD deaths
Peltomaa et al. (2002)	1986–1989	87	0.93	No excess CVD deaths
	1991–1993	63	1.62	
Established RA cohort-population based				
Jacobsson et al. (1993)	1965–1989	2979	1.28	Excess CVD deaths
Wolfe et al. (1994) (Santa Clara)	1978–1979	305	2.18	Excess CVD deaths
Bjornadal et al. (2002)	1964–1995	46,917	2.03	Excess CVD deaths
Established RA cohort-clinic based				
Symmons et al. (1998)	1968–1974	448	2.7	Excess CVD deaths
Wolfe et al. (1994) (Saskatoon)	1966–1974	905	2.24	Excess CVD deaths
Wolfe et al. (1994) (Wichita)	1973–1990	1,405	1.98	Excess CVD deaths
Wolfe et al. (2003) (Stanford)	1965–1990	886	3.08	Excess CVD deaths
Callahan et al. (1996)	1980–1990	1,384	1.54	Not reported
Wållberg-Jonsson et al. (1997)	1979	606	1.57	Excess CVD deaths
Kvalvik et al. (2000)	1977	147	1.49	Excess CVD deaths in Females
Riise et al. (2001)	1978–1982	187	2.0	No excess CVD deaths
Chehata et al. (2001)	1981–1985	309	1.65	Not reported

[a] Relative risk of mortality for women who developed RA.

improvements in the mortality rates of RA patients compared to the general population (Coste and Jougla, 1994; Gabriel et al., 1999b).

1.2.1. Causes of death in rheumatoid arthritis

It has been observed that patients with RA die of the same diseases as the general population only at younger ages. RA is rarely recorded as a cause of death on death certificates (Allebeck et al., 1981). RA patients die more frequently from infections, renal disease, gastrointestinal disorders and lymphoproliferative disease than do the general adult population (Pincus and Callahan, 1993). However, these causes of death represent only a small proportion of all RA deaths. The most commonly reported main cause of death in RA cohorts is cardiovascular disease (CVD), responsible for 35–50% of all RA deaths, whilst in the general UK adult population coronary heart disease (CHD) is responsible for 1 in 4 deaths that occur in males and 1 in 5 female deaths. It seems that CVD mortality is responsible for much of the excess mortality observed in RA cohorts. Symmons et al. (1998) reported that 34% of the excess deaths observed in a clinic-based cohort of RA patients were due to CVD and a similar proportion of excess CVD deaths were also observed in a Finnish, population-based, study of female RA patients (Myllykangas-Luosujärvi et al., 1995).

Many of these mortality studies examined established RA patients, identified in clinic-based settings, and therefore patient selection might be biased towards those with more severe disease. However, study of an inception cohort of inflammatory polyarthritis patients, identified in a community-based setting, revealed excess CVD mortality in seropositive patients during the early years of follow-up

(Goodson et al. 2001). This suggests that mechanisms that promote CVD mortality are present early in the RA disease process (Kaplan and Clune, 2003).

Why should RA patients have increased CVD mortality? There are several types of cardiac involvement in RA. It was previously highlighted that pericardial disease was a frequent cardiac manifestation in RA. However, pericardial disease is usually asymptomatic and benign in nature and is diagnosed as a coincidental finding on echocardiography or at autopsy. More recently there has been much interest in CHD in RA. This condition has been shown to be highly prevalent in RA cohorts. It is also often asymptomatic and is frequently diagnosed at autopsy. However, CHD in RA is not a benign disease and appears to be responsible for much of the observed excess mortality. Indeed, ischaemic heart disease (IHD) appears be the single largest cause of CVD deaths in RA populations (Myllykangas-Luosujärvi et al., 1995; Wållberg-Jonsson et al., 1997). Much is known about both primary and secondary prevention of CHD events from previous cardiovascular research. Therefore an understanding of cardiac involvement in RA is vital for clinicians caring for these patients.

In this chapter the recent literature pertaining to both traditional rheumatoid heart disease and CHD will be discussed.

2. Traditional rheumatoid heart disease

Cardiovascular involvement in RA is common although the true prevalence of cardiac involvement in RA is difficult to measure, as much disease remains clinically silent. Most studies examining cardiac involvement in RA are based either on autopsy data or on echocardiographic studies of RA patients. These studies tend to select RA patients identified from clinic-based settings and probably examine the more severe end of the RA disease spectrum. In particular most autopsy studies were carried out on patients who developed their RA over 50 years ago (Bonfiglio and Atwater, 1969; Cathcart and Spodick, 1962) and it may be that more recent advances in RA treatment will have influenced the degree and type of cardiac involvement detected in RA.

It seems that nearly all the structures of the heart can be involved in RA (Table 2). Pericarditis has been the most frequently reported cardiac manifestation although there are also reports of conduction disturbances (Leden et al., 1983), myocardial and endocardial involvement as well as coronary artery pathology including coronary arteritis (Guedes et al., 2001).

Table 2
Cardiac involvement in RA

Pericardium
Myocardium
Endocardium and heart valves
Conducting system and autonomic nervous system
Coronary arteries and vascular tree

In this section the manifestations of rheumatoid heart disease will be discussed in more detail.

2.1. Pericardial disease

2.1.1. Introduction

Rheumatoid pericarditis was first described by Charcot (1881) and subsequent postmortem (Bonfiglio and Atwater, 1969; Cathcart and Spodick, 1962) and echocardiographic studies (Mody et al., 1987) have confirmed that pericardial involvement is a common occurrence in RA. Although RA patients may rarely present with acute or recurrent pericarditis and occasionally constrictive pericarditis or tamponade, pericardial involvement in RA is usually clinically silent.

2.1.2. Prevalence

It is not known what the true prevalence of rheumatoid pericarditis is, as this condition is frequently only diagnosed as a coincidental finding on autopsy. Clinically evident RA pericarditis is reported infrequently affecting fewer than 2% of RA patients (Gordon et al., 1973; Hara et al., 1990). However, autopsy studies have reported a higher prevalence of pericardial disease in RA. One study reported a prevalence of pericardial involvement in 50% of seropositive patients undergoing autopsy (Bonfiglio and Atwater, 1969) More recent autopsy studies have reported much lower rates (Bely et al., 1992). It is difficult to ascertain rates of disease diagnosed at autopsy as most autopsy series are based on small numbers of patients, which are usually

Table 3
Echocardiographic studies of pericardial disease in RA

Study	*n*	Pericardial disease	Prevalence of disease (%)	Imaging modality
Nomeir et al. (1979)	30	Chronic pericardial effusion	20	Trans-thoracic echo
Mody et al. (1987)	101	Pericardial effusion	6	2D Trans-thoracic echo
Maione et al. (1993)	39	Pericardial effusion	7	2D Trans-thoracic echo
Tlustochowicz (1997)	100	Pericardial effusion	26	Trans-thoracic echo
Wislowska et al. (1999)	70	Pericardial effusion	4	2D Trans-thoracic echo
Dawson et al. (2000)	143	Pericardial effusion	1	2D Trans-thoracic echo
Guedes et al. (2001)	30	Pericarditis	13	Trans-oesophageal echo

selected from a hospital setting introducing selection bias towards more severe disease.

Pericardial disease is more common in male patients with active seropositive disease although it has been reported in seronegative cases (Sigal and Friedman, 1989).

More recent echocardiographic studies have suggested a lower prevalence of pericardial disease. Numerous studies have been carried out in RA cohorts and the reported prevalence of echocardiographic pericardial effusion ranges from 1 to 30% (Table 3).

A recent case control study utilised trans-oesophageal echocardiography to detect cardiac lesions in 30 randomly selected RA patients and controls; none were known to have CVD (Guedes et al., 2001). They found echocardiographic evidence of pericarditis in four patients and none of the controls. Trans-oesophageal echo is more sensitive than trans-thoracic echo as the higher frequency transducers enable imaging with higher resolution and one might expect this imaging modality to detect a higher prevalence of sub-clinical pericardial disease.

However, it is possible that the prevalence of pericarditis in RA may be reducing either because of more effective disease modifying anti-rheumatic drugs (DMARD) or possibly because RA is becoming a less severe disease (Silman, 1992).

2.1.3. *Aetiology of pericardial involvement in rheumatoid arthritis*

Pericarditis is an extra-articular manifestation of RA usually associated with increased disease severity. Patients are usually seropositive, and frequently have rheumatoid nodules and erosive disease. Systemic symptoms are common including fatigue, weight loss and other extra-articular system involvement (Hara et al., 1990). Extra-articular manifestations of RA were predicted by the early development of rheumatoid nodules and antinuclear antibodies in a retrospective clinic-based study. Male gender and rheumatoid factor seropositivity were not found to be predictors of pericarditis in this group (Turesson et al., 2000).

2.1.4. *Mortality*

Patients with RA have a reduced life expectancy and this is marked in those with extra-articular manifestations of RA (Turesson et al., 1999). Hara et al. (1990) observed that RA patients presenting with pericarditis had increased mortality during the first year of follow-up compared to the general population. Other mortality studies in RA cohorts have not reported large numbers of deaths from pericardial disease although many observe increased cardiovascular death. Given that this condition is frequently asymptomatic it is unlikely to significantly contribute to the excess CVD mortality observed in RA.

2.1.5. *Pathology*

The normal pericardium consists of two layers, a thin visceral inner layer and a thicker parietal layer, that are separated by a small amount of pericardial fluid. Inflammation of the pericardium may cause accumulation of pericardial fluid resulting in pericardial effusion. The RA pericardial fluid is classically exudative containing leukocytes, lactate dehydrogenase and a low concentration of glucose; however, these findings are not universal (Hara et al., 1990). Chronic inflammation can result in thickening of the pericardium that can result in constrictive pericarditis.

The pericardium becomes thickened and rigid and restricts cardiac filling. This is a rare sequelae of severe or recurrent pericarditis in RA (Thould, 1986). Calcification of the pericardium is rarely seen in RA pericarditis (Manji and Raven, 1990).

2.1.6. Clinical manifestations

Although usually asymptomatic RA pericarditis can present with symptoms of acute pericarditis with pericardial chest pain which is usually retrosternal, radiating to the neck, left shoulder, back, epigastrium and around the left scapular. The pain is often sharp and pleuritic in nature and is exacerbated by lying supine or on the left side. Dyspnoea is a common symptom. Peripheral oedema and ascites can occur. Examination during a clinical presentation frequently reveals tachycardia and the classical pericardial friction rub was evident in over half of patients in one study of 41 patients (Hara et al., 1990). Other clinical signs include elevation of the jugular venous pressure (JVP), additional heart sounds, pulsus paradoxus and peripheral oedema.

Cardial tamponade is the reduction of diastolic filling caused by the pressure of fluid in the pericardial space. This results in a drop in the cardiac output followed by hypotension and cardiovascular collapse. Clinical signs include tachycardia, pulsus paradoxus, hypotension, elevated JVP, heart sounds may be soft and the pericardial fiction rub may be audible.

Rapid accumulation of pericardial fluid can lead to cardiac tamponade with only modest increases in pericardial fluid volume. Pericardial effusions if chronic can usually be tolerated without generating symptoms. However, patients with very large chronic effusions can suddenly develop cardiac tamponade with rapid deterioration in cardiac function.

Constrictive pericarditis is a rare occurrence in RA. It can present with symptoms of right heart failure with dyspnoea, fatigue, peripheral oedema and hepatic congestion. Clinical signs include evidence of peripheral venous congestion and Kussmaul's sign may be present with paradoxical changes in the JVP during inspiration. A loud third heart sound due to rapid early diastolic ventricular filling in the restricted ventricle, 'pericardial knock', may be heard.

2.1.7. Diagnostic investigations

The postero-anterior chest radiograph provides little diagnostic information in RA pericardial involvement as abnormality in the cardiac outline is only observed with larger effusions (>250 ml). The calcification observed in constrictive pericarditis is rarely seen in RA pericarditis.

Currently trans-thoracic 2D Doppler echocardiography is the most frequently utilised investigation for diagnosing pericardial effusions and tamponade. This method can demonstrate moderate-sized effusions and Doppler examination can reveal decreased diastolic filling during inspiration. Trans-oesophageal echo can detect small effusions, but is not good at imaging the whole of the pericardium (Guedes et al., 2001).

The recent development of other imaging modalities, including spiral computerised tomography (CT) scanning and cardiac-gated magnetic resonance imaging (MRI) scanning, has enabled excellent high-resolution imaging of the whole pericardium (Breen, 2001). MRI has the advantage of distinguishing pericardial fluid from thickened pericardium. CT gives better estimation of pericardial calcification. Both modalities are useful when planning surgery on the pericardium. It may be that use of these newer imaging modalities would detect more pericardial disease in RA patients.

Other useful diagnostic information can be obtained from the electrocardiograph (ECG). In acute pericarditis the typical ECG changes include saddle-shaped ST segment elevation with no reciprocal changes or T wave inversion. The PR segment may be depressed. However, studies in RA patients have reported that ECG changes may be non-specific or absent in RA pericarditis (Hara et al., 1990).

Most patients with rheumatoid pericardial disease are seropositive and have active rheumatoid disease with associated elevations in acute phase reactants. Analysis of pericardial fluid should be undertaken if there is any suspicion of an infective cause of the effusion.

2.1.8. Differential diagnosis and management

For any patient presenting with chest pain, other differential diagnoses including cardiac ischaemia and pulmonary embolism should be considered. If investigation confirms pericarditis in a RA patient, causes other than RA pericarditis should be excluded. Particularly infective causes of pericardial effusion should be considered in patients receiving immunosuppressant. Cultures for TB and fungi as well as standard culture of pericardial fluid should be obtained if there is suspicion of an infective cause.

The treatment of the vast majority of patients presenting with acute pericarditis symptoms involves conservative treatment with non-steroidal anti-inflammatories for pain relief. Short courses of steroids may be used and DMARD therapy may be increased to control active rheumatoid disease. Colchicine has been used to treat recurrent non-RA pericarditis, however, it is not clear whether this is beneficial in RA pericarditis (Fernandez-Muixi et al., 1994).

Patients who have evidence of cardiovascular compromise with tachycardia, elevated JVP, hypotension, poor pain control or elevated cardiac enzymes, electrical or pulsus alternans should be admitted to hospital and closely monitored. Pericardiocentesis is indicated in those with large effusions or signs of tamponade. Although large effusions may be well tolerated these patients can rapidly deteriorate and thus treatment with pericardial fluid drainage is still required. Pericardectomy or creation of a pericardial window may be required in those with recurrent effusions. For constrictive pericarditis surgical pericardectomy is the treatment of choice, although cautious diuretic therapy may utilised to treat patients who are not candidates for surgery (Goyle and Walling, 2002).

2.2. Endocardial involvement in rheumatoid arthritis

2.2.1. Introduction

Endocardial and valve involvement in RA is divided into diffuse valve involvement and the rarer focal involvement of valves and endocardium with rheumatoid nodules.

Diffuse endocardial involvement in RA appears, from autopsy studies, to be a relatively common manifestation of RA (Bely et al., 1992; Liebowitz, 1963). Echocardiographic studies in RA patients have frequently reported valvular abnormalities and Bacon et al. (Bacon and Gibson, 1974) suggested that heart valve involvement may be a systemic effect of RA. Other more recent echocardiographic studies of small numbers of hospital-based RA cohorts have found that the non-specific aortic and or mitral valvular abnormalities are relatively common in RA affecting 5–30% of patients (Mody et al., 1987; Nomeir et al., 1979; Toumanidis et al., 1995). Most series report a higher prevalence of mitral valve abnormality with minimal mitral regurgitation being the most frequently reported abnormality (Dawson et al., 2000; Wislowska et al., 1998) Echocardiographic evidence of mitral valve insufficiency was detected more frequently in nodular RA patients than in those without nodules (Wislowska et al., 1999) suggesting that heart valve involvement may reflect more severe disease. It appears that the diffuse endocardial valve lesion is due to infiltration of inflammatory cells that lead to thickening and calcification at the base of the valve and valve ring (Bely et al., 1992; Liebowitz, 1963).

Symptomatic valve disease is a very rare manifestation of RA. There are reports in the literature of rheumatoid nodules affecting the endocardium or heart valves causing valve dysfunction. In particular there have been several reports of aortic valve nodulosis causing regurgitation requiring aortic valve replacement (Chand et al., 1999; Levine et al., 1999) and mitral valve nodules causing embolic disease (Mounet et al., 1997). There has also been one report in the literature of an endocardial nodule mimicking an atrial myxoma (Webber et al., 1995).

Therefore, although endocardial involvement is common in RA it does not usually lead to clinical symptoms.

2.3. Myocardial involvement and conduction system abnormalities in rheumatoid arthritis

Inflammation of the myocardium occurs in RA either as a result of focal granulomatous disease affecting the myocardium or due to more diffuse fibrosing lesions. Non-specific myocarditis is frequently asymptomatic (Liebowitz, 1963), but may lead to the development of cardiac failure or disruption of the conducting system of the heart. It seems that ECG evidence of abnormalities of the conducting system are common in patients with RA. One study reported that 50% of RA patients had evidence of cardiac arrhythmias on

24 h ECG monitoring, although this arrhythmia prevalence was similar to that seen in a hospital-based non-RA control group (Tlustochowicz et al., 1995). Another study reported a higher prevalence of abnormal ventricular repolarisation in RA patients compared to control patients (Goldeli et al., 1998). Complete heart block may also occur in association with RA possibly due to disruption of the atrio-ventricular node by rheumatoid granulomata (Ahern et al., 1983; Okada et al., 1983). Several studies have also demonstrated abnormalities in the autonomic nervous system in RA (Leden et al., 1983; Toussirot et al., 1993) which may be a risk factor for CVD events (Curtis and O'Keefe, 2002).

2.4. *Coronary arteritis*

Coronary arteritis has been reported in RA autopsy studies, affecting 10% of cases, but rarely presents as clinically apparent disease. The pathological lesion usually affects the medium and inter-mural vessels and has been associated with patchy myocardial necrosis and myocardial infarction in a small number of cases (Albada-Kuipers et al., 1986; Bely et al., 1992).

Thus, the structures of the heart are commonly involved in the systemic inflammatory process of RA. It is difficult to assess how much this 'rheumatoid heart disease' contributes to the excess CVD mortality observed in RA patients.

3. Coronary heart disease in RA

3.1. *Introduction*

Over recent years there has been increasing awareness of the association between inflammation and CVD and it is now accepted that inflammatory processes contribute to atherogenesis in CVD (Blake and Ridker, 2001). In this section the literature regarding CHD in RA will be discussed including the importance of traditional and emerging cardiovascular risk factors and their roles in RA.

3.2. *Epidemiology*

Most of the evidence for increased CHD in RA patients has been obtained from mortality studies. There have been relatively few reports measuring the prevalence of CHD in RA patients. If patients with RA have excessive CVD mortality one would assume that they also have increased prevalence of IHD. However, an alternative explanation could be that RA patients have the same prevalence of IHD, but are systematically more likely to die from the disease. Several studies have reported increased rates of CVD events in RA patients compared to the general population (del Rincon et al., 2001; Wållberg-Jonsson et al., 1997) and the risk of myocardial infarction in women with RA was twice that of women without RA in the Nurses' Health Study (Solomon et al., 2003). In another study, patient recall of CVD events was used to compare the prevalence of events in a large group of RA patients compared to patients with osteoarthritis. In this study RA patients reported a twofold increase in congestive heart failure and a 28% increase in ever reporting myocardial infarction. The prevalence of reported cerebrovascular accidents (CVA) was similar in both groups (Wolfe et al., 2003).

One of the problems with quantifying comorbid CHD is that, for many people, IHD remains clinically silent and is frequently only diagnosed at post-mortem examination. Banks et al. (2000) reported the prevalence of IHD, detected with myocardial perfusion scanning, to be 49% in a group of consecutive clinic-based RA patients.

Angina questionnaires have been used and validated in the general population to estimate the prevalence of IHD (Rose, 1967). However, these consist of questions about exertional chest pain, which may not be as valid in RA populations because of masking musculoskeletal symptoms or difficulty with mobility. Therefore, there is a need for a large population-based study to investigate the prevalence of IHD in RA patients.

3.3. *Aetiology of ischaemic heart disease in RA*

Epidemiological research in the last 30 years has identified several risk factors for CVD in the general population (Dawber, 1980). These 'traditional' risk factors are shown in Table 4. However, it has been shown that many patients in the general population

Table 4
Traditional risk factors for CVD

Increasing age
Male gender
Hypertension
Diabetes mellitus
Dyslipidaemia
Smoking
Family history of IHD
Physical inactivity
Obesity

who develop atherosclerotic disease do not have traditional CVD risk factors (Heller et al., 1984). Therefore more recently research has concentrated on 'novel' CVD risk factors that may contribute to the development of atherosclerotic disease (Kullo et al., 2000).

3.3.1. Traditional CVD risk factors

It seems that the prevalence of most CVD risk factors, measured prior to the onset of inflammatory polyarthritis, is similar to that observed in the general population (Goodson et al., 2002a). In established clinic-based RA cohorts there is evidence that RA patients have a high prevalence of classical CVD risk factors. McEntegart et al. (2001b) assessed CHD risk in 70 patients with established RA using the Joint Societies Coronary Risk Prediction Chart (Wood et al., 1998). They found that a third of their patients, eligible for primary prevention of CVD, had a predicted 15% risk of a CHD event over a 10-year period. Another study, assessing CVD risk in a hospital-based RA cohort, detected that 90% of patients had a moderate to high CVD event risk (Erb et al., 2001).

3.3.1.1. Hypertension

It has been shown in several studies (Berkanovic and Hurwicz, 1990; Gabriel et al., 1999a; Garnero et al., 1999) that RA patients frequently report co-existent hypertension and Kroot et al. reported that most RA patients with hypertension developed it after the onset of their joint disease (Kroot et al., 2001). One possible explanation for this could be that patients with RA are more likely to have their blood pressure measured after their RA has been diagnosed, as they will have increased contact with health care providers. An alternative explanation for the high prevalence of hypertension in RA patients is that the joint disease or its treatment gives rise to hypertension. It seems likely that the widespread chronic use of non-steroidal anti-inflammatory drugs (NSAIDS) may, in part, be responsible for this hypertension. McEntegart et al. (2001a) found that a cohort of established RA patients had higher diastolic blood pressure than age and gender-matched controls. Most of the patients in this study were using NSAIDs to treat symptoms of RA. However, previous research has suggested that NSAID usage is more likely to lead to an increase in systolic BP rather than diastolic BP (Frishman, 2002). It is possible that there is some other mechanism associated with RA that may have caused this rise in diastolic BP.

3.3.1.2. Smoking

Cigarette smoking has been identified by several studies to be a risk factor for the development of RA (Criswell et al., 2002; Heliövaara et al., 1993; Karlson et al., 1999; Reckner et al., 2001; Silman et al., 1996; Symmons et al., 1997). The amount and duration of smoking seems to influence both the risk of developing RA (Hutchinson et al., 2001) and the severity of RA (Saag et al., 1997). Studies have also shown that smoking has a dose-dependant relationship with RF production (Masdottir et al., 2000; Wolfe, 2000). Therefore it seems reasonable to hypothesise that smoking may increase the risk of CVD in RA patients. However, studies have failed to identify smoking as a predictor of CVD mortality in seropositive RA (Wållberg-Jonsson et al., 1997) and inflammatory polyarthritis (Goodson et al., 2002b).

3.3.1.3. Lipids

A population-based study suggested that serum cholesterol might be a risk factor for developing RA (Heliövaara et al., 1996) although no significant association was observed between lipid measurements and the subsequent development of inflammatory polyarthritis (Goodson et al., 2002a) and Jacobsson et al. (1993) reported that low cholesterol levels seem to predict the onset of RA in Pima Indians. Dyslipidaemia has been frequently reported in established RA cohorts (Situnayake and Kitas, 1997) and it seems that the lipid profile is modified by the acute phase response in RA (Lee et al., 2000). In RA the total cholesterol and low density lipoprotein (LDL) cholesterol levels may be reduced (Lazarevic et al., 1992; Rantapää-Dahlqvist et al., 1991) or increased (Lakatos and Harsagyi, 1988). However, the most consistent finding has been that high density lipoprotein (HDL) cholesterol is reduced in RA (Lakatos and Harsagyi, 1988; Lazarevic et al., 1992). This results in a high LDL/HDL lipid ratio, which represents an atherogenic lipid profile. Treatments with disease-modifying drugs can also modify the lipid profile and usually lead to elevation of lipids (Svenson et al., 1987). Hydroxychloroquine has been shown to have a more favourable effect on lipid profiles leading to preferential elevation of HDL cholesterol and reduction of LDL cholesterol in RA patients (Munro et al., 1997). This has also been observed in lupus patients (Wallace et al., 1990). The mechanism for this is not fully understood, but is postulated to be upregulation of LDL receptors or decreased synthesis of cholesterol by hepatocytes (Munro et al., 1997).

3.3.1.4. Other classical cardiovascular risk factors

The prevalence of diabetes in RA has not been extensively studied. One might expect a high prevalence of type 1 diabetes in RA as autoimmune diseases have a tendency to cluster in patients and there is evidence of a shared HLA locus (Payami et al., 1987). Type 2 diabetes might also be expected to be increased because of obesity, chronic steroid usage and increased insulin resistance observed in patients with established RA (Dessein et al., 2002; Svenson et al., 1988). However, a recent study carried out in a Spanish cohort of 788 established RA patients, found that the age and gender adjusted prevalence of diabetes mellitus (DM) (type 1 and type 2 combined) was less than that in the general population (Carmona et al., 2002). It therefore seems unlikely that excessive comorbid DM is responsible for accelerated atherosclerosis in RA.

It has previously been suggested that RA patients report a family history of premature maternal CVD mortality more frequently than the general population (Kaplan and Feldman, 1991). The conclusion from this study suggested that there might be a genetic predisposition to early CVD mortality in RA patients. However, a similar study carried out in the UK, comparing parental mortality between RA patients and osteoarthritis (OA) patients, found that the age of parental mortality was the same in both groups (Spector and Silman, 1988). The Nurses' Health Study found that a family history of parental myocardial infarction before the age of 60, was reported slightly more frequently by women who developed RA (42%) than by women who remained free from RA (36%) (Solomon et al., 2003). It is not clear whether there is actually a genetic or environmental predisposition to early CVD mortality in RA patients.

Several studies have examined the prevalence of traditional CVD risk factors in RA cohorts compared to controls and have found similar CVD risk rates in both groups. (del Rincon et al., 2000; Cisternas et al., 2002) (McEntegart et al. (2001a) found that a cohort of established RA patients reported significantly higher rates of previous smoking and had higher diastolic blood pressures than in control patients. However, these RA patients also had significantly lower cholesterol levels than controls and systolic blood pressure (SBP), current smoking history, exercise level, triglycerides and body mass index were not significantly different between the two groups. Despite the relative paucity of traditional CVD risk factors this group of patients were found to have a higher prevalence of CVD than their age and sex matched controls. A study in Chilean RA patients revealed similar rates of traditional CVD risk factors to that in a control population (Cisternas et al., 2002) and two studies that identified excess CVD events in RA patients did not find that these excess events were explained by increased traditional CVD risk factors (del Rincon et al., 2001; Solomon et al., 2003). Therefore it seems that the increased CVD mortality and morbidity in RA is not solely explained by elevations in traditional CVD risk factors.

3.3.2. Novel cardiovascular risk factors

Recent cardiovascular research has identified several factors, other than traditional CVD risk factors, that may contribute to CVD risk in the general population (Table 5). These include elevated levels of

Table 5
Novel risk factors for CVD

Abnormal Homocysteine metabolism	Elevated Homocysteine
Thrombotic markers	Elevated Fibrinogen Impaired Fibrinolysis
Lipoproteins and modified lipids	Elevated Lipoprotein (a) Small, dense, LDL Oxidised LDL
Markers of inflammation	Elevated CRP Soluble adhesion molecules Serum amyloid A

homocysteine, thrombotic markers, lipoprotein (a) and markers of inflammation.

3.3.2.1. Homocysteine

Homocysteine is an amino-acid intermediate formed during the metabolism of methionine to cysteine. In healthy people the fasting plasma level of homocysteine ranges between 5 and 15 μmol/l and factors including aging, menopause, chronic renal insufficiency and low plasma levels of vitamins B_6, B_{12}, and folate have all been associated with increase in plasma homocysteine levels (Kullo et al., 2000). There is also evidence that genetic abnormalities affecting homocysteine metabolism may also lead to elevation of homocysteine (Scheuner, 2001). There is considerable evidence to suggest that homocysteine is a potentially modifiable risk factor for CVD in the general population (Ridker et al., 1999; Ross, 1999). It is thought that hyperhomocysteinaemia may mediate endothelial dysfunction, LDL-cholesterol oxidation, cause vascular smooth muscle proliferation and affect haemostasis, all of which are involved in the pathogenesis of atherosclerosis (Booth and Wang, 2000).

Homocysteine has been shown to be elevated in patients with RA (Roubenoff et al., 1997) and was significantly higher in a group of RA patients with comorbid CVD than in controls (Cisternas et al., 2002). Long-term use of methotrexate or use of methotrexate and sulphasalazine in combination are associated with increased levels of homocysteine in RA (Haagsma et al., 1999). Concomitant folate supplementation with low-dose methotrexate prevents the rise in homocysteine levels associated with methotrexate use (Morgan et al., 1998; van Ede et al., 2002). One might expect that use of methotrexate would lead to increased CVD in RA patients. However, studies have reported that RA patients treated with methotrexate have a reduced mortality (Krause and Rau, 2000) and reduced CVD mortality (Choi et al., 2002). Further study is required to see whether increased homocysteine levels predict CVD events in RA patients.

3.3.2.2. Thrombotic markers

Fibrinogen has been identified as a cardiovascular risk factor in several studies. In a meta-analysis of six prospective epidemiological studies, patients in the highest tertile for levels of fibrinogen had a twofold increase in subsequent CVD events compared to those in the lowest tertile (Ernst and Resch, 1993). It is thought that fibrinogen may mediate atherosclerosis by increasing plasma viscosity, platelet aggregation and smooth muscle proliferation (Danesh et al., 1998). Fibrinogen levels are associated with other traditional CVD risk factors including smoking and obesity and are also increased in inflammatory states (Danesh et al., 1998). Other thrombotic markers, implicated as risk factors for CVD, include tissue plasminogen activator (tPA) and plasminogen activator inhibitor type 1 (PAI-1) (Kullo et al., 2000), D-dimer and von Willebrand factor (v-WF) (Koenig, 1998; Lee et al., 1995).

The levels of these thrombotic markers are increased in RA. One study reported that RA patients had significantly elevated fibrinogen, v-WF, t-PA antigen and D-dimer compared with population controls (McEntegart et al., 2001a). There is evidence that these thrombotic markers are associated with the level of RA disease activity (Ichikawa et al., 1998; Kamper et al., 2000; Kopeikina et al., 1997) and a Swedish study reported that RA patients with markers of haemostasis had increased rates of cardiovascular events (Wållberg-Jonsson et al., 2000).

3.3.2.3. Lipoproteins and oxidised LDL

Lipoprotein (a) are a group of lipoprotein particles with cholesterol rich cores that are associated with premature CVD in the general population. It is thought that levels of lipoprotein (a) are genetically determined. However, levels are increased in DM, during pregnancy and after oestrogen therapy (Kullo et al., 2000).

Patients with RA have increased lipoprotein (a) concentrations compared to controls (Asanuma and Mizushima, 1999; Rantapää-Dahlqvist et al., 1991) and it seems that this lipoprotein is not modified by disease activity (Lee et al., 2000) as it is observed in both active and treated RA (Park et al., 1999, 2002b).

Elevated levels of LDL-cholesterol have long been accepted as a risk factor for CVD. However, more recent evidence suggests that the size and density of LDL are important in CVD. It seems that the small, dense LDL particles are particularly atherogenic and have been shown to be predictors of CVD events (Kullo et al., 2000). This may possibly be because of their long half-life, reduced clearance by LDL receptors and their inability to resist oxidative stress (Chapman et al., 1998). These small, dense LDL particles are frequently seen with other lipid abnormalities including low HDL-cholesterol and high triglycerides. This combination has been termed the 'atherogenic lipoprotein phenotype' and has been shown to be associated with CVD in the general population (Austin, 2000). It seems that these atherogenic lipoprotein factors may be increased in RA patients. One study described an increased prevalence of small, dense LDL particles in RA patients compared to controls (Hurt-Camejo et al., 2001).

Oxidation of lipids appears to be an important mechanism in the progression of atherosclerosis with oxidised lipid products being observed in both atherosclerotic plaques and the plasma of patients with CVD (Berliner, 2002). Oxidised LDL has been detected in the RA synovial fluid and it is thought that the formation of oxidised LDL within joint fluid is influenced by the local inflammatory response (Dai et al., 2000). Paraoxonase 1 (PON1), an enzyme associated with HDL, breaks down oxidised LDL and reduces its pro-atherogenic effects. It has been suggested that increased activity of this enzyme may be protective against IHD in the general population (Mackness et al., 2001). It seems that RA patients have a reduced activity of paraoxonase compared to controls and thus are less protected against oxidised LDL promoted atherosclerosis (Tanimoto et al., 2003).

3.3.2.4. Inflammation and cardiovascular disease

Atherosclerosis is now accepted to be a chronic inflammatory process (Tracy, 1999) and prospective study has identified that inflammatory markers are powerful predictors of future CVD events in the general population (Pradhan et al., 2002; Ridker et al., 1997, 2000) and in patients with known IHD (Koukkunen et al., 2001; Liuzzo et al., 1994). C-reactive protein, in particular, has been widely studied in the general population and its associations with subsequent CVD events have been observed in several populations (Koenig et al., 1999; Ridker et al., 1997, 2000; Folsom et al., 2002). Other inflammatory biomarkers for atherosclerosis include serum amyloid A, IL-6 and cell adhesion molecules.

Ross (1999) proposed the hypothesis that atherosclerosis is a process that develops in the artery wall in response to injury. He described the atherosclerotic plaque as resembling a healing inflammatory lesion. It seems that this process starts with damage to endothelial cells and possible causes of endothelial dysfunction include smoking, hypertension, diabetes, elevated homocysteine concentrations, infection and high levels of LDL modified by oxidation. This endothelial dysfunction causes the endothelial cells to become permeable to inflammatory cells, to become procoagulant and to release inflammatory cytokines and vasoactive factors. Cellular adhesion molecules (CAM), P-selectin and E-selectin, encourage transport of leukocytes along the endothelium and vascular adhesion molecule-1 (VCAM-1) and intracellular adhesion molecule-1 (ICAM-1) enable leukocyte attachment to the endothelium (Blake and Ridker, 2002).

These leukocytes then migrate through the endothelial cell layer, attracted by monocyte chemotactic protein-1 (MCP-1), into the sub-endothelial space. Monocytes are converted to macrophage foam cells, which take up oxidised LDL. The leukocytes in the subendothelial space contribute to the local inflammatory response by secreting interleukin-1 (IL-1) and TNFα. This leads to stimulation and migration of smooth muscle cells into the intima. Smooth muscle cells produce interleukin-6 which is one of the main stimulants for CRP production. These processes lead to increases in the arterial intima media thickness

(IMT) and enlargement of the atherosclerotic plaque. With time the plaque can develop into a complicated lesion with a core of lipid and necrotic tissue covered by a fibrous tissue plaque.

CRP is an acute phase response protein and is usually produced in the liver in response to an elevation in IL-6 levels. It was previously thought that CRP levels were increased by acting as a downstream marker of the inflammatory cascade associated with development and progression of the atherosclerotic lesion (Rosenson and Koenig, 2002). However, recent evidence has turned this theory around and it has now been suggested that CRP may be directly involved in atherogenesis and that atherosclerotic plaques can produce CRP independent of hepatic production (Blake and Ridker, 2002). It is thought that CRP causes expression of CAMs (E-selectin, P-selectin, ICAM-1 and VCAM-1) on the vascular endothelium. Levels of the protein, MCP-1, are increased by CRP. CRP binds to receptors on smooth muscle cells to activate complement and also stimulates LDL-cholesterol uptake by macrophages to form foam cells that expand the atherosclerotic lesion. Fig. 1 illustrates the effects of CRP at the vascular wall. It seems that smooth muscle cells and macrophages in atherosclerotic arteries can produce CRP and that this production is not solely dependant on hepatic production (Yasojima et al., 2001).

In RA markers of inflammation, including CRP, have been shown to be predictors of persistent joint disease (Aman et al., 2000) and progressive radiological damage in early RA (Jansen et al., 2001; Listing et al., 2000). However, CRP measurement at baseline may not reflect the long-term burden of disease activity in RA. Several researchers have shown that it is the sustained inflammation over a prolonged period of time that is associated with both radiological (Plant et al., 2000) and disability outcomes (Devlin et al., 1997) in RA. Inflammatory markers have been examined as potential predictors of mortality and cardiovascular events in established populations of RA patients. Wållberg-Jonsson et al. (1999) found that baseline ESR did not predict CVD events or mortality in a retrospectively examined cohort of seropositive RA patients, but that ESR measurements were increased in the period prior to CVD events occurring. Chehata reported that individual measures of disease activity were poor predictors of mortality outcome in RA. However, sustained inflammation, measured serially using a

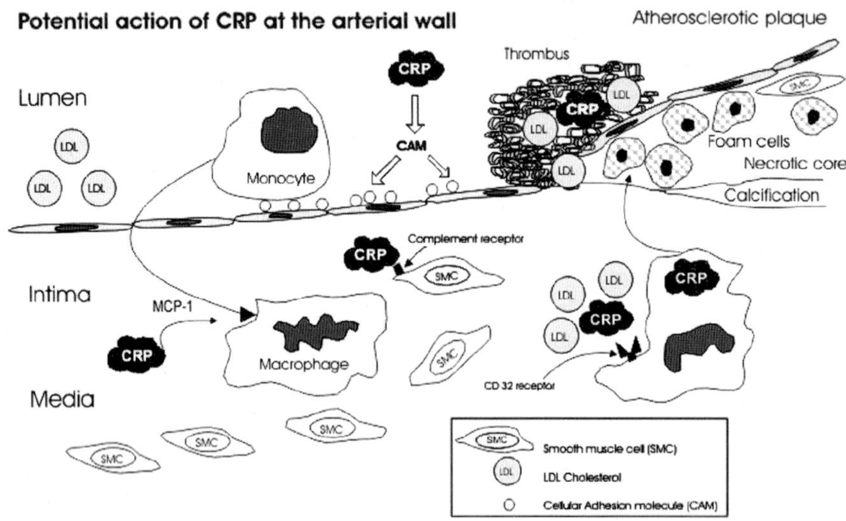

Figure 1. Actions of CRP at the vessel wall. CRP seems to be produced by smooth muscle cells and macrophages and has direct inflammatory effects on endothelial cells leading to expression of CAMs, IL6 and endothelin-1 (Pasceri et al., 2000). It also mediates monocyte chemoattractant protein-1 production and uptake of LDL by macrophages. CRP binds to complement receptors on smooth muscle cells and damaged cell membranes to release complement (Rosenson and Koenig, 2002).

composite disease activity score, was a strong predictor of all-cause mortality in established RA (Chehata et al., 2001). Baseline CRP has not been reported to be a predictor of CVD events in RA populations.

This previously reported research suggests that it is the sustained inflammation that is associated with adverse outcome and mortality in RA. It is possible that this systemic chronic inflammatory burden promotes atherosclerosis in RA patients.

CAMs, including E-selectin, P-selectin, ICAM-1 and VCAM-1, are proteins expressed on endothelial membranes in response to inflammation. They are found in atherosclerotic plaques and have been shown to be predictors of subsequent CVD events. In particular VCAM-1 seems to be a predictor of events in patients with known CVD whilst ICAM-1 is an independent predictor of primary CVD events in healthy individuals (Magliano et al., 2003). Patients with RA have increased levels of these soluble adhesion molecules and this suggests that continued endothelial activation occurs in RA. We know that activation of the vascular endothelium leads to the development of endothelial dysfunction and is one of the first steps in the pathogenesis of atherosclerosis (Bonetti et al., 2003). Inflammation and other cardiovascular risk factors appear to promote endothelial dysfunction in RA (Bacon et al., 2002). In vivo tests of vascular function have detected evidence of endothelial damage in RA patients (Van Doornum et al., 2003) and it seems that endothelial dysfunction develops early in the rheumatoid disease process (Bergholm et al., 2002). Interestingly endothelial dysfunction improves with treatment to suppress inflammation (Raza et al., 2000) and in particular tumour necrosis factor (TNF)-α antagonists have been shown to improve endothelial function in RA (Hurlimann et al., 2002).

3.4. Clinical presentation

CHD encompasses a broad spectrum of clinical manifestations including angina, myocardial infarction, congestive heart failure from coronary artery ischaemia, and sudden death. Many people with coronary artery disease have clinically silent disease without typical cardiac symptoms. Silent IHD may affect 2–6% of the general population (Lochen, 1992; Nalbantgil et al., 1998) and is more prevalent in people with diabetes (May et al., 1997) and hypertension (Lochen, 1992). The prevalence of silent IHD may also be increased in patients with RA. There have been two studies that have reported higher rates of silent ischaemia in RA populations compared to controls. Wislowska et al. (1998) performed non-invasive CVD assessments including echocardiography and ECG monitoring on a group of RA cases and controls all of whom were free from 'physician-diagnosed' CVD or hypertension. This study revealed that RA patients were more likely to experience ischaemic episodes diagnosed using ambulatory ECG monitoring than were controls. Of particular interest was the finding that in many cases these ischaemic episodes were not associated with typical angina symptoms suggesting an increased frequency of silent CVD. Banks et al. (1998) reported that 25% of a clinic-based RA cohort had clinically silent IHD detected using adenosine-stressed myocardial perfusion scanning. Thus if CVD in RA has a tendency to remain clinically silent it is likely that the increased incidence of CVD events reported by several studies, actually represents an underestimation of the comorbid CVD burden in these patients.

3.5. Diagnostic investigations

The presence and degree of severity of CHD can be assessed using many different diagnostic investigations. Investigation needs to be tailored to the individual patient and their stage of CVD. In the general population exercise ECG testing is a helpful functional tool for detecting and evaluating IHD. However, this investigation requires a degree of physical mobility that many RA patients are unable to achieve. Therefore ambulatory ECG monitoring may be a useful adjunct for detecting underlying CVD ischaemia in the RA patient. Alternatively the myocardium can be stressed using pharmacological agents to provoke ischaemia. Myocardial perfusion can then be assessed using single photon emission computerised tomography (SPECT) scanning after an intravenous injection of radiolabelled pharmaceutical. This test also provides information about the location and extent of myocardial ischaemia. Stress echocardiography can also be used to identify ventricular dysfunction induced by myocardial ischaemia and has been shown to have a similar sensitivity to myocardial perfusion scanning. Stress echocardiography also provides information about left ventricular function and valve abnormalities. Coronary artery imaging allows confirmation of the presence, extent and position of atheromatous lesions. This is essential for planning interventions. However, traditional coronary artery angiography is a relatively high-risk procedure. More recently other imaging modalities including magnetic resonance angiography (MRA) and computerised tomography angiography (CTA) have been developed to allow imaging of the coronary arteries (Gaylord, 2002). These modalities as well as being less invasive may allow better imaging of the atheromatous lesions and vessel wall in CAD than conventional coronary arteriography. Coronary calcification detected using CT scanning has also been shown to be a marker of underlying coronary artery disease in the general population. Other techniques that have recently been developed include intravascular ultrasound (Boersma et al., 2003) and contrast enhanced echocardiography (Ward and Lang, 2002). These tests enable the character of atherosclerotic lesions to be determined by detecting vulnerable macrophage laden atherosclerotic lesions that are prone to rupture. However, these recent advances in coronary artery imaging are not currently widely used in clinical practice.

Another non-invasive CVD imaging investigation is the measurement of carotid IMT using ultrasound. This has been shown to be a surrogate marker of CHD in several population-based studies (Sinha et al., 2002). Several studies have reported higher carotid IMT measurements in RA patients compared to controls (Kumeda et al., 2002; Park et al., 2002a; Rodriguez et al., 2002) and one study has reported higher carotid IMTs in association with dyslipidaemia in established RA patients compared to control patients (Wållberg-Jonsson et al., 2001). Trials have shown that treatment of dyslipidaemia retards the progression of IMT (Salonen et al., 1995) and it may be that screening high-risk patients for sub-clinical CVD would allow interventions to prevent progression of atherosclerosis.

Functional measures of endothelial dysfunction including brachial artery flow mediated dilatation and pulse wave analysis have been shown to be abnormal in RA patients (Van Doornum et al., 2003).

It is important to assess and treat classical cardiovascular risk factors in RA populations. Investigations include assessment of established CVD risk factors with the measurement of the fasting lipid profile including levels of HDL, LDL and triglycerides. Measurement of plasma glucose concentration to exclude diabetes is important. Current guidelines recommend use of composite CVD risk assessments that are based on the Framingham risk algorithm (Grundy et al., 1999) to guide primary prevention interventions. However, it is not known whether these risk assessments are appropriate for guiding intervention in RA patients.

There is evidence that the emerging thrombotic and inflammatory CVD risk factors may be independent predictors of CVD events in the general population. In particular, high-sensitivity CRP has been shown to be a stronger predictor of CVD events than LDL cholesterol and contributes prognostic information to the calculated Framingham CVD risk score (Ridker, 2003a). However, it is not clear whether CRP measurement contributes to CVD risk prediction in patients with known inflammatory conditions such as RA and further study is required to evaluate whether screening and treatment of emerging CVD risk factors leads to a reduction in CVD risk in RA patients.

Inflammatory markers have also been shown to be short-term predictors of adverse outcomes from acute coronary syndromes. An elevated CRP recorded at the time of presentation to hospital with chest pain was a strong diagnostic predictor of subsequent adverse CVD events (Magadle et al., 2002) and both CRP and serum amyloid A predicted adverse outcomes, including myocardial infarction and death, in patients with unstable angina (Liuzzo et al., 1994). Again it is difficult to assess the role of inflammatory markers as prognostic markers of outcome in patients with co-existent inflammatory conditions.

Investigations in the acute setting to diagnose myocardial infarction include measurement of serum creatine kinase-MB (CK-MB) as well as recording serial ECGs. However, CK-MB is not a sensitive marker of myocardial damage and measurement of cardiac troponin-T and I are now used in clinical practice to determine myocardial damage. These are highly sensitive and specific for myocardial damage. However, it must be noted that the presence of rheumatoid factor in the serum can lead to false positive troponin assay results (Bas et al., 2002; Dasgupta et al., 1999).

3.6. Treatment

It is not clear whether therapy used in the treatment of RA has a beneficial or detrimental effect on atherosclerosis. Many RA treatments have the potential to cause adverse side effects that could exacerbate CVD (Table 6). However, adequate disease suppression may actually reduce the risk of atherosclerosis by controlling inflammation.

3.6.1. Non-steroidal anti-inflammatory drugs

NSAIDs have been used to treat the symptoms of RA for many years. However, more recently the use of selective cyclooxygenase-2 inhibitors has become more widespread. Both traditional non-selective NSAIDs and selective COX-2 inhibitors are known to cause elevations in blood pressure through their effects on renal prostaglandins (Baigent and Patrono, 2003). They also lead to reduction in the glomerular filtration rate, which can exacerbate existing heart failure by causing fluid retention (FitzGerald and Patrono, 2001). Traditional NSAIDs inhibit both COX-1 and COX-2 and it is thought that inhibiting platelet COX-1 activity leads to a reduction in platelet aggregatability through inhibition of thromboxane A_2. This anti-platelet effect may prevent arterial thrombotic events and there are several reports that Naproxen, in particular, may have cardioprotective effects through its more persistent inhibition of platelet thromboxane A_2 (Solomon and Avorn, 2003; Watson et al., 2002). Ibuprofen appears to block the anti-platelet effect of aspirin and therefore should not be co-prescribed (Catella-Lawson et al., 2001). It is not clear whether specific COX-2 inhibitors are protective or have detrimental effects on the cardiovascular system. The VIGOR study reported an excess of myocardial infarction in the group of patients treated with rofecoxib (Bombardier et al., 2000). However, in this study, the comparison group was treated with Naproxen which has anti-platelet effects that may have provided this group with cardioprotection. Other studies comparing COX-2 inhibitors with other NSAIDS did not report increased risks of CVD events (Silverstein et al., 2000). There have also been concerns that selective COX-2 inhibitors may promote CVD through suppression of endothelial-derived prostacyclin. However, a study in healthy individuals found that selective COX-2 blockade did not result in significant impairment in endothelial function (Verma et al., 2001).

The role of corticosteroids in promoting CVD is controversial. The side effects of high-dose steroids are widely reported and include impaired glucose tolerance, hyperlipidaemia, obesity and hypertension all of which may potentially promote CVD. However, a Swedish study of seropositive RA patients reported that steroid usage did not predict CVD events or death (Wållberg-Jonsson et al., 1997). Another study found that steroid treatment combined with DMARD therapy actually resulted in an improved total/HDL cholesterol ratio in RA patients (Nurmohamed et al., 2002). These findings suggest that corticosteroid usage in RA patients could have a beneficial effect

Table 6
Potential cardiovascular side effects observed with RA medications

Medication	Potential CVD side effects
Conventional NSAIDS	Fluid retention Hypertension
Selective COX-2 inhibitors	Fluid retention Hypertension ?Prothrombotic
Steroids	?Dyslipidaemia Hyperglycaemia Hypertension
Gold	Increase LDL and HDL cholesterol
Sulphasalazine	?Hyperhomocysteineaemia
Leflunomide	Hypertension
Cyclosporin	Hypertension Dyslipidaemia
Methotrexate	Hyperhomocysteinaemia
Tumour necrosis factor α antagonists	?Exacerbate heart failure

on the cardiovascular system that may be the result of effective inflammatory disease suppression.

DMARDs also have the potential to modify CVD risk factors. Methotrexate can cause elevation in plasma homocysteine through its anti-folate actions and this has been described in RA cohorts (Haagsma et al., 1999; van Ede et al., 2002). The use of folic acid supplementation with methotrexate has been shown to prevent increases in homocysteine concentrations in RA patients (Jansen et al., 2001; Morgan et al., 1998; van Ede et al., 2002). Landewe reported that RA patients with known CVD had increased mortality if they were treated with methotrexate (Landewe et al., 2000). However, studies have also shown that methotrexate usage is associated with improved survival in RA patients (Krause and Rau, 2000) and in another study the risk of CVD death was reduced in methotrexate-treated RA patients (Choi et al., 2002). Methotrexate may reduce CVD mortality by reducing inflammation. However, supplementation with folic acid is advised to prevent increased homocysteine concentrations (Slot, 2001).

Both Leflunamide (Alldred and Emery, 2001) and cyclosporin can cause drug-induced hypertension in RA patients (Taler et al., 1999) and in addition, cyclosporin has been shown to cause dyslipidaemia in patients with transplants (Hilbrands et al., 1995). Other traditional DMARDs including Gold may also cause deterioration in lipid profiles of patients. However, hydroxychloroquine has been shown to have several potential cardio-protective effects including improving lipid profiles in RA patients (Munro et al., 1997; Wallace et al., 1990) and anti-platelet effects (Nosal' et al., 2000). Conversely there are a small number of case reports of chloroquine-induced cardiomyopathy (Roos et al., 2002; Stein et al., 2000) but this appears to be a very rare side effect.

Little is known about the effects of the biologic agents on the cardiovascular system in RA. One study has suggested that endothelial function, in active RA, may be improved by biologic therapy (Hurlimann et al., 2002). Studies have shown that non-RA patients with heart failure have elevated levels of TNFα and it has been suggested that anti-TNFα therapy may be an effective treatment for cardiac failure. However, two large randomised drug trials, examining the effects of Etanercept and Infliximab on heart failure, failed to show efficacy of these treatments. The trial using Infliximab also reported a significant excess of deaths in the high-dose Infliximab treatment arm (Anker and Coats, 2002). It is not clear whether these treatments will exacerbate heart failure in RA patients. However, current guidelines advise against the use of Infliximab in patients with congestive heart failure (Mikuls and Moreland, 2003). It is not clear whether these biological agents will improve the cardiovascular mortality outcomes in RA patients.

3.6.2. Treatment of CVD in RA

The cause of the increased CVD risk in RA is likely to be due to a combination of many factors including the effects of the inflammatory disease process and its treatment. Further research is required to investigate why RA patients die earlier from CVD to allow identification of interventions that will improve survival in these patients. The recognition that the RA patient is at high risk of CVD will encourage screening and treatment of CVD risk factors. It may also influence investigation of underlying CVD in these patients. In the first instance lifestyle advice should be given to all RA patients to encourage smoking cessation, dietary modification and to encourage weight control and exercise. However, this advice has been shown in clinical practice to induce only modest improvements in lifestyle risk factors (Gordon et al., 2002). In addition regular blood pressure monitoring and treatment of hypertension along with screening and treatment of hyperlipidaemia would seem sensible. Current guidelines for the general population recommend the use of composite CVD risk assessments, based on the Framingham CVD risk algorithm, to direct primary CVD prevention (1998). However, it is not known how applicable these assessments are in patients with RA as inflammation can lead to reductions in plasma cholesterol. Interestingly there is evidence that statins, used to treat hypercholesterolaemia, also have anti-inflammatory effects (Albert et al., 2001; Kent et al., 2003). They have been found to reduce CVD events in patients with elevated CRP concentrations even in the absence of hyperlipidaemia (Ridker et al., 2002; Ridker, 2003b). If inflammation in RA lowers plasma cholesterol, but promotes atherosclerosis, a drug that reduces inflammation and prevents CVD events in patients with 'normal' serum cholesterol might be very beneficial in the prevention and treatment of CHD in RA patients. Statins have also been shown, by lipid-independent mechanisms, to improve endothelial dysfunction. Other pharmaceutical interventions that improve the function of the endothelium include use of angiotensin converting enzyme (ACE) inhibitors, folic acid and anti-oxidants (Bonetti et al., 2003). It may be that reversing endothelial dysfunction with these interventions will lead to more favourable CVD outcomes. Further research is required to investigate whether these therapeutic strategies will reduce CVD in patients with inflammatory RA.

Key points

- RA patients have increased mortality.
- Much of this excess mortality is from CVD.
- IHD rather than rheumatoid heart disease seems to be responsible for this increased CVD mortality.
- CVD has a tendency to remain clinically silent in RA patients.
- Traditional CVD risk factors do not explain increased IHD events in RA.
- Emerging risk factors including inflammatory disease and homocysteine may be responsible for promoting IHD in RA patients.
- RA patients should be considered as being at high risk of IHD.
- Screening and treatment of CVD risk factors and underlying IHD should be considered when managing these patients.

References

Ahern, M., Lever, J.V., Cosh, J. 1983. Complete heart block in rheumatoid arthritis. Ann. Rheum. Dis. 42 (4), 389–397.

Albada-Kuipers, G.A., Bruijn, J.A., Westedt, M.L., et al. 1986. Coronary arteritis complicating rheumatoid arthritis. Ann. Rheum. Dis. 45 (11), 963–965.

Albert, M.A., Danielson, E., Rifai, N., et al. 2001. Effect of statin therapy on C-reactive protein levels: the pravastatin inflammation/CRP evaluation (PRINCE): a randomized trial and cohort study. JAMA 286 (1), 64–70.

Alldred, A., Emery, P. 2001. Leflunomide: a novel DMARD for the treatment of rheumatoid arthritis. Expert Opin. Pharmacother. 2 (1), 125–137.

Allebeck, P., Ahlbom, A., Allander, E. 1981. Increased mortality among persons with rheumatoid arthritis, but where RA does not appear on death certificate. Eleven-year follow-up of an epidemiological study. Scand. J. Rheumatol. 10 (4), 301–306.

Aman, S., Paimela, L., Leirisalo-Repo, M., et al. 2000. Prediction of disease progression in early rheumatoid arthritis by ICTP, RF and CRP. A comparative 3-year follow-up study. Rheumatology 39 (9), 1009–1013.

Anker, S.D., Coats, A.J. 2002. How to RECOVER from RENAISSANCE? The significance of the results of RECOVER, RENAISSANCE, RENEWAL and ATTACH. Int. J. Cardiol. 86 (2–3), 123–130.

Asanuma, Y., Mizushima, Y. 1999. Serum lipoprotein (a) and apolipoprotein (a) phenotypes in patients with rheumatoid arthritis. Arthritis Rheum. 42, 443–447.

Austin, M.A. 2000. Triglyceride, small, dense low-density lipoprotein, and the atherogenic lipoprotein phenotype. Curr. Atheroscler. Rep. 2 (3), 200–207.

Bacon, P.A., Gibson, D.G. 1974. Cardiac involvement in rheumatoid arthritis. An echocardiographic study. Ann. Rheum. Dis. 33 (1), 20–24.

Bacon, P.A., Raza, K., Banks, M., et al. 2002. The role of endothelial cell dysfunction in the cardiovascular mortality of RA. Int. Rev. Immunol. 21 (1), 1–17.

Baigent, C., Patrono, C. 2003. Selective cyclooxygenase 2 inhibitors, aspirin, and cardiovascular disease: a reappraisal. Arthritis Rheum. 48 (1), 12–20.
Review article appraising the effects of different NSAIDs on the cardiovascular system.

Banks, M., Flint, J., Bacon, P.A., et al. 2000. Rheumatoid arthritis is an independent risk factor for ischaemic heart disease. Arthritis Rheum. 43 (9), 1909.
Study using myocardial perfusion scanning and clinical assessments of IHD in a group of RA patients revealed a high prevalence of IHD but much was clinically silent.

Bas, S., Genevay, S., Mensi, N. 2002. False positive elevation of cardiac troponin I in seropositive rheumatoid arthritis. J. Rheumatol. 29 (12), 2665.

Bely, M., Apathy, A., Beke-Martos, E. 1992. Cardiac changes in rheumatoid arthritis. Acta Morphol. Hung. 40 (1–4), 149–186.

Bergholm, R., Leirisalo-Repo, M., Vehkavaara, S., et al. 2002. Impaired responsiveness to NO in newly diagnosed patients with rheumatoid arthritis. Arterioscler. Thromb. Vasc. Biol. 22 (10), 1637–1641.

Berkanovic, E., Hurwicz, M. 1990. Rheumatoid arthritis and comorbidity. J. Rheumatol. 17, 888–892.

Berliner, J. 2002. Introduction. Lipid oxidation products and atherosclerosis. Vasc. Pharmacol. 38 (4), 187–191.

Bjornadal, L., Baecklund, E., Yin, et al. 2002. Decreasing mortality in patients with rheumatoid arthritis: Results from a large population based cohort in Sweden, 1964–95. J. Rheumatol. 29 (5), 906–912.

Blake, G.J., Ridker, P.M. 2001. Novel clinical markers of vascular wall inflammation. Circ. Res. 89 (9), 763–771.

Blake, G.J., Ridker, P.M. 2002. Inflammatory bio-markers and cardiovascular risk prediction. J. Int. Med. 252 (4), 283–294.
Recent review of emerging inflammatory CVD risk factors and their mechanisms.

Boersma, E., Mercado, N., Poldermans, D., et al. 2003. Acute myocardial infarction. Lancet 361 (9360), 847–858.

Bombardier, C., Laine, L., Reicin, A., et al. 2000. Comparison of upper gastrointestinal toxicity of rofecoxib and naproxen in patients with rheumatoid arthritis. VIGOR Study Group. N. Engl. J. Med. 343 (21), 1520–1528.

Bonetti, P.O., Lerman, L.O., Lerman, A. 2003. Endothelial dysfunction: a marker of atherosclerotic risk. Arterioscler. Thromb. Vasc. Biol. 23 (2), 168–175.

Bonfiglio, T., Atwater, E.C. 1969. Heart disease in patients with seropositive rheumatoid arthritis; a controlled autopsy study and review. Arch. Int. Med. 124 (6), 714–719.

Booth, G.L., Wang, X.L. 2000. Preventative health care, 2000 update: screening and management of hyperhomocysteinemia for the prevention of coronary artery disease events. Can. Med. Assoc. J. 163 (1), 21–29.

Breen, J. 2001. Imaging of the pericardium. J. Thora. Imag. 16, 47–54.

Callahan, L.F., Cordray, D.S., Wells, G., et al. 1996. Formal education and five-year mortality in rheumatoid arthritis: mediation by helplessness scale score. Arthritis Care Res. 9 (6), 463–472.

Carmona, L., Balsa, A., Gonzalez-Alvaro, I., et al. 2002. Decreased prevalence of diabetes in rheumatoid arthritis patients compared to the general population after standardisation by age. Rheumatology 41, S71.

Catella-Lawson, F., Reilly, M.P., Kapoor, S.C., et al. 2001. Cyclooxygenase inhibitors and the antiplatelet effects of aspirin. N. Engl. J. Med. 345 (25), 1809–1817.
Study identified the potential for ibuprofen to reduce the antiplatelet effects of aspirin.

Cathcart, E.S., Spodick, D. 1962. Rheumatoid heart disease. N. Engl. J. Med. 266, 959–964.

Chand, E.M., Freant, L.J., Rubin, J.W. 1999. Aortic valve rheumatoid nodules producing clinical aortic regurgitation and a review of the literature. Cardiovasc. Pathol. 8 (6), 333–338.

Chapman, M.J., Guerin, M., Bruckert, E. 1998. Atherogenic, dense low-density lipoproteins. Pathophysiology and new therapeutic approaches. Eur. Heart J. 19, Suppl-30.

Charcot, J.M. 1881. Clinical Lectures on Senile and Chronic Disease. New Syddenham Society, London, p. 95.

Chehata, J.C., Hassell, A.B., Clarke, S.A., et al. 2001. Mortality in rheumatoid arthritis: relationship to single and composite measures of disease activity. Rheumatology (Oxford) 40 (4), 447–452.

Choi, H.K., Hernan, M.A., Seeger, J.D., et al. 2002. Methotrexate and mortality in patients with rheumatoid arthritis: a prospective study. Lancet 359 (9313), 1173–1177.

Cisternas, M., Gutierrez, M.A., Klaassen, et al. 2002. Cardiovascular risk factors in Chilean patients with rheumatoid arthritis. J. Rheumatol. 29 (8), 1619–1622.

Coste, J., Jougla, E. 1994. Mortality from rheumatoid arthritis in France, 1970–1990. Int. J. Epidemiol. 23 (3), 545–552.

Criswell, L.A., Merlino, L.A., Cerhan, J., et al. 2002. Cigarette smoking and the risk of rheumatoid arthritis among postmenopausal women: results from the Iowa Women's Health Study. Am. J. Med. 112 (6), 465–471.

Curtis, B.M., O'Keefe, J.H. Jr. 2002. Autonomic tone as a cardiovascular risk factor: the dangers of chronic fight or flight. Mayo Clinic Proc. 77 (1), 45–54.

Dai, L., Lamb, D.J., Leake, D.S., et al. 2000. Evidence for oxidised low density lipoprotein in synovial fluid from rheumatoid arthritis patients. Free Radical Res. 32 (6), 479–486.

Danesh, J., Collins, R., Appleby, P., Peto, R., 1998. Association of C-reactive protein, albumin, or leukocyte count with coronary heart disease: meta-analyses of prospective studies. JAMA 279 (18), 1477–1482.

Dasgupta, A., Banerjee, S.K., Datta, P. 1999. False-positive troponin I in the MEIA due to the presence of rheumatoid factors in serum—elimination of this interference by using a polyclonal antisera against rheumatoid factors. Am. J. Clin. Pathol. 112 (6), 753–756.

Dawber, T. 1980. The Framingham Study: The Epidemiology of Atherosclerotic Disease. Harvard University Press, Cambridge, MA.

Dawson, J.K., Goodson, N.G., Graham, D., et al. 2000. Raised pulmonary artery pressures measured with Doppler echocardiography in rheumatoid arthritis patients. Rheumatology 39 (12), 1320–1325.

del Rincon, I.D., Williams, K., Stern, M.P., et al. 2001. High incidence of cardiovascular events in a rheumatoid arthritis cohort not explained by traditional cardiac risk factors. Arthritis Rheum. 44 (12), 2737–2745.
Increased CVD events were identified in RA patients compared to control population. The prevalence of traditional CVD risk factors did not explain this excess.

Dessein, P.H., Joffe, B.I., Stanwix, A., et al. 2002. The acute phase response does not fully predict the presence of insulin resistance and dyslipidemia in inflammatory arthritis. J. Rheumatol. 29 (3), 462–466.

Devlin, J., Gough, A., Huissoon, A., et al. 1997. The acute phase and function in early rheumatoid arthritis. C-reactive protein levels correlate with functional outcome. J. Rheumatol. 24 (1), 9–13.

Doran, M.F., Pond, G.R., Crowson, C.S., et al. 2002. Trends in incidence and mortality in rheumatoid arthritis in Rochester, Minnesota, over a forty-year period. Arthritis Rheum. 46 (3), 625–631.
The incidence of RA reduced during this study. But mortality rates remained increased in RA patients compared to the general population.

Erb, N., Banks, M., Rowe, I.F.D., et al. 2001. Classical risk factors for ischaemic heart disease (IHD) and their modification in patients with rheumatoid arthritis (RA). Arthritis Rheum. 44 (9), S59.

Ernst, E., Resch, K. 1993. Fibrinogen as a cardiovascular risk factor: a meta-analysis. Ann. Intern. Med. 118, 956–963.

Fernandez-Muixi, J., Vidal, F., Bardaji, A., et al. 1994. Recurrent pericarditis and cardiac tamponade in rheumatoid arthritis: effectiveness of colchicine. Br. J. Rheumatol. 33 (6), 596–597.

FitzGerald, G.A., Patrono, C. 2001. The coxibs, selective inhibitors of cyclooxygenase-2. N. Engl. J. Med. 345 (6), 433–442.

Folsom, A.R., Aleksic, N., Catellier, D., et al. 2002. C-Reactive protein and incident coronary heart disease in the Atherosclerosis Risk In Communities (ARIC) study. Am. Heart J. 144 (2), 233–238.

Frishman, W.H. 2002. Effects of nonsteroidal anti-inflammatory drug therapy on blood pressure and peripheral edema. Am. J. Cardiol. 89 (6), 18–25.

Gabriel, S., Crowson, C., O'Fallon, M. 1999a. Comorbidity in arthritis. J. Rheumatol. 26, 2475–2479.

Gabriel, S.E., Crowson, C.S., O'Fallon, W.M. 1999b. Mortality in rheumatoid arthritis: have we made an impact in 4 decades? J. Rheumatol. 26 (12), 2529–2533.

Gabriel, S.E., Crowson, C.S., Kremers, H., et al. 2003. Survival in rheumatoid arthritis: a population-based analysis of trends over 40 years. Arthritis Rheum. 48, 54–58.

Garnero, A., Fasciolo, D., Accardo, S., Seriolo, B. 1999. Cardiac risk factors in patients with rheumatoid arthritis. Ann. Rheum. Dis. (Suppl.), 69–70, abstract.

Gaylord, G.M. 2002. Computed tomographic and magnetic resonance coronary angiography: are you ready? Radiol. Mgmt 24 (4), 16–20.

Goldeli, O., Dursun, E., Komsuoglu, B. 1998. Dispersion of ventricular repolarization: a new marker of ventricular arrhythmias in patients with rheumatoid arthritis. J. Rheumatol. 25 (3), 447–450.

Goodson, N.J., Pattison, D.J., Lunt, M., et al. 2002a. Cardiovascular risk factors are not increased prior to the onset of inflammatory polyarthritis. Rheumatology (Oxford) 41, 9, no. abstracts supplement.

Goodson, N.J., Wiles, N.J., Lunt, M., et al. 2002b. Mortality in early inflammatory polyarthritis: cardiovascular mortality is increased in seropositive patients. Arthritis Rheum. 46 (8), 2010–2019.

Gordon, D.A., Stein, J.L., Broder, I. 1973. The extra-articular features of rheumatoid arthritis: a systematic analysis of 127 cases. Am. J. Med. 54, 445–452.

Gordon, M.M., Thomson, E.A., Madhok, R., et al. 2002. Can intervention modify adverse lifestyle variables in a rheumatoid population? Results of a pilot study. Ann. Rheum. Dis. 61 (1), 66–69.

Goyle, K.K., Walling, A.D. 2002. Diagnosing pericarditis. Am. Family Phys. 66 (9), 1695–1702.

Grundy, S., Pasternak, R., Greenland, P., et al. 1999. Assessment of cardiovascular risk by use of multiple-risk-factor assessment equations: a statement for healthcare professionals from the American Heart Association and the American college of cardiology. Circulation 100, 1481–1492.

Guedes, C., Bianchi-Fior, P., Cormier, B., et al. 2001. Cardiac manifestations of rheumatoid arthritis: a case-control transesophageal echocardiography study in 30 patients. Arthritis Rheum. 45 (2), 129–135.

Haagsma, C.J., Blom, H.J., van-Riel, P.L.C.M., et al. 1999. Influence of sulphasalazine, methotrexate, and the combination of both on plasma homocysteine concentrations in patients with rheumatoid arthritis. Ann. Rheum. Dis. 58, 79–84.

Hara, K.S., Ballard, D.J., Ilstrup, D., et al. 1990. Rheumatoid pericarditis: clinical features and survival. Medicine 69 (2), 81–91.
Follow up study of 41 RA patients presenting with pericarditis. Describes clinical presentation and outcomes.

Heliövaara, M., Aho, K., Aromaa, A. 1993. Smoking as a risk of rheumatoid arthritis. J. Rheumatol. 20, 1830–1835.

Heliövaara, M., Aho, K., Knekt, P., Reunanen, A., Aromaa, A. 1996. Serum cholesterol and risk of rheumatoid arthritis in a cohort of 52800 men and women. Br. J. Rheumatol. 35, 255–257.

Heller, R.F., Chinn, S., Tunstall-Pedoe, H., et al. 1984. How well can we predict coronary heart disease? BMJ 288, 410–411.

Hennekens, C.H., Buring, J.E. 1987. Epidemiology in Medicine, first ed. Little, Brown and Company, Boston/Toronto.

Hilbrands, L.B., Demacker, P.N., Hoitsma, A., et al. 1995. The effects of cyclosporine and prednisone on serum lipid and (apo)lipoprotein levels in renal transplant recipients. J. Am. Soc. Nephrol. 5 (12), 2073–2081.

Hurlimann, D., Forster, A., Noll, G., et al. 2002. Anti-tumor necrosis factor-alpha treatment improves endothelial function in patients with rheumatoid arthritis. Circulation 106 (17), 2184–2187.

Hurt-Camejo, E., Paredes, S., Masana, L., et al. 2001. Elevated levels of small, low-density lipoprotein with high affinity for arterial matrix components in patients with rheumatoid arthritis: possible contribution of phospholipase A2 to this atherogenic profile. Arthritis Rheum. 44 (12), 2761–2767.

Hutchinson, D., Shepstone, L., Moots, R., et al. 2001. Heavy cigarette smoking is strongly associated with rheumatoid arthritis (RA), particularly in patients without a family history of RA. Ann. Rheum. Dis. 60 (3), 223–227.
Increasing amount of cigarette smoking is associated with increased odds of having RA.

Ichikawa, Y., Yamada, C., Horiki, T., et al. 1998. Serum matrix metalloproteinase-3 and fibrin degradation product levels correlate with clinical disease activity in rheumatoid arthritis. Clin. Exp. Rheumatol. 16 (5), 533–540.

Jacobsson, L.T.H., Knowler, W.C., Pillemer, S., et al. 1993. Rheumatoid-arthritis and mortality—a longitudinal-study in Pima-indians. Arthritis Rheum. 36 (8), 1045–1053.

Jansen, L.M., van der Horst-Bruinsma, I.E., Van schaardenburg, D., et al. 2001. Predictors of radiographic joint damage in patients with early rheumatoid arthritis. Ann. Rheum. Dis. 60 (10), 924–927.

Kamper, E.F., Kopeikina, L.T., Trontzas, P., et al. 2000. The effect of disease activity related cytokines on the fibrinolytic potential and cICAM-1 expression in rheumatoid arthritis. J. Rheumatol. 27 (11), 2545–2550.

Kaplan, D., Feldman, J. 1991. A Preliminary study of excess cardiovascular disease in the mothers of patients with RA. Am. J. Epidemiol. 133, 715–720.

Kaplan, M.J., Clune, W.J. 2003. New evidence for vascular disease in patients with early rheumatoid disease. Lancet 316, 1068–1069.

Karlson, E.W., Lee, I.M., Cook, N., et al. 1999. A retrospective cohort study of cigarette smoking and risk of rheumatoid arthritis in female health professionals. Arthritis Rheum. 42 (5), 910–917.

Kent, S.M., Flaherty, P.J., Coyle, L.C., et al. 2003. Effect of atorvastatin and pravastatin on serum C-reactive protein. Am. Heart J. 145 (2), e8.

Koenig, W. 1998. Haemostatic risk factors for cardiovascular diseases. Eur. Heart J. 19 (Suppl. 43).

Koenig, W., Sund, M., Frolich, M., et al. 1999. C-reactive protein, a sensitive marker of inflammation, predicts future risk of coronary heart disease in initially healthy middle-aged men: results from the MONICA (monitoring trends and determinants in cardiovascular disease) Augburg study 1984 to 1992. Circulation 99 (2), 237–242.

Kopeikina, L.T., Kamper, E.F., Koutsoukos, V., et al. 1997. Imbalance of tissue-type plasminogen activator (t-PA) and its specific inhibitor (PAI-1) in patients with rheumatoid arthritis associated with disease activity. Clin. Rheumatol. 16 (3), 254–260.

Koukkunen, H., Penttila, K., Kemppainen, A., et al. 2001. C-reactive protein, fibrinogen, interleukin-6 and tumour necrosis factor-alpha in the prognostic classification of unstable angina pectoris. Ann. Med. 33 (1), 37–47.

Krause, D., Rau, R. 2000. Response to methotrexate treatment is associated with reduced mortality in patients with severe rheumatoid arthritis. Arthritis Rheum. 43, 14–21.

Kroot, E.J.A., van Leeuwen, M.A., van Rijswijk, M.H., et al. 2000. No increased mortality in patients with rheumatoid arthritis: up to 10 years of follow up from disease onset. Ann. Rheum. Dis. 59 (12), 954–958.

Study of survival in RA patients with onset of disease in 1980s–1990s. Suggests an improved mortality outcome in RA over recent years.

Kroot, E.J.A., van Gestel, A.M., Swinkels, H.L., et al. 2001. Chronic comorbidity in patients with early rheumatoid arthritis: a descriptive study. J. Rheumatol. 28 (7), 1511–1517.

Kullo, I., Gau, G., Tajik, A. 2000. Novel risk factors for atherosclerosis. Mayo Clinic Proc. 75, 369–380.

Kumeda, Y., Inaba, M., Goto, H., et al. 2002. Increased thickness of the arterial intima-media detected by ultrasonography in patients with rheumatoid arthritis. Arthritis Rheum. 46 (6), 1489–1497.

Kvalvik, A.G., Jones, M.A., Symmons, D.P.M. 2000. Mortality in a cohort of Norwegian patients with rheumatoid arthritis followed from 1977 to 1992. Scand. J. Rheumatol. 29 (1), 29–37.

Lakatos, J., Harsagyi, A. 1988. Serum total, HDL, LDL cholesterol and triglyceride levels in patients with rheumatoid arthritis. Clin. Biochem. 21, 93–96.

Landewe, R.B., van den Borne, B.E., Breedveld, F.C., et al. 2000. Methotrexate effects in patients with rheumatoid arthritis with cardiovascular comorbidity. Lancet 355 (9215), 1616–1617.

Lazarevic, B., Vitic, J., Mladenovic, V., et al. 1992. Dyslipoproteinemia in the course of active rheumatoid arthritis. Semin. Arthritis Rheum. 22 (3), 172–180.

Leden, I., Eriksson, A., Lilja, B., et al. 1983. Autonomic nerve function in rheumatoid arthritis of varying severity. Scand. J. Rheumatol. 12 (2), 166–170.

Lee, A.J., Fowkes, F.G., Lowe, G.D., et al. 1995. Fibrin D-dimer, haemostatic factors and peripheral arterial disease. Thromb. Haemost. 74 (3), 828–832.

Lee, Y.H., Choi, S.J., Ji, J.D., et al. 2000. Lipoprotein (a) and lipids in relation to inflammation in rheumatoid arthritis. Clin. Rheumatol. 19 (4), 324–325.

Levine, A.J., Dimitri, W.R., Bonser, R.S. 1999. Aortic regurgitation in rheumatoid arthritis necessitating aortic valve replacement. Eur. J. Cardio-Thorac. Surg. 15 (2), 213–214.

Liebowitz, W.B. 1963. The heart in rheumatoid arthritis: a clinical and pathological study of 62 cases. Ann. Int. Med. 58, 102–110.

Lindqvist, E., Eberhardt, K. 1999. Mortality in rheumatoid arthritis patients with disease onset in the 1980s. Ann. Rheum. Dis. 58, 11–14.

Listing, J., Rau, R., Muller, B., et al. 2000. HLA-DRB1 genes, rheumatoid factor, and elevated C-reactive protein: independent risk factors of radiographic progression in early rheumatoid arthritis. Berlin Collaborating Rheumatological Study Group. J. Rheumatol. 27 (9), 2100–2109.

Liuzzo, G., Biasucci, L.M., Gallimore, J.R., Grillo, R.L., Rebuzzi, A.G., Pepys, M.B., Maseri, A. 1994. The prognostic value of C-reactive protein and serum amyloid a protein in severe unstable angina. N. Engl. J. Med. 331 (7), 417–424.

Lochen, M.L. 1992. The Tromso study: the prevalence of exercise-induced silent myocardial ischaemia and relation to risk factors for coronary heart disease in an apparently healthy population. Eur. Heart J. 13 (6), 728–731.

Mackness, B., Davies, G.K., Turkie, W., et al. 2001. Paraoxonase status in coronary heart disease: are activity and concentration more important than genotype? Arterioscler. Thromb. Vasc. Biol. 21 (9), 1451–1457.

Magadle, R., Weiner, P., Beckerman, M., et al. 2002. C-reactive protein as a marker for active coronary artery disease in patients with chest pain in the emergency room. Clin. Cardiol. 25 (10), 456–460.

Magliano, D.J., Liew, D., Ashton, E.L., et al. 2003. Novel biomedical risk markers for cardiovascular disease. J. Cardiovasc. Risk 10 (1), 41–55.

Maione, S., Valentini, G., Giunta, A., et al. 1993. Cardiac involvement in rheumatoid arthritis: an echocardiographic study. Cardiology 83 (4), 234–239.

Manji, H., Raven, P. 1990. Calcific constrictive pericarditis due to rheumatoid arthritis. Postgrad. Med. J. 66 (771), 57–58.

Masdottir, B., Jonsson, T., Manfredsdottir, V., et al. 2000. Smoking, rheumatoid factor iso types and severity of rheumatoid arthritis. Rheumatology 39 (11), 1202–1205.

May, O., Arildsen, H., Damsgaard, E.M., et al. 1997. Prevalence and prediction of silent ischaemia in diabetes mellitus: a population-based study. Cardiovasc. Res. 34 (1), 241–247.

McEntegart, A., Capell, H.A., Duncan, M.R., et al. 1997. Effect of social deprivation on disease severity and outcome in patients with rheumatoid arthritis. Ann. Rheum. Dis. 56, 410–413.

McEntegart, A., Capell, H.A., Creran, D., et al. 2001a. Cardiovascular risk factors, including thrombotic variables, in a population with rheumatoid arthritis. Rheumatology 40 (6), 640–644.

McEntegart, A., Capell, H.A., Madhok, R. 2001b. Predicting coronary risk in rheumatoid arthritis. Arthritis Rheum. 44 (9), s53.

Mikuls, T.R., Moreland, L.W. 2003. Benefit-risk assessment of infliximab in the treatment of rheumatoid arthritis. Drug Safety 26 (1), 23–32.

Mikuls, T.R., Saag, K.G., Criswell, L.A., et al. 2002. Mortality risk associated with rheumatoid arthritis in a prospective cohort of older women: results from the Iowa Women's Health Study. Ann. Rheum. Dis. 61 (11), 994–999.

Mody, G.M., Stevens, J.E., Meyers, O.L. 1987. The heart in rheumatoid arthritis—a clinical and echocardiographic study. QJM 65 (247), 921–928.

Morgan, S.L., Baggott, J.E., Lee, J.Y., et al. 1998. Folic acid supplementation prevents deficient blood folate levels and hyperhomocysteinemia during longterm, low dose methotrexate therapy for rheumatoid arthritis: Implications for cardiovascular disease. J. Rheumatol. 25, 441–446.

Mounet, F., Soula, P., Concina, P., et al. 1997. Specific valvular heart disease of rheumatoid arthritis: two case reports. Arch. Mal. Coeur Vaiss. 90 (7), 987–989.

Munro, R., Morrison, E., McDonald, A.G., et al. 1997. Effect of disease modifying agents on the lipid profiles of patients with rhuematoid arthritis. Ann. Rheum. Dis. 56, 374–377.

Study that revealed a favourable effect of hydroxychloroquine on lipid profiles in RA patients.

Myllykangas-Luosujärvi, R., Aho, K., Kautianen, H., et al. 1995. Cardiovascular mortality in women with rheumatoid arthritis. J. Rheumatol. 22, 1065–1067.

Nalbantgil, I., Onder, R., Nalbantgil, S., et al. 1998. The prevalence of silent myocardial ischaemia in patients with white-coat hypertension. J. Hum. Hypertens. 12 (5), 337–341.

Nomeir, A.M., Turner, R.A., Watts, L.E. 1979. Cardiac involvement in rheumatoid arthritis. Followup study. Arthritis Rheum. 22 (6), 561–564.

Nosal', R., Jancinova, V., Danihelova, E. 2000. Chloroquine: a multipotent inhibitor of human platelets in vitro. Thrombosis Res. 98 (5), 411–421.

Nurmohamed, M.T., van Halm, V.P., Dijkmans, B.A. 2002. Cardiovascular risk profile of antirheumatic agents in patients with osteoarthritis and rheumatoid arthritis. Drugs 62 (11), 1599–1609.

Review of cardiovascular effects of NSAIDs and DMARDs.

Okada, Y., Nakanishi, I., Kajikawa, K., et al. 1983. An autopsy case of rheumatoid arthritis with an involvement of the cardiac conduction system. Jpn. Circ. J. 47 (6), 671–676.

Park, Y.B., Lee, S.K., Lee, W.K., et al. 1999. Lipid profiles in untreated patients with rheumatoid arthritis. J. Rheumatol. 26 (8), 1701–1704.

Park, Y.B., Ahn, C.W., Choi, H.K., et al. 2002a. Atherosclerosis in rheumatoid arthritis: morphologic evidence obtained by carotid ultrasound. Arthritis Rheum. 46 (7), 1714–1719.

Park, Y.B., Choi, H.K., Kim, M.Y., et al. 2002b. Effects of antirheumatic therapy on serum lipid levels in patients with rheumatoid arthritis: a prospective study. Am. J. Med. 113 (3), 188–193.

Payami, H., Khan, M.H., Grennan, D.M., et al. 1987. Analysis of genetic interrelationship among HLA-associated diseases. Am. J. Hum. Genet. 41 (3), 331–349.

Peltomaa, R., Paimela, L., Kautiainen, H., et al. 2002. Mortality in patients with rheumatoid arthritis treated actively from the time of diagnosis. Ann. Rheum. Dis. 61 (10), 889–894.

Pincus, T., Callahan, L.F. 1993. What is the natural history of rheumatoid arthritis. Rheum. Dis. Clin. North Am. 19, 123–146.

Plant, M.J., Williams, A.L., O'Sullivan, M.M., et al. 2000. Relationship between time-integrated C-reactive protein levels and radiologic progression in patients with rheumatoid arthritis. Arthritis Rheum. 43 (7), 1473–1477.

Pradhan, A.D., Manson, J.E., Rossouw, J.E., et al. 2002. Inflammatory biomarkers, hormone replacement therapy, and incident coronary heart disease—prospective analysis from the Women's Health Initiative observational study. JAMA 288 (8), 980–987.

Rantapää-Dahlqvist, S., Wållberg-Jonsson, S., Dahlèn, G. 1991. Lipoprotein (a), lipids, and lipoproteins in patients with rheumatoid arthritis. Ann. Rheum. Dis. 50, 366–368.

Raza, K., Thambyrajah, J., Townend, J.N., et al. 2000. Suppression of inflammation in primary systemic vasculitis restores vascular endothelial function: lessons for atherosclerotic disease? Circulation 102 (13), 1470–1472.

Reckner, O.A., Skogh, T., Wingren, G. 2001. Comorbidity and lifestyle, reproductive factors, and environmental exposures associated with rheumatoid arthritis. Ann. Rheum. Dis. 60 (10), 934–939.

Reilly, P., Cosh, J.A., Maddison, P.J. 1990. Mortality and survival in rheumatoid arthritis: a 25 year study of 100 patients. Ann. Rheum. Dis. 49, 363–369.

Ridker, P.M. 2003a. Clinical application of C-reactive protein for cardiovascular disease detection and prevention. Circulation 107 (3), 363–369.

Ridker, P.M. 2003b. Connecting the role of C-reactive protein and statins in cardiovascular disease. Clin. Cardiol. 26 (4 Suppl. 3), III39–III44.

Ridker, P.M., Cushman, M., Stampher, M.J., et al. 1997. Inflammation, aspirin and the risk of cardiovascular disease in apparently healthy men. N. Engl. J. Med. 336, 973–979.

Ridker, P.M., Manson, J.E., Buring, J.E., et al. 1999. Homocysteine and risk of cardiovascular disease among postmenopausal women. JAMA 281 (19), 1817–1821.

Ridker, P.M., Hennikens, C.H., Buring, J.E., et al. 2000. C-reactive protein and other markers of inflammation in the prediction of cardiovascular disease in women. N. Engl. J. Med. 342, 836–843.

Ridker, P.M., Rifai, N., Rose, L., et al. 2002. Comparison of C-reactive protein and low-density lipoprotein cholesterol levels in the prediction of first cardiovascular events. N. Engl. J. Med. 347 (20), 1557–1565.

C-reactive protein identified as a stronger predictor of CVD events than LDL-cholesterol levels in apparently healthy women.

Riise, T., Jacobsen, B.K., Gran, J.T., et al. 2001. Total mortality is increased in rheumatoid arthritis. A 17-year prospective study. Clin. Rheumatol. 20 (2), 123–127.

Rodriguez, G., Sulli, A., Cutolo, M. 2002. Carotid atherosclerosis in patients with rheumatoid arthritis: a preliminary case-control study. Ann. NY Acad. Sci. 966, 478–482.

Roos, J.M., Aubry, M.C., Edwards, W.D. 2002. Chloroquine cardiotoxicity clinicopathologic features in three patients and comparison with three patients with Fabry disease. Cardiovasc. Pathol. 11 (5), 277–283.

Rose, G.A. 1967. The diagnosis of ischaemic heart pain and intermittent claudication in field studies. Bull. WHO 27, 645–658.

Rosenson, R.S., Koenig, W. 2002. High-sensitivity C-reactive protein and cardiovascular risk in patients with coronary heart disease. Curr. Opin. Cardiol. 17 (4), 325–331.

Ross, R. 1999. Mechanisms of disease: atherosclerosis—an inflammatory disease. N. Engl. J. Med. 340 (2), 115–126.

Roubenoff, R., Dellaripa, P., Nadeau, M., et al. 1997. Abnormal homocysteine metabolism in rheumatoid arthritis. Arthritis Rheum. 40 (4), 718–722.

Saag, K.G., Cerhan, J.R., Kolluri, S. 1997. Cigarette smoking and rheumatoid disease severity. Ann. Rheum. Dis. 56, 463–470.

Salonen, R., Nyyssonen, K., Porkkala, E. 1995. Kuopio atherosclerosis prevention study (KAPS). A population-based primary prevention trial of the effect of LDL lowering on atherosclerotic progression in carotid and femoral arteries. Circulation 92, 1758–1764.

Scheuner, M.T. 2001. Genetic predisposition to coronary artery disease. Curr. Opin. Cardiol. 16 (4), 251–260.

Sigal, L.H., Friedman, H.D. 1989. Rheumatoid pancarditis in a patient with well controlled rheumatoid arthritis. J. Rheumatol. 16 (3), 368–373.

Silman, A.J. 1992. Trends in the incidence and severity of rheumatoid arthritis. J. Rheumatol. Suppl. 32, 71–73.

Silman, A.J. 2002. The changing face of rheumatoid arthritis: why the decline in incidence? Arthritis Rheum. 46 (3), 579–581.

Silman, A.J., Newman, J., MacGregor, A.J. 1996. Cigarette smoking increases the risk of rheumatoid arthritis. Results from a nationwide study of disease-discordant twins. Arthritis Rheum. 39 (5), 732–735.

Silverstein, F.E., Faich, G., Goldstein, J.L., et al. 2000. Gastrointestinal toxicity with celecoxib vs nonsteroidal anti-inflammatory drugs for osteoarthritis and rheumatoid arthritis: the CLASS study: a randomized controlled trial. Celecoxib Long-term Arthritis Safety Study. JAMA 284 (10), 1247–1255.

Sinha, A.K., Eigenbrodt, M., Mehta, J.L. 2002. Does carotid intima media thickness indicate coronary atherosclerosis? Curr. Opin. Cardiol. 17 (5), 526–530.

Situnayake, R.D., Kitas, G. 1997. Dyslipidaemia and rheumatoid arthritis. Ann. Rheum. Dis. 56, 341–342.

Reviews the literature regarding lipid abnormalities associated with RA.

Slot, O. 2001. Changes in plasma homocysteine in arthritis patients starting treatment with low-dose methotrexate subsequently supplemented with folic acid. Scand. J. Rheumatol. 30 (5), 305–307.

Sokka, T., Mottonen, T., Hannonen, P. 1999. Mortality in early sawtooth treated rheumatoid arthritis patients during the first 8–14 years. Scand. J. Rheumatol. 28, 282–287.

Solomon, D.H., Avorn, J. 2003. Pharmacoepidemiology and rheumatic diseases: 2001–2002. Curr. Opin. Rheumatol. 15 (2), 122–126.

Solomon, D.H.M., Karlson, E.W.M., Rimm, E.B.S., et al. 2003. Cardiovascular morbidity and mortality in women diagnosed with rheumatoid arthritis. Circulation 107 (9), 1303–1307.

Study observed a threefold increase in rate of myocardial infarction in women diagnosed as having RA.

Spector, T.D., Silman, A.J. 1988. Parental mortality and rheumatoid-arthritis. J. Rheumatol. 15 (1), 150.

Stein, M., Bell, M.J., Ang, L.C. 2000. Hydroxychloroquine neuromyotoxicity. J. Rheumatol. 27 (12), 2927–2931.

Svenson, K.L., Lithell, H., Hallgren, R., et al. 1987. Serum lipoprotein in active rheumatoid arthritis and other chronic inflammatory arthritides. II. Effects of anti-inflammatory and disease-modifying drug treatment. Arch. Int. Med. 147 (11), 1917–1920.

Svenson, K.L., Pollare, T., Lithell, H., et al. 1988. Impaired glucose handling in active rheumatoid arthritis: relationship to peripheral insulin resistance. Metabolism 37 (2), 125–130.

Symmons, D.P.M. 2002. Epidemiolgy of rheumatoid arthritis: determinants of onset, persistence and outcome. Best Pract. Res. Clin. Rheumatol. 16 (5), 707–722.

Symmons, D.P.M., Bankhead, C.R., Harrison, B.J., et al. 1997. Blood transfusion, smoking and obesity as risk factors for development of rheumatoid arthritis: results from a primary care based incident case-control study in Norfolk, England. Arthritis Rheum. 40, 1955–1961.

Symmons, D.P.M., Jones, M.A., Scott, D.L., et al. 1998. Longterm mortality outcomes in patients with rheumatoid arthritis: early presenters continue to do well. J. Rheumatol. 25 (6), 1072–1077.

Taler, S.J., Textor, S.C., Canzanello, V.J., et al. 1999. Cyclosporin-induced hypertension: incidence, pathogenesis and management. Drug Safety 20 (5), 437–449.

Tanimoto, N., Kumon, Y., Suehiro, T., et al. 2003. Serum paraoxonase activity decreases in rheumatoid arthritis. Life Sci. 72 (25), 2877–2885.

Thould, A.K. 1986. Constrictive pericarditis in rheumatoid arthritis. Ann. Rheum. Dis. 45 (2), 89–94.

Tlustochowicz, W. 1997. Echocardiographic evaluation of cardiac structures in patients with rheumatoid arthritis. Polskie Archiwum Medycyny Wewnetrznej 97 (4), 352–358.

Tlustochowicz, W., Piotrowicz, R., Cwetsch, A., et al. 1995. 24-h ECG monitoring in patients with rheumatoid arthritis. Eur. Heart J. 16 (6), 848–851.

Toumanidis, S.T., Papamichael, C.M., Antoniades, L.G., et al. 1995. Cardiac involvement in collagen diseases. Eur. Heart J. 16 (2), 257–262.

Toussirot, E., Serratrice, G., Valentin, P. 1993. Autonomic nervous-system involvement in rheumatoid-arthritis—50 cases. J. Rheumatol. 20 (9), 1508.

Tracy, R.P. 1999. Inflammation markers and coronary heart disease. Curr. Opin. Lipidol. 10 (5), 435–441.

Turesson, C., Jacobsson, L., Bergstrom, U. 1999. Extra-articular rheumatoid arthritis: prevalence and mortality. Rheumatology 38, 668–674.

Turesson, C., Jacobsson, L., Bergstrom, U., et al. 2000. Predictors of extra-articular manifestations in rheumatoid arthritis. Scand. J. Rheumatol. 29 (6), 358–364.

Van Doornum, S., McColl, G., Jenkins, A., et al. 2003. Screening for atherosclerosis in patients with rheumatoid arthritis: comparison of two in vivo tests of vascular function. Arthritis Rheum. 48 (1), 72–80.

van Ede, A.E., Laan, R.F., Blom, H.J., et al. 2002. Homocysteine and folate status in methotrexate-treated patients with rheumatoid arthritis. Rheumatology 41 (6), 658–665.

Verma, S., Raj, S.R., Shewchuk, L., et al. 2001. Cyclooxygenase-2 blockade does not impair endothelial vasodilator function in healthy volunteers: randomized evaluation of rofecoxib versus naproxen on endothelium-dependent vasodilatation. Circulation 104 (24), 2879–2882.

Wallace, D.J., Metzger, A.L., Stetcher, V.J., et al. 1990. Cholesterol lowering effects of Hydroxychloroquine in patients with rheumatic disease: reversal of deleterious effects of steroids. Am. J. Med. 89, 322–326.

Wållberg-Jonsson, S., Öhman, M.L., Rantapää-Dahlqvist, S. 1997. Cardiovascular morbidity and mortality in patients with seropositive rheumatoid arthritis in northern Sweden. J. Rheumatol. 24, 445–451.

Study identified increased IHD events and CVD mortality in established RA patients.

Wållberg-Jonsson, S., Johansson, H., Ohman, M.L., et al. 1999. Extent of inflammation predicts cardiovascular disease and overall mortality in seropositive rheumatoid arthritis. A retrospective cohort study from disease onset. J. Rheumatol. 26 (12), 2562–2571.

Wållberg-Jonsson, S., Cederfelt, M., Rantapää-Dahlqvist, S. 2000. Hemostatic factors and cardiovascular disease in active rheumatoid arthritis: an 8 year follow-up study. J. Rheumatol. 27 (1), 71.

Wållberg-Jonsson, S., Backman, C., Johnson, O., et al. 2001. Increased prevalence of atherosclerosis in patients with medium term rheumatoid arthritis. J. Rheumatol. 28, 2597–2602.

Ward, M.M. 2001. Recent improvements in survival in patients with rheumatoid arthritis: better outcomes or different study designs? Arthritis Rheum. 44 (6), 1467–1469.

Ward, R.P., Lang, R.M. 2002. Myocardial contrast echocardiography in acute coronary syndromes. Curr. Opin. Cardiol. 17 (5), 455–463.

Watson, D.J., Rhodes, T., Cai, B., et al. 2002. Lower risk of thromboembolic cardiovascular events with naproxen among patients with rheumatoid arthritis. Arch. Int. Med. 162 (10), 1105–1110.

Webber, M.D., Selsky, E.J., Roper, P.A. 1995. Identification of a mobile intracardiac rheumatoid nodule mimicking an atrial myxoma. J. Am. Soc. Echocardiogr. 8 (6), 961–964.

Wislowska, M., Sypula, S., Kowalick, I. 1998. Echocardiographic findings, 24 hour electrocardiographic holter monitoring in patients with rheumatoid arthritis according to Steinbroker's criteria, functional index, value of Waaler-Rose titre and duration of disease. Clin. Rheumatol. 17, 369–377.

Wislowska, M., Sypula, S., Kowalik, I. 1999. Echocardiographic findings and 24-h electrocardiographic Holter monitoring in patients with nodular and non-nodular rheumatoid arthritis. Rheumatol. Int. 18 (5–6), 163.

Wolfe, F. 2000. The effect of smoking on clinical, laboratory, and radiographic status in rheumatoid arthritis. J. Rheumatol. 27, 630–637.

Wolfe, F., Mitchell, D.M., Sibley, J.T. 1994. The mortality of rheumatoid arthritis. Arthritis Rheum. 37, 481–494.

Large population and clinic based studies of mortality outcomes in RA patients.

Wolfe, F., Freundlich, B., Straus, W.L. 2003. Increase in cardiovascular and cerebrovascular disease prevalence in rheumatoid arthritis. J. Rheumatol. 30 (1), 36–40.

Wood, D., Durrington, P.N., Poulter, N., et al. 1998. Joint British recommendations on prevention of coronary heart disease in clinical practice. Heart 80 (2), S1–S29.

Yasojima, K., Schwab, C., McGeer, E.G., et al. 2001. Generation of C-reactive protein and complement components in atherosclerotic plaques. Am. J. Pathol. 158 (3), 1039–1051.

Handbook of Systemic Autoimmune Diseases, Volume 1
The Heart in Systemic Autoimmune Diseases
A. Doria and P. Pauletto, editors

CHAPTER 10

Cardiac Involvement in Systemic Lupus Erythematosus

Andrea Doria*[,a], Michelle Petri[b]

[a]*Division of Rheumatology, University of Padova, Via Giustiniani, 2, 35128 Padova, Italy*
[b]*Department of Medicine, The John Hopkins University School of Medicine, Baltimore, MD, USA*

1. Introduction

Systemic lupus erythematosus (SLE) is a chronic inflammatory disease with a still undefined etiology, characterized by the production of autoantibodies and autoreactive T cells which can trigger an inflammatory process in various organ systems. Among these, the most affected ones are skin, musculoskeletal, hematopoietic and nervous system, kidney, lung, blood vessels and heart. All the cardiac structures can be involved: pericardium, endocardium and valves, myocardium, coronary arteries and conduction tissue.

In the past, due to lack of sensitive tests, the diagnosis of SLE was made only in the most severe cases, where cardiac abnormalities were rather frequent, although in the majority of cases they were discovered only in the post-mortem examination (Harvey et al., 1954; Estes and Christian, 1971). Using more sensitive diagnostic tests, i.e. antinuclear and other autoantibody tests, SLE can be recognized in milder cases and in earlier stages of the disease. In spite of this, the prevalence of cardiac involvement does not seem to be decreased: in fact, very sensitive methods of cardiovascular investigation have found the prevalence of cardiac involvement in SLE to be higher than 50% (Mandell, 1987; Stevens, 1992; Moder et al., 1999; D'Cruz et al., 2001; Kao and Manzi, 2002).

2. Pericardial involvement

Pericarditis is one of the most characteristic manifestations of the disease and is included in the ARA/ACR classification criteria for SLE.

2.1. Prevalence

The prevalence of pericardial involvement varies between 11 and 83% (Tables 1 and 2). This variability depends on the type of study: post-mortem, clinical or echocardiographic. In post-mortem studies, the frequency of pericardial involvement varies between 43 and 83% (Table 1). Echocardiography finds pericardial abnormalities (effusion or thickening of the layers) in between 11 and 54% of SLE patients (Table 2).

2.2. Histopathologic findings/pathogenesis

In necroscopy studies, the pericardium was involved with acute and chronic inflammatory changes. Acute pericarditis can be serofibrinous or fibrinous; the latter form is also found in post-mortem, although less frequently than it was in the pre-corticosteroid era (Bulkley and Roberts, 1975). In chronic pericarditis, the fibrous or fibrofibrinous aspects prevail and the pericardial space may be obliterated by fibrous

* Corresponding author.
E-mail address: adoria@unipd.it (A. Doria).

DOI: 10.1016/S1571-5078(03)01010-9

Table 1
Prevalence of pericarditis in SLE patients: post-mortem studies

Reference	No. of patients	No. of positive cases (%)
Gross (1940)	23	14 (61)
Humphreys (1948)	21	9 (43)
Griffith and Vural (1951)	18	11 (61)
Jessar et al. (1953)	15	7 (47)
Copeland et al. (1958)	18	15 (83)
Shearn (1959)	16	7 (44)
Brigden et al. (1960)	27	20 (74)
Kong et al. (1962)	30	14 (47)
Hejtmancilk et al. (1964)	16	11 (69)
Bulkley and Roberts (1975)	36	19 (53)
Ropes (1976)	58	48 (83)
Total	278	175 (63)

adhesions (Kong et al., 1962). Very large effusions, leading to cardiac tamponade (Brigden et al., 1960; Kong et al., 1962), and constrictive pericarditis (Hejtmancilk et al., 1964; Jacobson and Reza, 1978) are very rare.

Table 2
Prevalence of pericarditis in SLE patients: echocardiographic studies

Reference	No. of patients	No. of positive cases (%)
Collins et al. (1978)	17	6 (35)
Ito et al. (1979)	48	22 (46)
Chia et al. (1981)	21	5 (23)
Klinkhoff et al. (1985)	47	10 (21)
Badui et al. (1985)	100	39 (39)
Doherty et al. (1988)	50	21 (42)
Crozier et al. (1990)	50	27 (54)
Leung et al. (1990a,b)	75	28 (37)
Kahl (1992)	395	75 (19)
Ramonda et al. (1992)	35	15 (43)
Cervera et al. (1992)	70	19 (27)
Sturfelt et al. (1992)	75	14 (19)
Rantapää-Dahlquist et al. (1997)	50	20 (40)
Castier et al. (2000)	325	107 (33)
Gentile et al. (2000)	91	19 (21)
Falcão et al. (2002)	70	8 (11)
Total	1519	435 (29)

The granular deposition of immunoglobulin and C3 demonstrated by direct immunofluorescence in surgical specimens of pericardial tissues from SLE patients (Jacobson and Reza, 1978; Bidani et al., 1980) supports the role of immunocomplexes in the development of pericarditis.

2.3. Clinical features

The most frequent symptoms of pericarditis are tachycardia, dyspnea, precordial or substernal chest pain that is emphasized by breathing, coughing, swallowing and worsened when lying flat. At clinical examination, an increase in the cardiac area and/or pericardial rub is classical, but rarely found in the modern era (Jessar et al., 1953; Copeland et al., 1958; Shearn, 1959; Hejtmancilk et al., 1964; Ropes, 1976; Cervera et al., 1993; D'Cruz et al., 2001).

Pericardial involvement appears more frequently during SLE relapses (Ramonda et al., 1992), and it is often associated with the involvement of other serous layers, leading to polyserositis.

The complications of pericarditis are rare. If the effusion is very large, it can lead to cardiac tamponade. This occurs in 1–2.5% of patients with pericarditis, considering all cases including asymptomatic ones (Doherty and Siegel, 1985; Kahl, 1992; Castier et al., 2000), and in 13% of cases with overt clinical manifestations (Kahl, 1992).

Constrictive pericarditis is even more rare. In the literature just a few cases have been reported (Jessar et al., 1953; Yurchak et al., 1965), some of which occurred in patients with drug-induced lupus from procainamide.

Purulent pericarditis, with or without tamponade (Doherty and Siegel, 1985), is extremely rare too; it represents an infectious complication of immunosuppressive therapy and it is often due to Staphylococcus aureus.

2.4. Diagnostic investigations

By means of a standard chest X-ray it is possible to recognize a pericardial effusion, documented by the widening of the cardiac silhouette, only when the effusion is large. Echocardiography demonstrates mild effusions and other abnormalities of the pericardial layers. Many patients with pericardial effusion and/or thickening of a moderate extent are asymptomatic (Doherty et al., 1988).

Pericardial effusion can also be detected by other investigations such as computer tomography (CT) and magnetic resonance imaging (MRI); these techniques allow a better definition of its extent.

In lupus pericarditis pericardial fluid, like pleural and synovial fluids, is an inflammatory exudate. Very seldom it is hemorrhagic. Acidity is high, which allows its differentiation from the effusions due to renal insufficiency, traumas or idiopathic effusions (Kindig and Goodman, 1983). In the pericardial exudate LE cells, antinuclear antibodies, anti-dsDNA antibodies, low levels of complement, immune complexes and rheumatoid factor may be detectable; glucose levels are normal (Moder et al., 1999).

2.5. Treatment

Non-steroidal anti-inflammatory drugs (NSAID) and/or corticosteroids (prednisone 0.5 mg/kg/day) are effective in mild pericarditis. In more severe cases or in tamponade a higher dose of corticosteroid is necessary, often given as an intravenous bolus (such as 1 g of methylprednisolone daily for 3 days).

In patients with recurring pericarditis chronic immunosuppression with azathioprine or mycophenolate mofetil may be beneficial. High dose intravenous immunoglobulins (IVIG) have also been reported to be effective (Meissner et al., 2000).

Invasive procedures such as pericardiocentesis, pericardial window or pericardial stripping are rarely needed.

3. Valvular disease

Anatomical and functional valvular abnormalities have been described in SLE (Mandell, 1987; Stevens, 1992; Moder et al., 1999; D'Cruz et al., 2001; Kao and Manzi, 2002). Libman–Sacks endocarditis (Libman and Sacks, 1924), also termed 'atypical verrucous endocarditis', is the most characteristic lesion.

3.1. Prevalence

In necroscopy studies the prevalence of valvular abnormalities ranges between 13 and 74% (Gross, 1940; Humphreys, 1948; Jessar et al., 1953; Harvey et al., 1954; Shearn, 1959; Brigden et al., 1960; Kong et al., 1962; Hejtmancilk et al., 1964; Dubois and Tuffanelli, 1964; Estes and Christian, 1971; Bulkley and Roberts, 1975; Lehman et al., 1989). Some authors have suggested that the frequency of valvular abnormalities decreased after the introduction of corticosteroids in treatment. A study by Doherty (1985) showed that the prevalence of these lesions was 59% before the use of corticosteroids and 35% after their introduction.

In Table 3 the prevalences of valvular verrucae and thickening observed in transthoracic and transesophageal echocardiography are reported.

3.2. Histopathologic findings/pathogenesis

Libman–Sacks endocarditis is characterized by ovoid verrucae, rather flat, smaller than those observed in rheumatic fever or in bacterial endocarditis, with a diameter ranging from 1 to 4 mm, consisting of fine granular material. The verrucae can be isolated, but they tend to gather together forming blackberry-shaped areas. These lesions can occur in any valve, but are observed more frequently in the mitral valve, on both surfaces of the valve. The simultaneous involvement of several valves is not uncommon.

In most post-mortem studies vegetations were observed in the recess between the posterior valvular leaflet and the ventricular wall (Doherty and Siegel, 1985), a location differing from that observed in infectious endocarditis, in which they are mostly found on the atrial aspect of the valve (Harvey et al., 1954; Bulkley and Roberts, 1975; Shearn, 1959; Tumulty and Harvey, 1949). The verrucae have also been described in the pockets of both atrioventricular and semilunar valves (pocket lesions) (Brigden et al., 1960).

In a recent study (Eiken et al., 2001), considering a surgical population, vegetations were found along the closing edges of the leaflets and along the atrial surfaces, without any involvement of the ventricular aspect—a pattern differing from that previously

Table 3
Prevalence of anatomical valvular abnormalities in SLE: echocardiographic studies

Reference	No. of patients	Valvular abnormalities		
		Verrucae no. (%)	Thickening no. (%)	Association with aPL
Transthoracic echocardiography				
Klinkhoff et al., 1985	47	0 (0)	10 (21)	–
Galve et al., 1988	74	7 (9)	6 (8)	–
Crozier et al., 1990	50	0 (0)	3 (6)	–
Khamashta et al., 1990	132	9 (7)	5 (4)	Yes
Nihoyannoupoulos et al., 1990	93	8 (9)	18 (19)	Yes
Leung et al., 1990	75	9 (12)	7 (9)	Yes
Cervera et al., 1992	70	3 (4)	12 (17)	Yes
Sturfelt et al., 1992	75	3 (4)	17 (23)	Yes
Ong et al., 1992	40	1 (2.5)	15 (38)	No
Ramonda et al., 1992	35	1 (3)	2 (6)	No
Giunta et al., 1993	75	0 (0)	9 (12)	Yes
Metz et al., 1994	52	3 (6)	4 (8)	No
Rantapää-Dahlquist et al., 1997	50	0 (0)	5 (10)	No
Total	868	44 (5)	113 (13)	
Transesophageal echocardiography				
Roldan et al., 1996	69	30 (43)	35 (51)	–
Omdal et al., 2001	35	12 (34)	10 (29)	No
Total	104	42 (29)	45 (43)	

APL: antiphospholipid antibodies.

reported in post-mortem investigations. Although rare, the vegetations can occur in chordae tendineae, papillary muscles and the parietal endocardium.

Histologic studies have shown two types of lesions (Bulkley and Roberts, 1975): (a) active lesions which consist of fibrin clumps, focal necrosis and mononuclear cell infiltrates, and (b) healed lesions characterized by vascularized fibrous tissue sometimes associated with calcifications; calcification of the mitral ring has also been described (Bulkley and Roberts, 1975; Barzizza et al., 1987; Doherty et al., 1988). These lesions have different prognostic implications. The active lesions have been more frequently observed in young patients with recent disease onset (Galve et al., 1988). These lesions can induce mild valve regurgitation, but they generally do not lead to a hemodynamically significant valvular lesion.

The healed lesions are found in patients with longstanding disease and who have taken corticosteroids for a long time. Healed lesions are frequently associated with functional valve abnormalities, especially valvular insufficiency (Humphreys, 1948; Doherty and Siegel, 1985).

According to some authors (Copeland et al., 1958; Galve et al., 1988; Carette, 1988) corticosteroid therapy can heal the valvular lesion with consequent retraction of the cusps and, in turn, valvular defect. Other authors (Doherty et al., 1988) did not observe any relationship between corticosteroid use and valvular abnormality.

In the last decade an association between valvular abnormalities and antiphospholipid antibodies (aPL) has been reported (Ford et al., 1988; Chartash et al., 1989; Nesher et al., 1997). It has also been shown that valvular lesions were more frequently observed in SLE patients with aPL syndrome (APS) than in those without APS or in patients with primary APS (PAPS) (Vianna et al., 1994). According to a recent study, the frequency of valvular abnormalities is 36% in patients with PAPS, 35% in those with SLE without APS and 48% in patients with SLE and APS (Nesher et al., 1997).

Therefore, it is likely that different mechanisms play a role in the development of valvular abnormalities in patients with SLE. These mechanisms need not be mutually exclusive.

There are two major pathogenetic hypothesis. The *primum movens* could be represented by a thrombus. According to this hypothesis, aPL and anti-endothelium antibodies could bind to endothelial cells which lead to their activation and, in turn, platelet aggregation and thrombus formation (Simantov et al., 1995; Del Papa et al., 1999; Yazici et al., 2001; Kaplanski et al., 2000). Alternatively, the *primun movens* could be immune complex deposition between the endothelium and the basal membrane, followed by the infiltration of inflammatory cells (Shapiro et al., 1977; Bidani et al., 1980; Ziporen et al., 1996; Amital et al., 1999).

3.3. Clinical features

Verrucous endocarditis is generally asymptomatic and only occasionally leads to a cardiac murmur (Griffith and Vural, 1951; Ropes, 1976; Straaton et al., 1988). In fact, the verrucae are near the edge of the valves, and therefore, tend not to deform the closing line, even when they are very large and protrude into the cardiac chambers.

Out of 13 SLE patients with a systolic murmur, only four had a Libman–Sacks endocarditis at the post-mortem investigation (Kong et al., 1962). However, it is rather common to find cardiac murmur in SLE patients. A systolic murmur has been reported with a frequency that varies between 20 and 70% in various surveys (Brigden et al., 1960; Shearn, 1959). It can be soft, holosystolic and of low tone, but occasionally it can be strong and rough, perceptible at the left cardiac thrust and/or at the base (Kong et al., 1962; Doherty et al., 1988; Barzizza et al., 1987; Comens et al., 1989). A diastolic murmur has been observed in 0.9% in Dubois' survey (1964) and in about 4% in another survey (Jessar et al., 1953).

However, it is difficult to evaluate the cause of a 'cardiac murmur' in SLE patients because often fever, tachycardia and anaemia may be present. Overlapping features between Libman–Sacks endocarditis and infectious endocarditis have also been reported (Jessar et al., 1953; Shearn, 1959). The prevalence of complications due to verrucous endocarditis is low: lesions are hemodynamically significant in only 3–4% of cases, making surgical treatment necessary in 1–2%. The indication for valve replacement rises to 9% in the subset of patients with valvular abnormalities (Roldan et al., 1996). Anatomical abnormalities are generally found in the mitral and aortic valves. Mitral and/or aortic insufficiency are more frequent than stenosis of the same valves (Griffith and Vural, 1951; Harvey et al., 1954; Brigden et al., 1960; Hejtmancilk et al., 1964; Ropes, 1976; Elkayam et al., 1977; Thandroyen et al., 1978; Kinney et al., 1980; Dajee et al., 1983; Doherty and Siegel, 1985; Roldan et al., 1996).

Among the complications of verrucous endocarditis, infectious endocarditis, embolism and rupture of chordae tendineae have to be considered. The prevalence of infectious endocarditis is 4.9% in post-mortem surveys and 1.3% in clinical studies (Doherty and Siegel, 1985). It was observed in 3 (7%) out of 45 patients with valvular disease in the study of Roldan et al. (1996). It is facilitated by dental surgical treatments carried out without an appropriate antibiotic prophylaxis. In the setting of such surgical procedures, antibiotics should be taken by all SLE patients with valvular abnormalities (including mitral prolapse), especially if they are taking immunosuppressants (Griffith and Vural, 1951; Klinkhoff et al., 1985; Doherty and Siegel, 1985; Comens et al., 1989; Luce et al., 1990). Fever, cardiac murmur and splinter haemorrhages are common clinical manifestations in infectious endocarditis.

Stroke or peripheral embolism were observed in 13% of patients with valvular abnormalities (Roldan et al., 1996). It has also been suggested that aPL positivity could increase the risk of cardioembolism (Fox et al., 1980). Finally, the rupture of chordae tendinae has occasionally been observed (Kinney et al., 1980).

Jensen-Urstad et al. (2002) recently reported a close association between valvular abnormalities and cardiovascular disease as well as raised levels of homocysteine and triglycerides in SLE patients.

Therefore, patients with valvular disease should be screened for clinical and subclinical atherosclerotic features.

3.4. Diagnostic investigations

Echography has been shown to be much more sensitive than clinical examination in the detection of Libman–Sacks endocarditis and/or its complications. This procedure allows the visualization of verrucae, thickening and calcification of valvular rings and, when it is completed by Doppler investigation, can show valvular regurgitation (Kahan et al., 1985; Klinkhoff et al., 1985; Galve et al., 1988; Crozier et al., 1990; Leung et al., 1990a,b; Khamashta et al., 1990; Nihoyannopoulos et al., 1990; Sturfelt et al., 1992; Ramonda et al., 1992; Cervera et al., 1992; Ong et al., 1992; Giunta et al., 1993; Metz et al., 1994). The transesophageal technique is more sensitive than the transthoracic one in revealing these abnormalities (Table 3) (Roldan et al., 1996; Shively, 2000; Omdal et al., 2001).

3.5. Treatment

Since Libman–Sacks endocarditis is clinically silent in the majority of cases, it is not treated generally. When it is found in an early active stage, corticosteroids (prednisone 1 mg/kg/day) are recommended, especially if antiphospholipid antibodies and lupus anticoagulant are negative. It has been reported that valvular abnormalities frequently resolved over time (Roldan et al., 1996). Although no direct relationship between treatment and changes in valvular disease was demonstrated, these data support the hypothesis that active valvular lesions may be modifiable by therapy.

When endocarditis is detected at a later stage during the course of the disease, careful clinical surveillance is necessary and, if the lesion becomes hemodynamically significant, valve surgery is needed (Comens et al., 1989; Hakim et al., 2001). It is necessary to carefully evaluate the type of surgical treatment: valve repair, replacement with mechanical valve or bioprosthetic porcine graft. The current trend is towards anatomic valve repair which is a more conservative surgical treatment with no need for anticoagulation. However, valve repair often leads to repeated surgery and later valve replacement (Hakim et al., 2001). Moreover, SLE patients who need valve surgery have, in the majority of cases, an associated APS, which itself requires anticoagulation. Bioprosthetic porcine valves have also been hindered by complications such as valvulitis relapse (Gordon et al., 1996). Therefore, mechanical valve replacement seems to be the best choice in lupus patients (Hakim et al., 2001). In contrast with previous reports (Dajee et al., 1983), more recent data suggest that valve replacement is generally uneventful and makes surgery a feasible option without posing a major risk to patients with compensated organ dysfunction (Morin et al., 1996).

4. Myocarditis

The most characteristic feature of myocardial involvement in SLE is myocarditis. However, myocardial dysfunction may be the result not only of clinical or subclinical myocarditis, but the consequence of other non-inflammatory features including ischemic heart disease, hypertension, renal failure, valvular disease and toxicity from medications, especially cyclophosphamide and chloroquine (Ratliff et al., 1987; Moder et al., 1999; D'Cruz et al., 2001; Kao and Manzi, 2002). Myocardial dysfunction may progress to dilated cardiomyopathy, characterised by enlargement of all chambers, or hypertrophic cardiomyopathy involving the left ventricle (Kao and Manzi, 2002). This last feature typically develops in patients with long-standing hypertension.

4.1. Prevalence

The prevalence of lupus myocarditis has very much decreased since the introduction of steroid therapy (Kong et al., 1962; Bulkley and Roberts, 1975; Ropes, 1976) and nowadays clinically overt myocarditis is uncommon.

In post-mortem studies myocarditis prevalence varied from 40 to 50% (Griffith and Vural, 1951; Shearn, 1959; Hejtmancilk et al., 1964; Badui et al., 1985; Doherty and Siegel, 1985); although in some recent reports (Bulkley and Roberts, 1975; Bidani et al., 1980; Roberts and High, 1999) the overall prevalence was 7%.

The prevalence of clinical manifestations due to myocarditis is 10% (Harvey et al., 1954; Estes and Christian, 1971; Brigden et al., 1960; Hejtmancilk et al., 1964; Ropes, 1976; Badui et al., 1985; Dubois and Tuffanelli, 1964; Borenstein et al., 1978), however, as for other cardiac manifestations, subclinical involvement is probably more frequent.

4.2. Histopathologic findings/pathogenesis

Histological findings include small foci of fibrinoid necrosis with infiltrates of plasma cells and lymphocytes and, more rarely, diffuse interstitial inflammatory changes. Hematoxylin bodies, monocyte infiltrates and foci of myocyte necrosis have also been found; however, this last feature is rare. In patients treated with corticosteroids, the finding of small foci of myocardial fibrosis is common (Griffith and Vural, 1951; Brigden et al., 1960; Bulkley and Roberts, 1975; Doherty and Siegel, 1985; Bidani et al., 1980; Fairfax et al., 1988).

Immunofluorescence studies demonstrate fine granular immune complexes and complement deposition in the walls and perivascular tissues of myocardial blood vessels (Bidani et al., 1980). Moreover, foci of immune deposits are observed along or within the myocyte bundles (Bidani et al., 1980). These observations support the hypothesis that lupus myocarditis is primarily an immune complex-mediated vascular phenomenon. However, the association between myocarditis and some circulating autoantibodies including anti-Ro/SSA (Logar et al., 1990), anti-U1RNP (Borenstein et al., 1978; Lash et al., 1986) and anti-heart (Das and Cassidy, 1973) antibodies has been reported. Although there is some evidence supporting the role of anti-Ro/SSA in the foetal development of myocarditis, the pathogenetic effects of these antibodies in adult myocarditis remain uncertain.

4.3. Clinical features

The signs and symptoms are similar to those of myocarditis due to other causes, i.e. viral myocarditis (Wijetunga and Rockson, 2002): fever, dyspnea, palpitations, resting tachycardia which is disproportionate to the patient's temperature, cardiomegaly, gallop rhythms, rarely extrasystoles or other arrhythmias, increase of creatinephosphokinase (CPK), particularly CPK MB, and troponin release (Feldman et al., 2000).

In some patients, myocarditis progresses to ventricular dysfunction, dilated cardiomyopathy and heart failure (Hejtmancilk et al., 1964). Heart failure can develop if other factors such as valvulitis, pericarditis, anaemia and hypertension concomitantly occur (Del Rio et al., 1978; Borenstein et al., 1978; Berg et al., 1985; Badui et al., 1985).

4.4. Diagnostic investigations

Nonspecific ST-T wave changes, conduction abnormalities, frequent premature complexes, and supraventricular and ventricular tachycardia may be noted on the electrocardiogram (ECG) (Shearn, 1959; Brigden et al., 1960; Hejtmancilk et al., 1964; Estes and Christian, 1971; Borenstein et al., 1978; Badui et al., 1985).

Echocardiography is a useful procedure (Feldman et al., 2000), because it is able to show findings that, although not specific, are indicative of myocardial inflammation and/or dysfunction. The most relevant findings are global, regional, or segmental wall motion abnormalities, decreased ejection fraction, increased chamber size, and prolonged isovolumic relaxation time (Klinkhoff et al., 1985; Doherty et al., 1988; Crozier et al., 1990; Leung et al., 1990a,b; Nihoyannopoulos et al., 1990; Sturfelt et al., 1992; Giunta et al., 1993). Obviously echocardiography cannot distinguish the causes of myocardial inflammation and/or dysfunction.

Endomyocardiac biopsy is useful not just in confirming the diagnosis of lupus myocarditis (Feldman et al., 2000), but also in ruling out other causes of cardiomyopathy. Moreover, it can give some information about the severity and the extent of cardiac involvement (Fairfax et al., 1988). There are several promising non-invasive investigations for diagnosing myocarditis. Scintigraphy using gallium citrate 67 (Jolles and Tatum, 1996) or indium 111-labeled Fab fragments of antimyosin antibody (Mourguet et al., 1995) may be useful in the diagnosis of myocardial involvement in lupus. MRI with T1 spin echo may be another helpful tool in supporting a diagnosis of myocarditis (Roditi et al., 2000).

However, the diagnosis of myocarditis depends largely on clinical suspicion rather than on definitive diagnostic tests (Feldman et al., 2000).

4.5. Treatment

Myocarditis, although mild, has to be treated immediately with high-dose corticosteroids (Moder et al., 1999; Wijetunga and Rockson, 2002). In the most severe forms it is necessary to use intravenous pulse corticosteroid (methylprednisolone 1 g/day for three consecutive days) followed by high doses of oral prednisone. The use of immunosuppressants, cyclophosphamide or azathioprine, is particularly recommended for patients in whom active myocarditis has been histologically confirmed (Fairfax et al., 1988; Naarendorp et al., 1999). IVIG may be beneficial in the treatment of myocarditis (Disla et al., 1993; Sherer et al., 1999).

In patients with heart failure additional supportive pharmacologic therapy, such as inotropics, afterload-reducing agents and diuretics are used; moreover, factors which can worsen heart failure such as anaemia, hypertension and infections have to be resolved.

5. Coronary artery disease (CAD)

Angina pectoris and acute myocardial infarction (MI), which once represented rare SLE manifestations (Harvey et al., 1954; Humphreys, 1948; Brigden et al., 1960; Shearn, 1959), are now more frequently observed (Jonsson et al., 1989; Manzi et al., 1997).

5.1. Prevalence

CAD is described with a prevalence ranging from 6 to 10% (Petri et al., 1992; Abu-Shakra et al., 1995; Manzi et al., 1997; Petri, 2000a) and the risk of developing this manifestation is 4–8 times higher than normal. Manzi's study shows an increase of 50-fold in women between 35 and 44 years of age. However, subclinical manifestations are also frequent.

Abnormalities of the coronary circulation have been reported in 40% of SLE patients using scintigraphy with Tallium-201 (Hosepund et al., 1984; Bruce et al., 2000a,b; Ishida et al., 2000) and even a higher percentage using single photon emission computed tomography (SPECT) dual isotope myocardial perfusion imaging (DIMPI) (Schillaci et al., 1999; Sun et al., 2001).

In post-mortem studies, a significant narrowing of coronary arteries was observed in 25–45% of cases (Bulkley and Roberts, 1975; Haider and Roberts, 1981; Fukumoto et al., 1987).

5.2. Histopathology/pathogenesis

Different mechanisms can play a part in the development of CAD. These include atherosclerosis, coronary arteritis, thrombotic events with or without aPL, vasospasm or embolization of valvular material and hypertension (Bulkley and Roberts, 1975; Doherty and Siegel, 1985; Meller et al., 1975; Rosenthal et al., 1980; Pritzker et al., 1980; Lerman et al., 1982; Englund and Lucas, 1983; Matayoshi et al., 1999).

Histologically, two major findings occur: (a) large transmural infarctions: in this case a remarkable reduction of the lumen of at least one of the three major extramural coronary arteries has been reported, more frequently due to atherosclerotic plaque and more seldom to embolism; (b) small areas of necrosis, detectable only histologically, adjacent to small intramural coronary arteries the lumen of which appear restricted and walls infiltrated by inflammatory cells.

The lesions of the major coronary arteries are predominantly of an atherosclerotic nature and, histologically, are not different from those seen in non-SLE subjects.

The minor coronary arteries can be affected by a vasculitic process. Histologically, a fibrinoid reaction of the intima and the media layers with partial interruption of the elastic layer, swelling and scaling of the endothelial cells (which can be followed by thrombosis) and perivascular inflammatory infiltrates of lymphocytes and plasma cells can be detected. The evolution is towards healing, sclerosis of all the arterial layers and fibrous hyperplasia of the intima with remarkable reduction of the lumen.

5.3. Clinical features

The clinical manifestations of CAD in SLE are angina pectoris and MI. The distinction between atherosclerosis and coronary vasculitis is a difficult, but very important issue for therapeutic decisions. Ischemia due to vasculitis is more frequent in young people with active disease, often of short duration. Moreover, in these patients the detection of vasculitic abnormalities in other organs is not uncommon; however, the absence of these last features does not rule out coronary arteritis (Wilson et al., 1992). Ischemia due to atherosclerosis, although occurring earlier in SLE patients than in the normal population, affects more frequently older SLE patients, with long-standing disease and a longer period of corticosteroid intake.

Ischemic cardiopathy could be due to APS (Asherson et al., 1989; Murpy and Leach, 1989; Leung et al., 1990a,b; MacGregor et al., 1992; Kattwinkel et al., 1992), and in this case could develop at any age and in any stage of the course of the disease.

In SLE patients, acute MI was the cause of death in between 3 and 25% in different surveys (Jonsson et al., 1989; Wallace et al., 1981; Rosner et al., 1982; Cervera et al., 1999; Bruce et al., 2000a,b). Urowitz et al. (1976) described a bimodal distribution of the causes of death in SLE: an 'early' peak due to SLE severity/activity or infections, and a 'late' peak due to atherosclerotic CAD; this trend has been confirmed in more recent studies too (Rubin et al., 1985; Abu-Shakra et al., 1995). Some authors found that 21% of the patients with previous MI, younger than 45 years, had aPL. Other authors did not confirm this association (De Catenina et al., 1990; Phadke et al., 1993).

Premature atherosclerosis. Many studies have been published showing premature atherosclerosis in SLE patients (Gladman and Urowitz, 1987; Petri et al., 1992; Manzi et al., 1997; Ward, 1999; Manzi et al., 1999; Esdaile et al., 2001; Roman et al., 2001; Svenungsson et al., 2001).

Since early atherosclerotic lesions cannot be explained by Framingham risk factors alone, i.e. age, male sex, arterial hypertension, hypercholesterolemia, diabetes, obesity, sedentary life and smoke, (Manzi et al., 1999; Esdaile et al., 2001; Rahman et al., 1999; Bruce et al., 1999), it has been attributed to complex interactions between traditional risk factors and factors associated with the disease per se or its treatment (Ward, 1999; Bruce et al., 2000a,b; Roman et al., 2001; Svenungsson et al., 2001).

Many studies have shown abnormality of lipids in SLE patients with an increase in total cholesterol, VLDL and triglycerides and a decrease of HDL and LDL cholesterol. These abnormalities seem to be influenced by disease activity (Ilowite et al., 1988; Borba and Bonfa, 1997; Borba et al., 1998), corticosteroid therapy (Ettinger et al., 1987; MacGregor et al., 1992; Petri et al., 1992b; Leong et al., 1994), nephrotic syndrome (Leong et al., 1994) and diabetes mellitus. The prevalence of diabetes in SLE patients is approximately 7% (Manzi et al., 1997; Gladman and Urowitz, 1987; Petri et al., 1992a). A beneficial effect of hydroxychloroquine on the lipid profile in SLE patients has also been reported (Wallace et al., 1990; Petri et al., 1994), with a reduction of total cholesterol, LDL and triglycerides.

Other studies (Kannel and Sorlie, 1979; Clarke et al., 1991; Fermo et al., 1995; Petri et al., 1996; Manzi et al., 1999; Petri et al., 1992a,b; Doria et al., 2003) have shown an important role of hypertension, sedentary life style and hyperhomocysteinemia in the development of atherosclerosis. Hypertension can be secondary to renal involvement, corticosteroid therapy, insulin resistance induced by corticosteroid therapy and, therefore, it is a common feature in SLE patients. A study by Petri et al. (1996) has also shown that corticosteroids and nephropathy could lead to an increase in homocysteine, which is significantly associated with arterial thrombosis and vascular events such as TIA and stroke.

Among the non-traditional risk factors, besides cumulative dosage and/or length of corticosteroid therapy, disease duration, high scores of activity (measured by scoring systems such as SLAM, SLEDAI or ECLAM) or damage (SLICC DI) (Gladman and Urowitz, 1987; Petri et al., 1992a; Petri et al., 1994; Manzi et al., 1997; Manzi et al., 1999; Petri, 2000a,b; Doria et al., 2003), some other inflammatory and immunologic parameters have been recently proposed which could contribute to the development of atherosclerotic plaque. In fact, some experimental data seem to confirm the role of inflammation and autoimmunity in the development of atherosclerotic plaque: (a) deposits of immunoglobulins and complement have been demonstrated within the plaque; (b) mononuclear cells are involved in the early stage of plaque formation, particularly T lymphocytes and monocytes which turn into foamy cells; (c) inflammation could induce the formation of oxidized LDL (Wick et al., 1995).

The aPL can also contribute to the development of the atherosclerotic plaque. Some studies point out that aPL cross-react with oxidized LDL (Vaarala et al., 1993); it seems that LDL contain phospholipids and apolipoprotein B which could become 'antigenic' after lipoprotein oxidation. According to another hypothesis, β2-GPI could bind with oxidized LDL turning them into a target for anti-β2GPI (Bruce et al., 2000a,b; Witztum, 1994; Matsuura et al., 1994). In both cases the binding of oxidized LDL to anti-β2GPI antibodies facilitates phagocytosis in the macrophage, which turns into foamy cells.

It has been noted that in SLE as well as in non-SLE population atherosclerotic plaques are associated with an increase of inflammatory parameters such as CRP and fibrinogen (Lahita et al., 1993; Ridker et al., 1997; Manzi et al., 1999; Ridker, 2001) and with some autoantibodies such as anti-HSP65, anti-oxidized LDL and anti-β2GPI (Shoenfeld et al., 2001).

However, Doria et al. (2003) in a recent 5-year prospective study did not observe any convincing relationship between the new inflammatory and immunologic parameters and subclinical atherosclerosis in SLE. The conclusion of the study was that in SLE the predictive value of the new parameters is overwhelmed by other factors such as corticosteroid cumulative dosage and nephropathy.

5.4. Diagnostic investigations

Resting and exercise electrocardiography represent standard non-invasive techniques that can be used to routinely investigate CAD in SLE.

Moreover, in recent years, several advances in nuclear cardiac imaging have occurred. Thallium-201 scintigraphy was the first technique used for detecting perfusion abnormalities in SLE patients (Hosepund et al., 1984; Bruce et al., 2000a,b; Ishida et al., 2000). More recently, the technique of DIMPI has been introduced which employs two isotopes: thallium-201 and technetium 99m sestamibi (Schillaci et al., 1999; Sun et al., 2001). This technique has several advantages in comparison with thallium scintigraphy including a better image resolution. However, both thallium scintigraphy and DIMPI are more sensitive than specific; therefore, their results have to be considered with caution.

Coronary scanning by electron beam CT detects coronary calcification which is considered to be a marker of coronary atherosclerosis (von Felt, 1998).

In some cases angiography can be useful in differentiating coronary vasculitis from atherosclerosis. In fact, aneurysms and/or rapidly progressive narrowing of coronary arteries, showed by serial angiographies, although not pathognomonic, support the diagnosis of coronary vasculitis (Heibel et al., 1976; Homcy et al., 1982; Englund and Lucas, 1983; Wilson et al., 1992; Nobrega et al., 1996).

For the investigation of subclinical atherosclerosis, carotid color Doppler ultrasonography (US) has been widely used (Manzi et al., 1999; Roman et al., 2001; Svenungsson et al., 2001; Doria et al., 2003). Although carotid US directly investigates only the carotid artery, this technique provides an accurate measurement of subclinical atherosclerosis (Li et al., 1996). In fact, people with asymptomatic carotid abnormalities are at an increased risk for CAD (O'Leary et al., 1999).

5.5. Treatment

The therapeutical approach to SLE patients with CAD depends on the nature of the underlining pathological process. If it is due to vasculitis, corticosteroid therapy at high dosage is recommended (prednisone 1–1.5 mg/kg/day); if it is due to aPL and/or atherosclerosis, the use of anticoagulation and/or platelet antiaggregation as well as vasodilatator drugs is suggested (Moder et al., 1999; D'Cruz et al., 2001; Kao and Manzi, 2002).

6. Rhythm and conduction abnormalities

6.1. Prevalence

Sinus tachycardia is the most frequent rhythm abnormality and is quite common in SLE patients. Atrioventricular block and bundle branch block are the most common conduction defects, however, they are rare both in adult (Logar et al., 1990; Martinez-Costa et al., 1991; Fonseca et al., 1994; Comín-Colet et al., 2001; Gómez-Barrado et al., 2002) and in neonatal (Brucato et al., 2001) lupus patients. Some occasional surveys in adults showed a prevalence of any abnormalities higher than 10% (James et al., 1965; Bulkley and Roberts, 1975). In a recent prospective study congenital heart block occurred in 2% of children born from mothers with anti-Ro/SSA antibodies (Brucato et al., 2001; Brucato et al., 2002).

6.2. Histopathology/pathogenesis

Sinus tachycardia can be due to fever, anaemia or cardiac abnormalities including pericarditis and myocarditis. Recently it has been hypothesized that in some patients an autonomic dysfunction could account for heart rate variability in SLE (Louthrenoo et al., 1999; Hogarth et al., 2002). Conduction defects may result from different pathological processes leading to structural damage of the conduction system. Histopathologic studies showed inflammatory abnormalities caused by arteritis or degenerative and necrotic changes due to ischemia. In both cases small blood vessels and capillaries of nodal and conduction tissue were involved. Inflammatory and ischemic lesions resulted in fibrous tissue formation (James et al., 1965; Bulkley and Roberts, 1975; Bharati et al., 1975). However, conduction defects can also be the result of antimalarial use (Comín-Colet et al., 2001) or simply represent a coexisting idiopathic conduction system disease.

The pathogenesis of congenital heart block has not been completely elucidated (Brucato et al., 1999), however, there is clear evidence that anti-Ro/SSA antibodies play a definite role. Some cases of heart block in adult patients with anti-Ro/SSA have been reported (Biazarian et al., 1989; Martinez-Costa et al., 1991; Mevorach et al., 1993; Fonseca et al., 1994; Comín-Colet et al., 2001).

6.3. Clinical findings

Signs and symptoms of rhythm and conduction abnormalities depend on the type of defect and its severity. However, they are mostly asymptomatic or may lead to some mild complaints such as palpitation or fatigue. They are recognized during follow-up clinical examination and/or by routine electrocardiography. In some cases syncope may occur.

6.4. Diagnostic investigations

In the case of a patient with rhythm and conduction abnormalities, examinations including 24 h Holter monitoring, echocardiography, gallium scintigraphy, electrolyte balance and thyroid hormonal status should be considered.

6.5. Treatment

Arrhythmia therapy depends on the type of rhythm or conduction abnormality. Common antiarrhythmic drugs can be used, but in the most severe cases the implant of a pacemaker is necessary. All potential causes of the rhythm or conduction abnormality (i.e. pericarditis, myocarditis, cardiac ischemia, etc.) have to be resolved.

Acknowledgements

Dr Petri's Hopkins Lupus Cohort is supported by NIH RO-I AR43727 and the General Clinical Research Center MOI-RR 00082.

Key points

- Cardiac abnormalities are common in SLE patients. Pericarditis is the most common, but lesions of the valves, myocardium and coronary vessels may all occur.
- In the past cardiac manifestations were severe and life threatening, often leading to death. Therefore, they were frequently found in post-mortem examinations.
- Nowadays cardiac manifestations are often mild and asymptomatic. However, they can be frequently recognised by echocardiography and other non-invasive tests.

- Echocardiography is a sensitive and specific technique in detecting cardiac abnormalities, particularly mild pericarditis, valvular lesions and myocardial dysfunction. Therefore, echocardiography should be performed periodically in SLE patients.
- Vascular occlusion, including coronary arteries, may develop due to vasculitis, premature atherosclerosis or antiphospholipid antibodies associated with SLE.
- Premature atherosclerosis is the most frequent cause of CAD in SLE patients, Efforts should be made to control traditional risk factors as well as all other factors which could contribute to atherosclerotic plaque development.

References

Abu-Shakra, M., Urowitz, M.B., Gladman, D.D., et al. 1995. Mortality studies in systemic lupus erythematosus. Results from a single centre. I. Causes of death. J. Rheumatol. 22, 1259.

Amital, H., Langevitz, P., Levy, Y., et al. 1999. Valvular deposition of antiphospholipid antibodies in the antiphospholipid syndrome: a clue to the origin of the disease. Clin. Exp. Rheumatol. 17, 99.

Asherson, R.A., Khamashta, M.A., Baguley, E., et al. 1989. Myocardial infarction and antiphospholipid antibodies in SLE and related disorders. Q. J. Med. 73, 1100.

Badui, E., Garcia-Rubi, D., Robles, E., et al. 1985. Cardiovascular manifestations in systemic lupus erythematosus. Prospective study of 100 patients. Angiology 36, 452.

Barzizza, F., Venco, A., Grandi, A.M., et al. 1987. Mitral valve prolapse in systemic lupus erythematosus. Clin. Exp. Rheumatol. 5, 59.

Berg, G., Bodet, J., Webb, K., et al. 1985. Systemic lupus erythematosus presenting as isolated congestive heart failure. J. Rheumatol. 12, 1182.

Bharati, S., de la Fuente, D.J., Kallen, R.J. 1975. Conduction system in systemic lupus erythematosus with atrioventricular block. Am. J. Cardiol. 35, 299.

Biazarian, S.D., Taylor, A.J., Brezinski, D., et al. 1989. High grade atrioventricular heart block in an adult with systemic lupus erythematosus: the association of nuclear RNP (U1 RNP) antibodies, a case report, and a review of the literature. Arthritis Rheum. 32, 1170.

Bidani, A.K., Roberts, J.L., Schwartz, M.M., et al. 1980. Immunopathology of cardiac lesions in fatal systemic lupus erythematosus. Am. J. Med. 69, 849.

Borba, E.F., Bonfa, E. 1997. Dyslipoproteinemias in systemic lupus erythematosus: influence of disease, activity and anticardiolipin antibodies. Lupus 6, 533.

Borba, E.F., Bonfa, E., Vinagre, C.G. 1998. Impaired metabolism of artificial chylomicronis in systemic lupus erythematosus (abstract). Arthritis Rheum. 41, S79.

Borenstein, D.G., Fye, W.B., Arnett, F.C., et al. 1978. The myocarditis of systemic lupus erythematosus: association with myositis. Ann. Intern. Med. 89, 619.

Brigden, W., Bywaters, E.G.L., Lessof, M.H., et al. 1960. The heart in systemic lupus erythematosus. Br. Heart J. 22, 1.

Brucato, A., Buyon, J.P., Horsfall, A.C., et al. 1999. Fourth international workshop on neonatal lupus syndromes and the Ro/SSA-La/SSB System. Clin. Exp. Rheumatol. 17, 130.

Brucato, A., Frassi, M., Franceschini, F., et al. 2001. Risk of congenital complete heart block in newborns of mothers with anti-Ro/SSA antibodies detected by counterimmunoelectrophoresis: a prospective study of 100 women. Arthritis Rheum. 44, 1832.

Brucato, A., Doria, A., Frassi, M., et al. 2002. Pregnancy outcome in 100 women with autoimmune diseases and anti-Ro/SSA antibodies: a prospective controlled study. Lupus 11, 716.
It is the first prospective study on the risk of CCHB in newborns of mothers with anti-Ro/SSA antibodies.

Bruce, I.N., Urowitz, M.B., Galdman, D.D., et al. 1999. Natural history of hypercholesterolemia in systemic lupus erythematosus. J. Rheumatol. 26, 2137.

Bruce, I.N., Burns, R.J., Gladman, D.D., et al. 2000a. Single photon emission computed tomograpy dual isotope myocardial perfusion imaging in women with systemic lupus erythematosus. I. Prevalence and distribution of abnormalities. J. Rheumatol. 27, 2372.

Bruce, I.N., Gladman, D.D., Urowitz, M.B. 2000b. Premature atherosclerosis in systemic lupus erythematosus. Rheum. Dis. Clin. N. Am. 26, 257.
Bruce and co-authors extensively reviewed clinical and subclinical atherosclerosis in SLE as well as traditional and non-traditional risk factors for coronary artery disease.

Bulkley, B.H., Roberts, W.C. 1975. The heart in systemic lupus erythematosus and the changes induced in it by corticosteroid therapy: a study of 36 necropsy patients. Am. J. Med. 58, 243.
This paper is a milestone in the modern history of SLE. It deals with the histopathologic changes of lupus carditis including those induced by corticosteroids.

Carette, S. 1988. Cardiopulmonary manifestations of systemic lupus erythematosus. Rheum. Dis. Clin. N. Am. 14, 135.

Castier, M.B., Albuquerque, E.M., Menezes, M.E., et al. 2000. Cardiac tamponade in systemic lupus erythematosus. Report of four cases. Arq. Bras. Cardiol. 75, 446.

Cervera, R., Font, J., Pare, C., et al. 1992. Cardiac disease in systemic lupus erythematosus: prospective study of 70 patients. Ann. Rheum. Dis. 51, 156.

Cervera, R., Khamashta, M.A., Font, J., et al. 1993. Systemic lupus erythematosus: clinical and immunonologic patterns of disease expression in a cohort of 1000 patients. The European working party on systemic lupus erythematosus. Medicine (Baltimore) 72, 113.

Cervera, R., Khamashta, M.A., Font, J., et al. 1999. Morbidity and mortality in systemic lupus erythematosus during a 5 year period. A multicenter prospective study of 1000 patients. European Working Party on Systemic lupus erythematosus. Medicine (Baltimore) 778, 167.

This paper is a 5-year prospective study on clinical manifestations in a very large group of patients.

Chartash, E.K., Lans, D.M., Paget, S.A., et al. 1989. Aortic insufficiency and mitral regurgitation in patients with systemic lupus erythematosus and the antiphospholipid syndrome. Am. J. Med. 86, 407.

Chia, B.L., Mah, E.P., Feng, P.H. 1981. Cardiovascular abnormalities in systemic lupus erythematosus. J. Clin. Ultrasound 9, 237.

Clarke, R., Daly, L., Robinson, K., et al. 1991. Hyperhomocysteinemia. An independent risk factor for vascular disease. N. Engl. J. Med. 324, 1149.

Collins, R.L., Turner, R.A., Nomeir, A.M., et al. 1978. Cardiopulmonary manifestations of systemic lupus erythematosus. J. Rheumatol. 5, 299.

Comens, S.M., Alpert, M.A., Sharp, G.C., et al. 1989. Frequency of mitral valve prolapse in systemic lupus erythematosus, progressive systemic sclerosis and mixed connective tissue disease. Am. J. Cardiol. 63, 369.

Comín-Colet, J., Sánches-Corral, M.A., Alegre-Sancho, J.J., et al. 2001. Complete heart block in an adult with systemic lupus erythematosus and recent onset of hydroxychloroquine therapy. Lupus 10, 59.

Copeland, G.D., Von Capeller, D., Stern, T.N. 1958. Systemic lupus erythematosus: a clinical report of 47 cases with pathologic findings in 18. Am. J. Med. Sci. 236, 318.

Crozier, I.G., Li, E., Miline, M.J., et al. 1990. Cardiac involvement in systemic lupus erythematosus detected by echocardiography. Am. J. Cardiol. 65, 1145.

Dajee, H., Hurley, E.J., Szarnicki, R.J. 1983. Cardiac valve replacement in systemic lupus erythematosus: a review. J. Thorac. Cardiovasc. Surg. 85, 718.

Das, S.K., Cassidy, J.T. 1973. Anti-heart antibodies in patients with systemic lupus erythematosus. Am. J. Med. Sci. 265, 275.

D'Cruz, D., Khamashta, M., Huges, G. 2001. Cardiovascular manifestation of systemic lupus erythematosus. In: D. Wallace, B.H. Hahn (Eds.), Dubois' lupus erythematosus. Lippincott Williams & Wilkins, Philadelphia, p. 645.

De Catenina, R., d'Ascanio, A., Mazzone, A., et al. 1990. Prevalence of anticardiolipin antibodies in coronary artery disease. Am. J. Cardiol. 65, 922.

Del Papa, N., Raschi, E., Moroni, G., et al. 1999. Anti-endothelial cell IgG fractions from systemic lupus erythematosus patients bind to human endothelial cells induce a pro-adhesive and a pro-inflammatory phenotype in vitro. Lupus 8, 423.

Del Rio, A., Vazquez, J.J., Sobrino, J.A., et al. 1978. Myocardial involvement in systemic lupus erythematosus. A noninvasive study of left ventricular function. Chest 74, 414.

Disla, E., Rhim, H.R., Reddy, A., et al. 1993. Reversible cardiogenic shock in a patients with lupus myocarditis. J. Rheumatol. 20, 2174.

Doherty, N.E., Siegel, R.J. 1985. Cardiovascular manifestation of systemic lupus erythematosus. Am. Heart J. 110, 1257.

Doherty, N.E. III, Feldman, G., Maurer, G., et al. 1988. Echocardiographic findings in systemic lupus erythematosus. Am. J. Cardiol. 61, 1144.

Doria, A., Shoenfeld, Y., Wu, R., et al. 2003. Risk factors for subclinical atherosclerosis in a prospective cohort of patients with Systemic Lupus Erythematosus. Ann. Rheum. Dis. 62, 1071.

In this paper the first prospective evaluation of risk factors for subclinical atherosclerosis has been carried out.

Dubois, E.L., Tuffanelli, D.L. 1964. Clinical manifestation of systemic lupus erythematosus. Computer analysis of 520 cases. JAMA 190, 104.

Eiken, P.W., Edwards, W.D., Tazelaar, H.D., et al. 2001. Surgical pathology of nonbacterial thrombotic endocarditis in 30 patients, 1985–2000. Mayo Clin. Proc. 76, 1204.

Elkayam, U., Weiss, S., Laniado, S. 1977. Pericardial effusion and mitral valve involvement in systemic lupus erythematosus: echocardiographic study. Ann. Rheum. Dis. 36, 349.

Englund, J.A., Lucas, R.V. Jr 1983. Cardiac complications in children with systemic lupus erythematosus. Pediatrics 72, 724.

Esdaile, J.M., Abrahamowicz, M., Grodzicky, T., Li, Y., et al. 2001. Traditional Framingham risk factors fail to fully account for accelerated atherosclerosis in systemic lupus erythematosus. Arthritis Rheum. 44, 2231.

Estes, D., Christian, C.L. 1971. The natural history of systemic lupus erythematosus by prospective analysis. Medicine (Baltimore) 50, 85.

This paper is a milestone in the modern history of lupus. It is a clinical study.

Ettinger, W.H., Glodberg, A.P., Applebaum-Bowden, D., et al. 1987. Dyslipoproteinemia in systemic lupus erythematosus. Effect of corticosteroids. Am. J. Med. 83, 503.

Fairfax, M.J., Osborn, T.G., Williams, G.A., et al. 1988. Endomyocardial biopsy in patients with systemic lupus erythematosus. J. Rheumatol. 15, 593.

Falcão, C.A., Alves, I.C., Chahade, W.H., et al. 2002. Echocardiographic abnormalities and antiphospholipid antibodies in patients with systemic lupus erythematosus. Arq. Bras. Cardiol. 79, 285.

Feldman, A.M., McNamara, D., Myocarditis, N. 2000. Engl. J. Med. 343, 1388.

Fermo, I., D'Angelo, S.V., Paroni, R., et al. 1995. Prevalence of moderate hyperhomocysteinemia in patients with early onset venous and arterial occlusive disease. Ann. Intern. Med. 123, 747.

Fonseca, E., Crespo, M., Sobrino, J.A. 1994. Complete heart block in an adult with systemic lupus erythematosus. Lupus 3, 129.

Ford, P.M., Ford, S.E., Lillicrap, D.P. 1988. Association of lupus anticoagulant with severe valvular heart disease in systemic lupus erythematosus. J. Rheumatol. 15, 597.

Fox, I.S., Spence, A.M., Wheelis, R.F., et al. 1980. Cerebral embolism in Libman–Sacks endocarditis. Neurology 30, 487.

Fukumoto, S., Tsumagari, T., Kinjo, M., et al. 1987. Coronary atherosclerosis in patients with systemic lupus erythematosus at autopsy. Acta Pathol. Jpn 37, 1.

Galve, E., Candell-Riera, J., Pigrau, C., et al. 1988. Prevalence, morphologic types and evolution of cardiac valvular disease in systemic lupus erythematosus. N. Engl. J. Med. 319, 817.

Gentile, R., Laganaà, B., Tubani, M., et al. 2000. Assessment of echocardiographic abnormalities in patients with systemic lupus erythematosus: correlation with levels of antiphospholipid antibodies. Ital. Heart J. 1, 487.

Giunta, A., Picillo, U., Maione, S., et al. 1993. Spectrum of cardiac involvement in systemic lupus erythematosus: echocardiographic, echo-Doppler observations and immunologivcal investigation. Acta. Cardiol. 48, 183.

Gladman, D.D., Urowitz, M.B. 1987. Morbidity in systemic lupus erythematosus. J. Rheumatol. 14, 223.

Gómez-Barrado, J.J., García-Rubira, J.C., Polo Ostáriz, M.A., et al. 2002. Complete atrioventricular block in a woman with systemic lupus erythematosus. Int. J. Cardiol. 82, 289.

Gordon, R.J., Weilbaecher, D., Davy, S.M., et al. 1996. Valvulitis involving a bioprosthetic valve in a patients with systemic lupus erythematosus. J. Am. Soc. Echocardiogr. 9, 104.

Griffith, G.C., Vural, I.L. 1951. Acute and subacute disseminated lupus erythematosus: a correlation of clinical and post-mortem findings in eighteen cases. Circulation 3, 492.

Gross, L. 1940. Cardiac lesions in Libman–Sacks disease, with consideration of its relationship to acute diffuse lupus erythematosus. Am. J. Pathol. 16, 375.

Haider, Y.S., Roberts, W.C. 1981. Coronary arterial disease in systemic lupus erythematosus: quantification of degrees of narrowing in 22 necropsy patients (21 women) ages 16 to 37 years. Am. J. Med. 70, 775.

Hakim, J.P., Mehta, A., Jain, A.C., et al. 2001. Mitral valve replacement and repair. Report of 5 patients with systemic lupus erythematosus. Tex. Heart Inst. J. 28, 47.

Harvey, A.M., Shulman, L.E., Tumulty, P.A., et al. 1954. Systemic lupus erythematosus: review of the literature and clinical analysis of 138 cases. Medicine 33, 291.
This is the oldest clinical study of the modern era in the history of SLE.

Heibel, R.H., O'Toole, J.D., Curtiss, E.I., et al. 1976. Coronary arteritis in systemic lupus erythematosus. Chest 69, 700.

Hejtmancilk, M.R., Wright, J.C., Quint, R., et al. 1964. The cardiovascular manifestation of systemic lupus erythematosus. Am. Heart J. 68, 119.

Hogarth, M.B., Judd, L., Mathias, C.J., et al. 2002. Cardiovascular autonomic function in systemic lupus erythematosus. Lupus 11, 308.

Homcy, C.J., Libertson, R.R., Fallon, J.T., et al. 1982. Ischemic heart coronary vasculitis in systemic lupus erythematosus in the young patient: report of six cases. Am. J. Cardiol. 49, 478.

Hosepund, J.D., Montanaro, A., Hart, M.V., et al. 1984. Myocardial perfusion abnormalities in asymptomatic patients with systemic lupus erythematosus. Am. J. Med. 77, 286.

Humphreys, E.M. 1948. The cardiac lesions of acute disseminated lupus erythematosus. Ann. Intern. Med. 28, 12.

Ilowite, N.T., Samuel, P., Ginzler, E., et al. 1988. Dyslipoproteinemia in pediatric systemic lupus erythematosus. Arthritis Rheum. 31, 859.

Ishida, R., Murata, Y., Sawada, Y., et al. 2000. Thallium-201 myocardial SPECT in patients with collagen disease. Nucl. Med. Commun. 21, 729.

Ito, M., Kagiyama, Y., Omura, I., et al. 1979. Cardiovascular manifestation of systemic lupus erythematosus. Jpn. Circ. J. 43, 985.

Jacobson, E.J., Reza, M.J. 1978. Constrictive pericarditis in systemic lupus erythematosus: demonstration of immunoglobulins in the pericardium. Arthritis Rheum. 21, 972.

James, T.N., Rupe, C.E., Monto, R.W. 1965. Pathology of the cardiac conduction system in systemic lupus erythematosus. Ann. Intern. Med. 63, 402.

Jensen-Urstad, K., Svenungsson, E., de Faire, U., et al. 2002. Cardiac valvular abnormalities are frequent in systemic lupus erythematosus with manifest arterial disease. Lupus 11, 744.

Jessar, R.A., Lamont-Havers, R.W., Ragan, C. 1953. Natural history of lupus erythematosus disseminatus. Ann. Intern. Med. 38, 717.

Jolles, P.R., Tatum, J.L. 1996. SLE myocarditis. Detection by Ga-67 citrate scintigraphy. Clin. Nucl. Med. 21, 284.

Jonsson, H., Nived, O., Surfelt, G. 1989. Outcome in systemic lupus erythematosus: a prospective study of patients from a defined population. Medicine 68, 141.

Kahan, A., Amor, B., De Vernejoul, F., et al. 1985. Libman–Sacks endocarditis. The diagnostic importance of two-dimensional echocardiography. Br. J. Rheum. 24, 187.

Kahl, L.E. 1992. The spectrum of pericardial tamponade in systemic lupus erythematosus: report of ten patients. Arthritis Rheum. 35, 1343.

Kannel, W.B., Sorlie, P. 1979. Some health benefits of physical activity. Arch. Intern. Med. 139, 857.

Kao, A.H., Manzi, S. 2002. How to manage patients with cardiopulmonary disease? Best Pract. Res. Clin. Rheumatol. 16, 211.

Kaplanski, G., Cacoub, B., Farnarier, C., et al. 2000. Increased soluble vascular cell adhesion molecule 1 concentration in patients with primary or lupus erythematosus related antiphospholipid syndrome: correlation with the severity of thrombosis. Arthritis Rheum. 43, 55.

Kattwinkel, N., Villanueva, A.G., Labib, S.B., et al. 1992. Myocardial infarction caused by cardiac microvasculopathy in a patient with the primary antiphospholipid syndrome. Ann. Intern. Med. 116, 974.

Khamashta, M.A., Cervera, R., Asherson, R.A., et al. 1990. Association of antibodies against phospholipid with heart valve disease in systemic lupus erythematosus. Lancet 335, 1541.

Kindig, J.R., Goodman, M.R. 1983. Clinical utility of pericardial fluid pH determination. Am. J. Med. 75, 1077.

Kinney, E.L., Wynn, J., Ward, S., et al. 1980. Ruptured chordae tendinae: its association with systemic lupus erythematosus. Arch. Pathol. Lab. Med. 104, 595.

Klinkhoff, A.V., Thompson, C.R., Reid, G.D., et al. 1985. M-mode and two-dimensional echocardiogrphic abnormalities in systemic lupus erythematusus. JAMA 253, 3273.

Kong, T.Q., Kellum, R.E., Haserich, J.R. 1962. Clinical diagnosis of cardiac involvement in systemic lupus erythematosus: a correlation of clinical and autopsy findings in thirty. Circulation 26, 7.

Lahita, R.G., Rivkin, E., Cavanagh, I., et al. 1993. Low levels of total cholesterol, high-density lipoprotein, and apolipoprotein A1 in association with anticardiolipin antibodies in patients with systemic lupus erythematosus. Arthritis Rheum. 36, 1566.

Lash, A.D., Wittman, A.L., Quisimoro, F.P. Jr 1986. Myocarditis in mixed connective tissue disease: clinical and pathologic study of three cases and review of literature. Semin. Arthritis Rheum. 15, 288.

Lehman, T.J.A., Mc Curdy, D.K., Bernstein, B.H., et al. 1989. Systemic lupus erythematosus in the first decade of life. Pediatrics 83, 235.

Leong, K.H., Koh, E.T., Feng, P.H., et al. 1994. Lipid profiles in patients with systemic lupus erythematosus. J. Rheumatol. 21, 1264.

Lerman, B.B., Thomas, L.C., Abrams, G.D., et al. 1982. Aortic stenosis associated with systemic lupus erythematosus. Am. J. Med. 72, 707.

Leung, W.H., Wong, K.L., Lau, C.P., et al. 1990a. Cardiac abnormalities in systemic lupus erythematosus: a prospective M-mode, cross-sectional and Doppler echocardiographic study. Int. J. Cardiol. 27, 367.

Leung, W.H., Wong, K.L., Llau, C.P., et al. 1990b. Association between antiphospholipid antibodies and cardiac abnormalities in patients with systemic lupus erythematosus. Am. J. Med. 89, 411.

Li, R., Cai, J., Tegeler, C., Sorlie, P., et al. 1996. Reproducibility of extracranial carotid atherosclerotic lesion assessed by B-mode ultrasound: the Artherosclerosis Risk in Communities Study. Ultrasound Med. Biol. 22, 791.

Libman, E., Sacks, B. 1924. A hitherto undescribed form of valvular and mural endocarditis. Arch. Intern. Med. 33, 701.
It is the first original description of verrucous endocarditis, later termed Libman–Sacks endocarditis.

Logar, D., Kveder, T., Rozman, B., et al. 1990. Possible association between anti-Ro antibodies and myocarditis or cardiac conduction defects in adults with systemic lupus erythematosus. Ann. Rheum. Dis. 49, 627.

Louthrenoo, W., Ruttanaumpawan, P., Aramrattana, A., et al. 1999. Cardiovascular autonomic nervous system dysfunction in patients with rheumatoid arthritis and systemic lupus erythematosus. Q. J. Med. 92, 97.

Luce, E.B., Montgomery, M.T., Redding, S.W. 1990. The prevalence of cardiac valvular pathosis in patients with systemic lupus erythematosus. Oral Surg. Oral Med. Oral Pathol. 70, 590.

MacGregor, A.J., Dhillon, V.B., Binder, A., et al. 1992. Fastings lipids and antiacardiolipin antibodies as risk factors for vascular disease in systemic lupus erythematosus. Ann. Rheum. Dis. 51, 152.

Mandell, B.F. 1987. Cardiovascular involvement in systemic lupus erythematosus. Semin. Arthritis Rheum. 17, 126.

Manzi, S., Meilahn, E.N., Rairie, J.E., et al. 1997. Age-specific incidence rates of myocardial infarction and angina in women with systemic lupus erythematosus: comparison with Framingham Study. Am. J. Epidemiol. 145, 408.
This study reports the incidence of coronary artery disease in a very large cohort of lupus patients and an extensive evaluation of risk factors.

Manzi, S., Selzer, F., Sutton-Tyrrel, K., et al. 1999. Prevalence and risk factors of carotid plaque in women with systemic lupus erythematosus. Arthritis Rheum. 42, 51.
In this study, Manzi and co-authors examined the prevalence of subclinical atherosclerosis in SLE. The evaluation of risk factors was also reported.

Martinez-Costa, X., Ordi, J., Barbera, J., et al. 1991. High grade atrioventricular heart block in 2 adults with systemic lupus erythematosus. J. Rheumatol. 18, 1926.

Matayoshi, A.H., Dhond, M.R., Laslett, L.J. 1999. Multiple coronary aneurysms in a case of systemic lupus erythematosus. Chest 116, 1116.

Matsuura, E., Igarashi, Y., Yasuda, T., et al. 1994. Anticardiolipin antibodies recognize (2-glycoprotein I structure altered by interacting with an oxigen modified solid phase surface. J. Exp. Med. 179, 457.

Meissner, M., Sherer, Y., Levy, Y., et al. 2000. Intravenous immunoglobulin therapy in a patient with lupus serositis and nephritis. Rheumatol. Int. 19, 199.

Meller, J., Conde, C.A., Deppisch, L.M., et al. 1975. Myocardial infarction due to coronary atherosclerosis in three young adults with systemic lupus erythematosus. Am. J. Cardiol. 35, 309.

Metz, D., Jolly, D., Graciet-Richard, J., et al. 1994. Prevalence of valvular involvement in systemic lupus erythematosus and association with antiphospholipid syndrome: a matched echocardiographic study. Cardiology 85, 129.

Mevorach, D., Raz, E., Shalev, O., et al. 1993. Complete heart block and seizure in an adult with systemic lupus erythematosus. Arthritis Rheum. 36, 259.

Moder, G.K., Miller, T.D., Tazelaar, H.D. 1999. Cardiac involvement in Systemic lupus erythematosus. Mayo Clin. Proc. 74, 275.

Morin, A.M., Boyer, A.S., Nataf, P., et al. 1996. Mitral insufficiency caused by systemic lupus erythematosus requiring valve replacement: three case reports and a review of the literature. Thorac. Cardiovasc. Surg. 44, 313.

Mourguet, A.J., Sandrock, D., Stille-Siegener, M., et al. 1995. Indium-111-antimyosin Fab imaging to demonstrate myocardial involvement in systemic lupus erythematosus. J. Nucl. Med. 36, 1432.

Murpy, J.J., Leach, I.H. 1989. Findings at necropsy in the heart of patients with the primary antiphospholipid syndrome. Br. Heart J. 62, 61.

Naarendorp, M., Kerr, L.D., Khan, A.S., et al. 1999. Dramatic improvement of left ventricular function after cytotoxic therapy in lupus patients with acute cardiomyopathy: report of 6 cases. J. Rheumatol. 26, 2257.

Nesher, G., Ilany, J., Rosemann, D., et al. 1997. Valvular dysfunction in antiphospholipid syndrome: prevalence, clinical features, and treatment. Semin. Arthritis Rheum. 27, 27.

Nihoyannopoulos, P., Gomez, P.M., Joshi, J., et al. 1990. Cardiac abnormalities in systemic lupus erythematosus. Association with raised anticardiolipin antibodies. Circulation 82, 369.

Nobrega, T.P., Klodas, E., Breen, J.F., et al. 1996. Giant coronary artery aneurysm in systemic lupus erythematosus. Cathet. Cardiovasc. Diagn. 39, 75.

O'Leary, D.H., Polak, J.F., Kronmal, R.A., et al. 1999. Carotid-artery intima and media thickness as a risk factor for myocardial infarction and stroke in older adults. Cardiovascular Health Study Collaborative Research Group. N. Eng. J. Med. 340, 14.

Omdal, R., Lunde, P., Rasmussen, K., et al. 2001. Transesophageal and trans thoracic echocardiography and Doppler-examination in systemic lupus erythematosus. Scand. J. Rheumatol. 30, 275.

Ong, M.L., Veerapen, K., Chambers, J.B., et al. 1992. Cardiac abnormalities in systemic lupus erythematosus: prevalence and relationship to disease activity. Int. J. Cardiol. 34, 69.

Petri, M., Perez-Gutthann, S., Spence, D., et al. 1992a. Risk factors for coronary artery disease in patients with systemic lupus erythematosus. Am. J. Med. 93, 513.
Petri and co-authors studied the risk factors for coronary artery disease in a very large cohort of lupus patients.

Petri, M., Spence, D., Bone, L.R., et al. 1992b. Coronary artery disease risk factors in the Johns Hopkins Lupus Cohort: Prevalence, recognition by patients and preventing pratices. Medicine 71, 291.

Petri, M., Lakatta, C., Magder, L., et al. 1994. Effect of prednisone and hydroxychloroquine on coronary artery disease risk factors in systemic lupus erythematosus: a longitudinal data analysis. Am. J. Med. 96, 254.

Petri, M., Roubenoff, R., Dallal, G.E., et al. 1996. Plasma homocysteine as a risk factor for atherothrombotic events in systemic lupus erythematosus. Lancet 348, 1120.

Petri, M. 2000a. Detection of coronary artery disease and the role of traditional risk factors in the Hopkins Lupus Cohort. Lupus 9 (3), 170.

Petri, M. 2000b. Hopkins Lupus Cohort. 1999 update. Rheum. Dis. Clin. N. Am. 26, 199.

Phadke, K.V., Phillips, R.A., Clarke, D.T., et al. 1993. Antiacardiolipin antibodies in ischemic heart disease: marker or myth? Br. Heart J. 69, 391.

Pritzker, M.R., Ernst, J.D., Caudill, C., et al. 1980. Acquired aortic stenosis in systemic lupus erythematosus. Ann. Intern. Med. 93, 434.

Rahman, P., Urowitz, M.B., Galdman, D.D., et al. 1999. Contribution of traditional risk factors to coronary artery disease in patients with systemic lupus erythematosus. J. Rheumatol. 26, 2363.

Ramonda, R., Doria, A., Villanova, C., et al. 1992. Évaluation de l'atteinte cardiaque au cours du lupus érythémateux disséminé: étude clinique et échocardiographique. Rev. Rhum. Mal. Ostéoartic. 59 (12), 790.

Rantapää-Dahlquist, S., Neumann-Andersen, G., Backman, C., et al. 1997. Echocardiographic findings, lipids and lipoprotein (a) in patients with systemic lupus erythematosus. Clin. Rheumatol. 16, 140.

Ratliff, N.B., Estes, M.L., Myles, J.L., et al. 1987. Diagnosis of chloroquine cardiomyopathy by endomyocardial biopsy. N. Engl. J. Med. 316, 191.

Ridker, P.M. 2001. High-sensitivity C-reactive protein: potential adjunct for global risk assessment in the primary prevention of cardiovascular disease. Circulation 103, 1813.

Ridker, P.M., Cushman, M., Stampfer, M.J., et al. 1997. Inflammation, aspirin and the risk of cardiovascular disease in apparently healthy men. N. Engl. J. Med. 336, 973.

Roberts, W.C., High, S.T. 1999. The heart in systemic lupus erythematosus. Curr. Probl. Cardiol. 24, 1.

Roditi, G.H., Hartnell, G.C., Cohen, M.C. 2000. MRI changes in myocarditis—evaluation with spin echo, cine MR angiography and contrast enhanced spin echo imaging. Clinical Radiology 55, 752.

Roldan, C.A., Shively, B.K., Crawford, M.H. 1996. An echocardiographic study of valvular heart disease associated with systemic lupus erythematosus. N. Eng. J. Med. 335, 1424.

Roman, M.J., Salmon, J.E., Sobel, R., et al. 2001. Prevalence and relation to risk factors of carotid atherosclerosis and left ventricular hypertrophy in systemic lupus erythematosus and antiphospholipid antibody syndrome. Am. J. Cardiol. 87, 663.

Ropes M.W. (Ed.), 1976. Systemic lupus erythematosus. Harvard University Press, Cambridge, MA.

Rosenthal, T., Neufeld, H., Kishon, Y., et al. 1980. Myocardial infarction in a young woman with systemic lupus erythematosus. Angiology 31, 573.

Rosner, S., Ginzler, E.M., Diamond, H.S., et al. 1982. A multicenter study of outcome in systemic lupus erythematosus. II. Causes of death. Arthritis Rheum. 25, 612.

Rubin, L.A., Urowitz, M.B., Gladman, D.D. 1985. Mortality in systemic lupus erythematosus: the bimodal pattern revisited. Q. J. Med. 55, 87.

Schillaci, O., Laganà, B., Danieli, R., et al. 1999. Technetium-99m sestamibi single-photon emission tomography detects subclinical myocardial perfusion abnormalities in patients with systemic lupus erythematosus. Eur. J. Nucl. Med. 26, 713.

Shapiro, R.F., Gamble, C.N., Wiesner, K.B., et al. 1977. Immunopathogenesis of Libman–Sacks endocarditis. Assessment by light and immunofluorescent microscopy in two cases. Ann. Rheum. Dis. 36, 508.

Shearn, M.A. 1959. The heart in systemic lupus erythematosus. Am. Heart J. 58, 452.

Sherer, Y., Levy, Y., Shoenfeld, Y. 1999. Marked improvement of severe cardiac dysfunction after one course of intravenous immunoglobulin in a patient with systemic lupus erythematosus. Clin. Rheumatol. 18, 238.

Shively, B.K. 2000. Transesophageal echocardiography (TEE) evaluation of the aortic valve, left ventricular outflow tract, and pulmonic valve. Cardiol. Clin. 18, 711.

Shoenfeld, Y., George, J., Sherer, Y., et al. 2001. Atherosclerosis: evidence for the role of autoimmunity. In: Y. Shoenfeld, D. Harats, G. Wick (Eds.), Atherosclerosis and Autoimmunity. Elsevier Science, pp. 139–142.
In this chapter autoimmune mechanisms involved in atherosclerosis have been extensively reviewed.

Simantov, R., LaSale, S.M., Lo, S.K., et al. 1995. Activation of cultured vascular endothelial cells by antiphospholipid antibodies. J. Clin. Invest. 96, 2211.

Stevens, M.B. 1992. Systemic lupus erythematosus and the cardiovascular system: the heart. In: R.G. Lahita (Ed.), Systemic lupus erythematosus. Churcill Livingstone, New York, p. 707.

Straaton, K.V., Chatham, W.W., Reveille, J.D., et al. 1988. Clinically significant valvular heart disease in systemic lupus erythematosus. Am. J. Med. 85, 645.

Sturfelt, G., Eskilsson, J., Nived, O., et al. 1992. Cardiovascular disease in systemic lupus erythematosus: a study of 75 patients from a defined population. Medicine 71, 216.

Sun, S.S., Shiau, Y.C., Tsai, S.C., et al. 2001. The role of technetium-99m sestamibi myocardial perfusion single-photon emission tomography (SPECT) in the detection of cardiovascular involvement in systemic lupus erythematosus patients with non-specific chest complaints. Rheumatology 40, 1106.

Svenungsson, E., Jensen-Urstad, K., Heimbürger, M. 2001. Risk factors for cardiovascular disease in systemic lupus erythematosus. Circulation 104, 1887.

In this study, many novel risk factors for subclinical atherosclerosis have been evaluated.

Thandroyen, F.T., Matisonn, R.E., Weir, E.K. 1978. Severe aortic incompetence caused by systemic lupus erythematosus: a case report. S. Afr. Med. J. 54, 166.

Tumulty, P.A., Harvey, A.M. 1949. The clinical course of disseminated lupus erythematosus: an evaluation of Osler's contribution. Bull. Johns Hopkins Hosp. 85, 47.

Urowitz, M.B., Bookman, A.A.M., Koehler, B.E., et al. 1976. The bimodal mortality pattern of systemic lupus erythematosus. Am. J. Med. 60, 221.

This is the paper which provides the first clinical evidence of early atherosclerosis.

Vaarala, O., Alfthan, G., Jauhiainen, M., et al. 1993. Cross-reaction between antibodies to oxidized low-density lipoprotein and to cardiolipin in systemic lupus erythematosus. Lancet 341, 923.

Vianna, J.L., Khamashta, M.A., Ordi-Ros, J., et al. 1994. Comparison of the primary and secondary antiphospholipid syndrome: an European Multicenter Study of 114 patients. Am. J. Med. 96, 3.

Von Felt, J.M. 1998. Coronary electron beam computed tomography (EBCT) in 13 patients with 2 or more cardiovascular risk factors. Arthritis Rheum. 41, S139.

Wallace, D.J., Podell, T., Weiner, J., et al. 1981. Systemic lupus erythematosus—survival patterns. Experience with 609 patients. JAMA 245, 934.

Wallace, D.J., Metzger, A.L., Stecher, V.J., et al. 1990. Cholesterol-lowering effect of hydroxychloroquine in patients with rheumatic disease: effects on lipid metabolism. Am. J. Med. 89, 322.

Ward, M.M. 1999. Premature morbidity from cardiovascular and cerebrovascular disease in women with systemic lupus erythematosus. Arthritis Rheum. 42, 338.

Wick, G., Schett, G., Amberger, A., et al. 1995. Is atherosclerosis an immunologically mediated disease? Immunol. Today 16, 27.

Wijetunga, M., Rockson, S. 2002. Myocarditis in systemic lupus erythematosus. Am. J. Med. 113, 419.

Wilson, V.E., Eck, S.L., Bates, E.R. 1992. Evaluation and treatment of acute myocardial infarction complicating systemic lupus erythematosus. Chest 101, 420.

Witztum, J.L. 1994. The oxidation hypothesis of atherosclerosis. Lancet 344, 793.

Yazici, Z.A., Raschi, E., Patel, A., et al. 2001. Human monoclonal anti-endothelial cell IgG-derived from a systemic lupus erythematosus patient bind and activates human endothelium in vitro. Int. Immunol. 13, 349.

Yurchak, P.M., Levine, S.A., Gorlin, R. 1965. Constrictive pericarditis in procainamide induced lupus erythematosus. Circulation 31, 113.

Ziporen, L., Goldberg, I., Arad, M., et al. 1996. Libman–Sacks endocarditis in the antiphospholipid syndrome. Immunopathologic findings in deformed heart valves. Lupus 5, 196.

Handbook of Systemic Autoimmune Diseases, Volume 1
The Heart in Systemic Autoimmune Diseases
A. Doria and P. Pauletto, editors

CHAPTER 11

Neonatal Lupus Syndromes: Clinical Features

Antonio Brucato[*,a], Jill P. Buyon[b]

[a]*Department of Medicine, Ospedale Niguarda Ca' Granda, Milano, Italy*
[b]*Hospital for Joint Diseases, New York University School of Medicine, New York, NY, USA*

1. Introduction

In 1901, congenital complete heart block (CHB) was first reported by Morquio (1901) and in 1945 was diagnosed antepartum by Plant and Steven (1945). Congenital CHB can occur in association with structural heart diseases such as AV septal defects, left atrial isomerism, and abnormalities of the great arteries (Machado et al., 1988), tumors such as mesotheliomas (Carter et al., 1974), or as an isolated defect. In 1928, Aylward reported the occurrence of CHB in two children whose mother 'suffered from Mikulicz's disease' (Aylward, 1928). This curious clinical observation was further solidified in the 1970s with reports of CHB in children whose mothers had autoimmune diseases (McCue et al., 1977; Chameides et al., 1977; Winkler et al., 1977) and by the finding that the maternal sera contained antibodies to Ro/SSA ribonucleoproteins (Scott et al., 1983; Lee et al., 1983; Harley et al., 1985). It was subsequently noted that many mothers also had antibodies to La/SSB (Buyon et al., 1989a, 1993; Silverman et al., 1991). Other abnormalities affecting the skin, liver, and blood elements were reported to be associated with anti-Ro/SSA-La/SSB antibodies in the maternal and fetal circulation and are now grouped under the heading of neonatal lupus syndromes (NLSs) (Watson et al., 1988; Laxer et al., 1990; Lee, 1990; Lee et al., 1993; Buyon et al., 1998). Neonatal lupus was so termed because the cutaneous lesions of the neonate resembled those seen in systemic lupus erythematosus (SLE) (McCuistion and Schoch, 1954; Kephardt et al., 1987). Notably, this might be a misleading name, because the baby does not have systemic lupus, and usually the mother too does not have SLE.

The biology of human viviparity involves a wide variety of fetal–maternal relationships, several of which may facilitate the occurrence of passively acquired autoimmunity (Buyon et al., 1996). Tissue injury in the fetus is presumed to be dependent on the IgG IIb (CD32) Fc receptor (Lin et al., 1994) mediated transplacental passage of maternal IgG autoantibodies from the mother who has an autoimmune process but who may be clinically asymptomatic. Disease in the offspring parallels the presence of maternal antibodies in the fetal and neonatal circulation and disappears, except for CHB, with the clearance of the maternal antibodies by the eighth month of postnatal life. The transient hematologic abnormalities and skin disease of the neonate reflect the effect of passively acquired autoantibodies on those organ systems which have the capacity of continual regeneration. In contrast, these regenerative processes apparently do not occur in cardiac tissue; complete block is irreversible to date. Curiously, the transient manifestations of this passively acquired

---

Abbreviations: ANA, anti-nuclear antibodies; AV, atrioventricular; CHB, complete heart block; ECG, electrocardiogram; NLS, neonatal lupus syndromes; SLE, systemic lupus erythematosus; SS, primary Sjogren's syndrome; UCTD, undifferentiated connective tissue disease.

*Corresponding author.
E-mail address: abrucato@ospedaleniguarda.it (A. Brucato).

DOI: 10.1016/S1571-5078(03)01011-0

autoimmune syndrome closely mimic the disease manifestations observed in adolescents or adults with SLE, while heart block is rarely, if ever, present in these same patients.

2. Definitions and implications

Immunologists and rheumatologists understand as congenital a block 'existing at or dating from birth' (Tseng and Buyon, 1997). In contrast, cardiologists often use Yater's criteria: "heart block established in a young patient. There must be some evidence of the existence of the slow pulse at a fairly early age and absence of a history of any infection which might cause the condition after birth: notably diphteria, rheumatic fever, chorea and congenital syphilis" (Yater, 1929). Thus it is evident that when immunologists, cardiologists, and obstetricians write about CHB they may not be describing the same clinical or pathological entity (Brucato, 1997a,b).

To reduce the existing confusion in the literature, we recommend a change from the existing definition (Yater, 1929). We propose a new definition of isolated congenital complete AV block, acceptable to cardiologists, rheumatologists, immunologists, obstetricians, pediatricians: "an AV block is defined as congenital if it is diagnosed in utero, at birth, or within the neonatal period (0–27 days after birth)" (Brucato et al., 2003). Accumulated data reveal that the large majority of cases detected in utero and not associated with structural heart defects causally linked with CHB are associated with the presence of anti-Ro/SSA antibodies in the mothers (Brucato et al., 1997a,b; Brucato et al., 1999; Scott et al., 1983; Julkumen et al., 1993b; Waltuk et al., 1994; Dorner et al., 1995; Frohn-Mulder et al., 1994; Reichlin et al., 1994; Hubscher et al., 1995; Silverman et al., 1995; Brucato et al., 1995a; Groves et al., 1996; Press et al., 1996; Shinohara et al., 1999; Udink ten Cate et al., 2001; Jaeggi et al., 2002; Buyon et al., 1989; Julkunen et al., 1993; Buyon et al., 1993; Machado et al., 1988). The percentages of anti-Ro/SSA positivity vary according to the laboratory method employed (counterimmunoelectrophoresis, immunoblot, ELISA—commercial kits, ELISA—home made), since different methods have different sensitivities and different specificities. Immunological studies using the most sensitive and advanced methods approach 100% of positivity (Julkunen et al., 1993a; Buyon et al., 1993; Brucato et al., 1995a; Dorner et al., 1995; Silverman et al., 1995; Colombo et al., 1999; Jaeggi et al., 2002). In these studies, there may have been a selection bias; in fact mothers may have been selected based on a diagnosed or suspected connective tissue disease, since these cases were collected mainly from rheumatological centers. On the other hand cardiological studies generally report lower percentages of anti-Ro/SSA positive cases (e.g. 65%), but details of methods employed to detect the antibodies often are lacking (Schmidt et al., 1991). In contrast, the study by Hubscher supports that heart block diagnosed after birth is only rarely associated with maternal anti-Ro/SSA antibodies (Hubscher et al., 1995).

Congenital CHB is then defined 'isolated CHB' in the absence of structural heart disease that may be causally related to heart block such as heterotaxia, single ventricle, endocardial cushion defects, and congenitally corrected transposition of the great arteries (ventricular inversion), but it may include lesions such as patent ductus arteriosus, secundum atrial septal defect, small ventricular septal defect, etc. Furthermore, it would be worthwhile to subdivide isolated CHB into categories related to the current degree of functional disease, i.e. (1) *complete* vs. (2) *incomplete*. The latter category may be further divided into first degree, second degree (Type I or II), or intermittent third degree. In this way, each case is characterized by major category (*congenital or non-congenital*), associated structural anomalies or the absence of anatomical disease (*isolated*), and the degree of conduction system disease at diagnosis (*complete or incomplete*). This may help in future research efforts regarding separating out etiologies, pathogeneses, and prognoses. Furthermore a dichotomous definition (isolated CHB vs. non-immune late-onset isolated heart block) will open the door for further research and more appropriate clinical care of the latter group as well. In fact, isolated heart block detected later in childhood may be associated with specific genetic markers or other pathogenic mechanisms such as long QT syndrome (Benson et al., 1999; Mehdirad et al., 1999; Wang et al., 2002), as well as acquired mechanisms in the modern era including Lyme disease (Gildein et al., 1993) or viral diseases, although it is of interest that in Lyme disease, the heart block is generally transient unlike CHB (see chapter on pathogenesis of CHB).

3. Prevalence and incidence

The incidence of isolated CHB is not well established. A generally accepted figure is 1 in 23,000–25,000 live births, based on two studies mostly done before the 1960s, each reporting a very limited number of affected children (Michaelsson and Engle, 1972). More recently, Siren et al. (1998) conducted a nationwide search for all cases of CHB born in Finland between 1970 and 1995. Patients with CHB were identified by using the registries of hospitalized patients and pacemaker insertions in all 5 university hospitals in Finland, as well as the registry of congenital abnormalities in Finland. Patients included had isolated CHB, i.e. there was no evidence of major cardiac structural malformations causally linked to CHB. In 73 patients, heart block had been diagnosed during pregnancy; in 24 additional patients, heart block was diagnosed after birth but before 5 yr of age. Considering an annual birth rate of about 65,000, according to the Office of Statistics in Finland, the mean incidence of the CHB in Finland between 1970 and 1995 was 1:17,000 live births (95% confidence interval 1:14,000–1:21,000). Furthermore the incidence of CHB showed a tendency to increase: in 1970s, 1:24,000, and in the first half of the 1990s, 1:11,000 ($P < 0.05$). This increase in incidence may be due to the increasing number of successful pregnancies in women with connective tissue diseases. It is also possible that the diagnostic accuracy has changed or fetuses diagnosed in utero with CHB may now survive better due to more effective antenatal care. In fact, approximately 20% of fetuses with CHB die in utero, so they are not included in statistics focusing on live birth.

4. Epidemiology

Good epidemiological data exist in USA, derived from the Research Registry for Neonatal Lupus, and in Finland, derived from the work of Julkunen's group. The Research Registry for Neonatal Lupus was established by the National Institute for Arthritis, Musculoskeletal and Skin Diseases (NIAMS) in September 1994, under the directorship of Dr Buyon. The purpose of this registry is to document cases of neonatal lupus for basic and/or clinical research. Cases are considered potential candidates for enrollment if a mother has a child with any manifestation of neonatal lupus such as AV block, characteristic skin rash, hemolytic anemia, leukopenia, thrombocytopenia, or cholestatic liver disease. Following review of medical records, a case is considered to be definite neonatal lupus if the following two criteria are met: (1) maternal antibodies to the 52 kDa Ro, 60 kDa Ro/SSA, or 48 kDa La/SSB ribonucleoproteins are identified; and (2) CHB or characteristic skin rash is diagnosed. The affected births occurred from 1970 to the present. Referrals to the Registry are generally from obstetricians, pediatricians, rheumatologists, and pediatric cardiologists. As of September 1997, 105 mothers whose sera were documented to contain anti-Ro/SSA and/or -La/SSB antibodies and their 113 infants diagnosed with CHB between 1970 and 1997 were enrolled in the Registry: 56 were males and 57 females. In Finland, 97 children with CHB were studied: 60% were female and 40% male (this difference is not statistically significant) (Siren et al., 1998).

5. Clinical manifestations

5.1. Conventional clinical features

5.1.1. Cardiac manifestations

Congenital atrioventricular (AV) block is the most severe manifestation of NLSs, since if complete it is probably irreversible and carries a high morbidity and mortality rate. It is usually a complete (i.e. third degree) block, although lesser degree blocks have been described (Geggel et al., 1988; Brucato et al., 1995b; Buyon et al., 1998; Saleeb et al., 1999). The presence of signs or symptoms is mainly related to the ventricular rate, which usually ranges between 30 and 100 beats/min (Schmidt et al., 1991; Vignati et al., 1999), but may be also related to the cardiac contractility and to the ratio between atrial and ventricular contractions; heart rate usually declines during pregnancy (Vignati et al., 1997); the lower the rate, the higher the possibility of fetal hydrops and neonatal cardiac failure, and fetal or neonatal death correlates with a ventricular rate in utero less than or equal to 55 bpm (Schmidt et al., 1991; Vignati et al., 1999). CHB is most frequently detected in utero by prenatal ultrasound, between 18 and 24 wk of gestational age. This 'window' occurs after the passage of maternal autoantibodies and after the structural development of the heart. In the majority of cases CHB requires pacemaker implantation, frequently in the neonatal period (Michaelsson et al., 1995; Eronen et al., 2000).

5.1.2. Skin disease

A skin rash can be present in the neonatal period, but more frequently appears between the second and third month of life (Weston et al., 1999; Neiman et al., 2000). Unlike CHB, it is transient since it disappears with the clearance of maternal autoantibodies from the baby's circulation, usually without any residua. The rash is erythematous and scaly, frequently annular in shape, and mostly located in sun-exposed areas with a characteristic predilection for the periorbital area. Ultraviolet exposure may be an initiating factor and can exacerbate an existing rash. Histologically the lesions are similar to subacute cutaneous lupus, with hyperkeratosis, epidermal atrophy, basal degeneration, interstitial edema, and perivascular mononuclear infiltrate (Bangert et al., 1984). On immunofluorescence, immunoglobulin and complement deposition at the dermo-epidermal junction have been demonstrated (Lee, 1993). Since these lesions are self-limiting, usually no treatment is required.

5.1.3. Hepatobiliary disease

Neonatal cholestasis has been a finding in several cases of neonatal lupus (Laxer et al., 1990; Lee et al., 1993). A recent review of cases in the Research Registry for Neonatal Lupus revealed three types of hepatobiliary disease: (1) liver failure occurring at birth or in utero, often having the phenotype of neonatal iron storage disease or neonatal 'hemochromatosis'; (2) transient conjugated hyperbilirubinemia occurring in the first few weeks of life; and (3) transient transaminase elevations occurring in the first few months of life (Lee et al., 2002). The latter two categories were associated with a good prognosis, with spontaneous resolution of disease activity and no evidence of long-term sequelae. It is not yet known if all three types of hepatobiliary disease are definitely manifestations of neonatal lupus, but their presence in children with other manifestations of neonatal lupus certainly raises that possibility. Hepatobiliary disease attributable or possibly attributable to neonatal lupus occurred in about 10% of cases in the Registry.

5.1.4. Hematologic abnormalities

Hematologic abnormalities have been described, usually consisting of anemia and/or thrombocytopenia (Watson et al., 1988). Similar to the rash, these manifestations are transient and usually do not need medical treatment. Even severe neutropenia associated with mildly abnormal liver functions has been reported (Kanagasegar et al., 2002).

5.2. Novel clinical aspects

5.2.1. Spectrum and progression of conduction abnormalities in infants born to mothers with anti-Ro/SSA-La/SSB antibodies

In considering the pathologic process of injury, it may be that tissue damage results in a range of conduction abnormalities. Identification of less-advanced degrees of block or fibrosis around the AV node without any conduction abnormality on ECG would support this pathologic model, and serve as a potential marker for treatment if the conduction defect could be shown to progress. To ascertain the spectrum of arrhythmias associated with maternal anti-Ro/SSA-La/SSB antibodies, records of all the children enrolled in the Research Registry for Neonatal Lupus were reviewed (Askanase et al., 2002). Of 187 children with CHB whose mothers have anti-Ro/SSA-La/SSB antibodies, 9 had a prolonged PR interval on ECG at birth, 4 of whom progressed to more advanced AV block. A child whose younger sibling had third degree block was diagnosed with first degree block at 10 yr of age, at the time of surgery for a broken wrist. Two children diagnosed in utero with second degree block were treated with dexamethasone and reverted to normal sinus rhythm by birth, but ultimately progressed to third block. Four children had second degree block at birth: of these, two progressed to third degree block. These data have important research and clinical implications.

Perhaps many fetuses sustain mild inflammation, but resolution is variable, as suggested by the presence of incomplete AV block. Since subsequent progression of less-advanced degrees of block can occur, an ECG should be performed on all infants born to mothers with anti-Ro/SSA-La/SSB antibodies.

In contrast to the AV node, evidence for atrial slowing is quite rare (see below).

5.2.2. Late-onset dilated cardiomyopathy

Recently evidence has emerged that a subset of patients with CHB may develop dilated cardiomyopathy (Eronen et al., 2000; Udink ten Cate et al., 2001; Moak et al., 2001), even if the risk seems low (6%) (Udink ten Cate et al., 2001). A multicenter study reported recently on the development of late-onset cardiomyopathy in CHB (Moak et al., 2002). They found 16 infants with CHB who developed late-onset dilated cardiomyopathy despite early pacing. The authors estimated that the total incidence of late cardiomyopathy was 5–11% in all cases of CHB. Twelve of 16 cases were diagnosed in utero, 6 with pericardial effusions. All the cases had normal in utero myocardial function, and 15/16 had normal left ventricular function at birth; one had a low shortening fraction (SF) of 20%. One neonate had a rash, and two had elevated liver enzymes and low platelet counts. Fifteen of the 16 were paced within the first 2 wk, 1 at 7 months. The SF fell to 9–5% from 2 wk to 9.3 yr after diagnosis. Twelve of the 16 developed congestive heart failure by 2 yr of age. Biopsies showed hypertrophy, fibrosis, and myocyte degeneration, but none had antibody deposition or an active inflammatory infiltrate. Four of the 16 died of congestive heart failure, 7/16 had transplantation (1 is waiting), and only 4/16 recovered a normal SF. The cardiomyopathy was not felt to be due to simply a slow heart rate (it occurred despite adequate pacing) or underlying structural heart disease, present in 3/16 patients. The authors recommend that all cases of CHB need close follow-up, not only for rate and rhythm disorders, but also with echocardiograms for myocardial disease.

Eronen et al. (2000) confirmed these findings. Their cohort included 91 infants with CHB. Dilated cardiomyopathy was found in 21 (23%), of whom 13 died. It was associated with intrauterine hydrops, low fetal and neonatal heart rate, low birth weight, male sex, and neonatal problems attributable to prematurity or neonatal lupus.

Udink ten Cate et al. (2001) sought to identify the risk factors predicting the development of dilated cardiomyopathy in patients with CHB. In a retrospective study of 149 patients, 9 patients (6%) developed dilated cardiomyopathy at the age of 6.5 ± 5 yr. No definite cause could be identified. In these 9 patients, CHB was diagnosed in 8 at 23 ± 2.3 wk gestation and in 1 at birth. Maternal anti-Ro/SSA antibodies were confirmed in seven of the nine patients. Pacemakers were implanted in eight patients in the first month and in one patient at 5 yr of age. Two patients with dilated cardiomyopathy died within 2 months of diagnosis; one patient is neurologically compromised; two patients received a heart transplant; and four patients are listed for heart transplantation. The authors conclude that risk factors for the development of dilated cardiomyopathy may be an increased heart size at initial evaluation, and the absence of pacemaker-associated improvement of the left ventricular end-diastolic dimension and of the cardiothoracic ratio.

Abbot et al. (1998) reviewed the prevalence of cardiomyopathy in patients recorded in the Research Registry for Neonatal Lupus. In this study, data from the Registry were analyzed to determine the prevalence of cardiomyopathy as defined by the evidence of cardiac dysfunction or the need for anti-congestive medications or treatments. Patients with primary structural defects or who died within the first month of life were excluded from analysis. A total of 163 NLS patients were identified. Of this population 134 were found to have CHB, 75 of whom required pacemaker implantation. Nine (5.5%) of the patients with CHB developed a cardiomyopathy, and among those with pacemakers, 12% developed a cardiomyopathy. The 9 observed cases, consisting of 2 males and 7 females, presented with symptoms between birth and the age of 11 yr, and among these, 3 died and 1 required transplantation.

5.2.3. Endocardial fibroelastosis

CHB may be associated with endocardial fibroelastosis, and recently it has been reported that isolated endocardial fibroelastosis may be independently related to maternal anti-Ro/SSA and anti-La/SSB antibodies. Nield et al. (2002) identified three cases (one fetus and two infants, all female) of isolated endocardial fibroelastosis in infants born to anti-Ro/SSA positive mothers in the absence of CHB. Two cases died and one received a cardiac transplant. All three cases had histologically confirmed endocardial fibroelastosis and demonstrated significant diffuse IgG infiltration. To a lesser extent, myocardial tissue was also positive for IgM, CD43, and Granzyme B. None of the specimens were TUNEL positive. These are the first reported cases of isolated endocardial fibroelastosis associated with maternal anti-Ro/SSA and anti-La/SSB antibodies in the absence of CHB. The diffuse deposition of IgG and the presence of a T-cell infiltrate throughout the myocardium suggest that the transplacental passage of maternal autoantibodies induces an immune reaction within the myocardium, leading to isolated endocardial fibroelastosis. Autoantibody-mediated endocardial fibroelastosis may be an etiologic factor in cases of fetal and neonatal 'idiopathic' dilated cardiomyopathy. The absence of apoptosis remains unexplained given the observation of exaggerated apoptosis observed by Clancy and colleagues in the septal region of two fetuses with CHB (see chapter 4 on pathogenesis of CHB).

5.2.4. QT interval prolongation

Although the main feature of the NLSs is complete or incomplete CHB, other electrocardiographic abnormalities have been recently reported by several groups. Specifically, alterations in ventricular repolarization have been found to be associated with transplacental transmission of anti-Ro/SSA antibodies (Cimaz et al., 2000). We have seen one of these infants—born from an anti-Ro/SSA positive mother—who presented a marked QT prolongation in the absence of AV conduction abnormalities. Since a prolonged QT interval in the neonatal period and during infancy is a risk factor for sudden infant death (Schwartz et al., 1998), we have then analyzed the ECG tracings for QT interval measurement of other anti-Ro/SSA positive infants who did not have CHB, as well as those of a control group of anti-Ro/SSA negative infants born from mothers with autoimmune diseases but negative for these autoantibodies. The study was performed in 21 anti-Ro/SSA positive and 7 anti-Ro/SSA negative infants. The 20 anti-Ro/SSA positive mothers, one of whom gave birth to twins, were affected by SLE (8/20), Sjogren's syndrome (SS) (3/20), or undifferentiated connective tissue disease (UCTD) (9/20). None of the infants had a family history of long QT syndrome or sudden unexpected death during infancy, and none had experienced an apparently life-threatening event. All had been delivered without complications and were apparently healthy. A standard 12 lead-ECG, recorded during the first 6 months of life (mostly at the third month), was analyzed for each subject. QT and RR intervals were measured in lead two from five non-consecutive beats by a single investigator who was blinded to the infant's antibody status. Corrected QT (QTc) was automatically calculated according to the Bazett's formula. Sixteen of 21 infants were positive for antibodies against 52 and 60 kDa Ro/SSA proteins, 4 of 21 were positive for anti-60 kDa, and 1 of 21 for anti-52 kDa only. Five sera were also positive for anti-La/SSB antibodies. Positive and negative infants did not differ significantly for PR interval and QRS duration, whereas QTc interval was significantly greater in the group with anti-Ro/SSA antibodies (442 ± 35 vs. 403 ± 16 ms, $P = 0.001$). When we analyzed the individual values of QTc, we observed that 9/21 (43%) of the infants with anti-Ro/SSA had a QTc greater than 440 ms, the upper normal limit (97.5th percentile) established in the previously mentioned large prospective study of more than 33,000 infants (Schwartz et al., 1998). By contrast, all infants without anti-Ro/SSA antibodies had a QTc within the normal limits. Thus, a significant proportion of infants with anti-Ro/SSA antibodies of maternal origin have a prolongation of QTc interval but children born to mothers with autoimmune diseases but without anti-Ro/SSA (Cimaz et al., 2000) do not. We have followed the children with prolonged QTc, in order to evaluate the relationship between electrocardiographic abnormalities and the disappearance of autoantibodies from the babies' circulation. Interestingly, we observed a concomitant disappearance of electrocardiographic abnormalities and acquired maternal autoantibodies during the first year of life (Cimaz et al., 2003). In agreement with these findings, Gordon et al. (2001a,b) have described that the QTc is longer in children of anti-Ro/SSA positive mothers, and even longer in those with siblings with CHB.

Clinical and experimental studies demonstrated that a prolongation of the QT interval on the baseline surface electrocardiogram is associated with an increased electrical instability and can favor the development of malignant ventricular arrhythmias. Specifically, it has recently been shown in a study of more than 33,000 infants that the risk of sudden infant death is 41 times greater when QTc > 440 ms (Schwartz et al., 1998). The observation of a prolonged QT interval in infants born to positive mothers suggests that anti-Ro/SSA antibodies may interfere with ventricular repolarization during development, even if the pathogenetic mechanism is unknown. Different studies have demonstrated that anti-Ro/SSA antibodies inhibit L-type calcium currents (Boutjdir et al., 1997, 1998; Xiao et al., 2001) but do not affect some of the ionic currents, i.e. the potassium currents Ik1, Ito, and Iks and the sodium current, involved in the control of repolarization in ventricular myocytes (Boutjdir et al., 1998; Qu et al., 2001). However, the effects of anti-Ro/SSA antibodies on other important potassium currents involved in ventricular repolarization, e.g. Ikr, have not been tested. It is worth noting that mutations of the gene encoding for these potassium currents are responsible for one form of congenital long QT syndrome (Priori et al., 1999). Thus, we cannot exclude that the presence of anti-Ro/SSA antibodies in infants might interfere with these types of potassium currents during development and induce QT interval prolongation. This transient alteration in ventricular repolarization in some anti-Ro/SSA positive infants may temporarily predispose them to lethal arrhythmias. These findings further emphasize that ECG screening of babies born to anti-Ro/SSA positive mothers should become a required element of the neonatal evaluation. Prophylactic treatment may be required during the first year of life for those who have a prolonged QT interval, given the increased risk for sudden cardiac death.

5.2.5. *Sinus bradycardia*

Mazel reported that passive transfer of human anti-Ro/SSA and anti-La/SSB autoantibodies into naive pregnant mice induced bradycardia and first degree AV block in pups, suggesting a possible sinoatrial node involvement (Mazel et al., 1999). Recently Xiao et al. (2001) observed that IgG containing anti-Ro/SSA antibodies inhibited both L-type and T-type calcium channels expressed in *Xenopus* oocytes. Because T-type channels have been implicated in the pacemaker activity in the heart, these findings may provide, at least in part, an ionic basis for the sinus bradycardia reported in murine models (Xiao et al., 2001). We observed similar findings in humans (Brucato et al., 2000; Cimaz et al., 1997). In the last 4 yr, we prospectively performed 24 ECGs in our centers in newborns from anti-Ro/SSA positive mothers, in the first days after birth. In four cases (16.7%), a significant transient sinus bradycardia was observed (heart rate < 3rd percentile for age) (Brucato et al., 2001). Prenatal ultrasound fetal heart rate was normal; no perinatal complication (in particular, no metabolic or thermal problems) were observed, and possible causes of bradycardia in newborns were excluded, e.g. electrolyte abnormalities and drug interferences. In all cases, bradycardia disappeared within 10 days after birth, with no sequelae. Two mothers had SLE and two had UCTD. Notably, three mothers had a fine specificity directed against the 60 kDa component alone of the Ro/SSA antigen in immunoblot, and the fourth was positive for both anti-52 and anti-60 kDa. Our observations indicate that sinus bradycardia and sinus node dysfunction not only occur in experimental animals passively transfused with anti-Ro/SSA antibodies, but also that they might be detectable in rare cases in human newborns. In the Research Registry for Neonatal Lupus, data on atrial rates were sought among the 187 records reviewed. Atrial rates of 78 fetuses were recorded in utero by echocardiogram; the mean rate was 138 bpm ± 17 SD, range 68–160. Three fetuses (3.8%) had atrial rates less than 100 bpm. The rate of the first increased from 68 to 158 on postnatal ECG. The rate of the second increased minimally from 95 to 104 on postnatal ECG. The third had a rate of 95 bpm in utero and a postnatal ECG was not provided. Atrial rates from postnatal ECGs were available for 40 neonates; the mean rate was 137 bpm ± 20 SD, range 75–200. The one slow rate of 75 bpm was obtained during sleep and increased to 140 bpm when awake. In an additional child, the records stated sinus bradycardia; however, no ECG was available and subsequent records were not sent to the Registry (Askanase et al., 2002).

Several groups are assessing the presence of PR prolongation, i.e., first degree AV block, in the newborns from anti-Ro/SSA positive mothers, but data are not available at present.

5.2.6. Central nervous system involvement and learning disabilities

There is recent evidence that central nervous system involvement may be observed in neonatal lupus. Computerized tomography of the brain was performed in 10 of 11 consecutive infants with neonatal lupus erythematosus (five boys and six girls) (Prendiville et al., 2003). Ten of the 11 infants had brain neurosonography. Nine of 10 infants had abnormal computerized tomography scans. There was diffuse, markedly reduced attenuation of the cerebral white matter in four infants studied in the first week of life, and also in an infant 5 wk of age. Patchy reduced subcortical white matter attenuation was observed in another 5 wk old infant. Basal ganglia calcifications were present in two infants at 2 months of age, one of whom also had mild ventriculomegaly. A patient with macrocephaly studied at 4 months of age had enlarged ventricles and subarachnoid spaces consistent with benign macrocephaly of infancy. Cerebral ultrasound examination was abnormal in all five infants studied in the first week of life and in one infant at 2 months of age. Findings included subependymal cysts (4), echogenic white matter (3), and echogenic lenticulostriate vessels (3). Apart from one case of macrocephaly, there was no clinical evidence of neurologic disease and the subsequent development of these infants has been normal. The investigators' hypothesis is that subclinical central nervous system disease in NLS is likely to be a transient phenomenon that resolves as maternal antibodies are cleared from the infant's circulation. It is important to be aware of these neuroimaging abnormalities to avoid misdiagnosis of congenital viral infection in a newborn with multisystem NLS. The potential for neurologic sequelae is uncertain.

Ross et al. (2003) have recently reported in a case-controlled study whether children (and particularly sons) of women with SLE during pregnancy are more likely to have learning disabilities and be non-right-handed, and if maternal disease variables (i.e. presence of maternal antibodies, disease activity level, and use of corticosteroids) predict the prevalence of learning disabilities in offspring; 58 children whose mothers had SLE during pregnancy and 58 children of healthy mothers were assessed. All children took a standardized intelligence test (Wechsler Intelligence Scale for Children—III) and completed a modified version of the Edinburgh Hand Preference Questionnaire. They also took standardized tests of reading, arithmetic, and writing achievement. Learning disability was defined as having an academic achievement score of at least 1.5 SDs below the full-scale IQ. Sons of women with SLE were significantly more likely to have learning disabilities than daughters of women with SLE or children of either sex in the control group. Maternal SLE was not associated with non-right-handedness in sons or daughters. The presence of anti-Ro/La/SSB antibodies and disease activity (flare) in mothers during pregnancy were significantly related to higher prevalence of learning disabilities in offspring. The authors hypothesize that maternal antibodies, particularly anti-Ro/La, likely affect the fetal brain of male offspring and result in later learning problems (Ross et al., 2003). These findings are very preliminary and the observed difference between sons and daughters is puzzling. However, these provocative findings should promote greater awareness of the risk for learning disabilities in sons of women with autoimmune disease and the possible need for early educational intervention in those children.

6. Diagnostic investigations

6.1. Fetal echocardiography

Instrumental monitoring includes fetal echocardiography and Doppler velocimetry. Fetal echocardiograms have become the most useful non-invasive means for detection, diagnosis, and monitoring of fetal arrhythmias. The diagnosis of congenital CHB is obtained during fetal life with the echocardiographic demonstration of AV dissociation. Fetal echocardiogram is essential to diagnose (fetal ECGs are not available) and also follow the course of disease and may suggest the presence of an associated myocarditis by the finding of decreased contractility in addition to the secondary changes associated with myocarditis such as an increase of cardiac size, pericardial effusions, and tricuspid regurgitation. The obstetric management should be guided by the degree of cardiac failure noted on the ultrasound images.

6.1.1. The mechanical PR interval

By placing M-mode sampling cursors through both the fetal atrium and ventricle imaged by two-dimensional echocardiography, the relative timing of atrial and ventricular contractions can be determined. Hence, electrical activity can be inferred from the timing of the mechanical events. However, fetal echocardiographic M-mode tracings are limited in their ability to detect and distinguish between milder levels of AV block, specifically first and second degree (Wenkebach) AV block. Gated-pulsed Doppler studies of the AV and semilunar valves have been described in helping to identify rhythm disturbances in fetal hearts. By using the gated-pulsed Doppler technique, time intervals from the onset of the mitral A wave (atrial systole) to the onset of the aortic pulsed Doppler tracing (ventricular systole) within the same left ventricular cardiac cycle may be measured. This time interval represents the 'mechanical' PR interval. Its validity was confirmed by neonatal electrocardiographic correlation to the pulsed Doppler mechanical PR interval (Glickstein et al., 2000). The normal mechanical PR interval in the fetus is 0.12 ± 0.02 s (95% confidence intervals 0.10–0.14). There was no variation of the mechanical PR interval with heart rate or gestational age. The measurement of mechanical PR interval of the fetal heart might be the earliest reliable non-invasive echocardiographic marker of AV nodal dysfunction (first degree AV block) and/or myocardial injury, and for this reason it might be an excellent means of monitoring pregnant anti-Ro/SSA positive women.

6.1.2. The Tei index

A useful, non-invasive, Doppler-derived myocardial performance tool which can be used to assess aspects of systolic and diastolic function has been validated and is called the Tei index (TI) (Friedman et al., 2003). The normal TI in the second- and early third-trimester fetuses (18–31 wk gestation) was 0.53 ± 0.13. This index can be easily obtained in the fetus without the need for precise anatomic imaging and may be a useful tool to explore fetal myocardial function in pregnant anti-Ro/SSA positive women.

6.2. Serology/immunology: evaluation of the fine specificities of the maternal autoantibody response

Can our rapidly expanding knowledge of anti-Ro/SSA and -La/SSB autoantibodies and their cognate antigens help define the mother at the highest risk for having a pregnancy complicated by NLS? While seemingly straightforward, the task is a challenging one. Several laboratories from the US and abroad have tackled this problem using various techniques including immunodiffusion, immunoblot of various tissues and cell lysates, ELISA employing recombinant and purified proteins, and immunoprecipitation of radiolabeled in vitro translation products and cell lysates. Large series of CHB patients have showed that anti-52 kDa Ro/SSA and anti-La/SSB might be more strongly associated with CHB than other specificities, at least as tested by immunoblot (Julkunen et al., 1993a; Buyon et al., 1993; Dorner et al., 1995; Colombo et al., 1999), even if one group did not find this association (Meilof et al., 1993). Buyon's laboratory has used gel separation methods which vary the quantity of acrylamide to bis-acrylamide to obtain a more precise molecular characterization of the relevant antigenic structures identified by the immune response in women whose children have NLS (Buyon et al., 1989a,b, 1993).

Specifically, increasing the ratio of monomer to crosslinker from 37.5 (used in a standard Laemmli buffer system (Laemmli, 1970)) to 172.4 in a 15% acrylamide solution readily separates the 48 kDa La/SSB polypeptide from the 52 kDa Ro/SSA component. We have employed this method of gel separation for immunoblot, as well as ELISA, to evaluate antibody frequency, titer, and fine specificity in the sera from four groups of mothers segregated according to the status of the child: 57 whose children had CHB, 12 whose children had transient dermatologic or hepatic manifestations of NLS but no detectable cardiac involvement, 152 with SLE and related autoimmune diseases who gave birth to healthy children, and 30 with autoimmune diseases whose pregnancy resulted in miscarriage, fetal demise, or early postpartum death unrelated to NLS (Buyon et al., 1993). Anti-Ro/SSA antibodies were identified by ELISA in 100, 91, 47, and 43% of mothers of infants with CHB, transient NLS, healthy children, and fetal demise, respectively. High titers of anti-Ro/SSA antibodies were more often present in mothers of children with cardiac or cutaneous manifestations of NLS than in either of the other two groups. Maternal antibodies to La/SSB were detected by ELISA in 76% of the CHB group, 73% of the cutaneous/hepatic group, 15% with healthy children, and 7% with fetal demise. On immunoblot, 91% of the heart block group who had antibodies to Ro/SSA but not to La/SSB recognized at least one Ro/SSA antigen, with significantly greater reactivity against the 52 kDa component. In contrast, 62% of the anti-Ro/SSA-positive La/SSB-negative responders in the healthy group recognized either the 52 kDa and/or 60 kDa components. Although there was no profile of anti-Ro/SSA response unique to the mothers of children with heart block or cutaneous manifestations of NLS, only 1% of normal infants were born of mothers with antibodies directed to both the 52 kDa Ro/SSA and 48 kDa La/SSB antigens and not to the 60 kDa Ro/SSA antigen, compared to 21% with cardiac and 25% with cutaneous manifestations of NLS.

Dorner et al. (1995) investigated quantitative and qualitative differences of anti-Ro/SSA-La/SSB antibodies by ELISA in sera from 16 infants with CHB and their mothers compared to 8 healthy anti-Ro/SSA positive infants born to SLE mothers. No serum sample contained IgM autoantibodies. All 16 (100%) CHB infants had anti-52 kDa Ro/SSA antibodies, 14 (88%) had anti-La/SSB, and 9 (56%) had anti-60 kDa Ro/SSA compared to 6 (75%) anti-52 kDa, 3 (38%) anti-48 kDa, and 2 (25%) anti-60 kDa in the control infants. The anti-52 kDa Ro/SSA and anti-La/SSB antibody levels were significantly higher in CHB infants than in the controls. The anti-60 kDa Ro/SSA IgG levels of sera from infants and mothers from the CHB and control groups were similar.

Based on analysis by immunoblot and ELISA of sera from 14 mothers of children with CHB and 12 lupus patients with healthy offspring, Meilof et al. (1993) concluded that the fine specificity of the autoantibody response to Ro/SSA and La/SSB proteins does not predict the occurrence of CHB. These results are not surprising, since it can be predicted from the disparity of disease expression in twins and the low recurrence rate in subsequent pregnancies (see below) that another factor (probably fetal) is operative, and that the discovery of a unique risk profile is unlikely.

In a study of sera from 31 mothers of children with CHB, Julkunen et al. (1993a,b) demonstrated 97% reactivity with 52 kDa Ro/SSA by ELISA, 77% with 60 kDa Ro/SSA and 39% with La/SSB. Compared to 45 mothers with SLE and healthy children, mothers of CHB children had higher titers of antibodies to recombinant 52 and 60 kDa Ro/SSA proteins. However, compared to 19 mothers with primary SS and healthy offspring, the autoantibody responses were similar. No differences in the titer of anti-La/SSB antibodies were found between mothers within any of these three groups. In agreement with previous data, these investigators did not find a specific antibody profile unique to CHB.

Silverman et al. (1995) evaluated the maternal antibody profile in two groups of sera, 41 obtained from mothers whose children had manifestations of NLS (21 CHB, 20 cutaneous) and 19 from lupus patients known to have anti-Ro/SSA and/or anti-La/SSB antibodies and healthy children. Significantly higher levels of anti-La/SSB and anti-52 kDa Ro/SSA antibodies were demonstrated in the mothers of affected children. Mothers whose children had cutaneous manifestations had higher titers of anti-La/SSB antibodies than mothers whose children had CHB. Fine delineation of the anti-La/SSB responses revealed that a small carboxyl terminus polypeptide of recombinant La/SSB, DD, was recognized by 30% of mothers whose children had NLS but none who had healthy children.

Salomonsson et al. (2002) evaluated the maternal antibody profile in 9 Ro/SSA-La/SSB-positive mothers who gave birth to affected children, their 8 newborns with CHB, and 26 Ro/SSA-La/SSB-positive mothers whose children were healthy. Antibodies against 52 kDa Ro/SSA, 60 kDa Ro/SSA, and La/SSB were analyzed by enzyme-linked immunosorbent assay and immunoblotting, using recombinant proteins and synthetic peptides. IgG anti-52 kDa Ro/SSA antibodies were detected in all mothers who gave birth to children with CHB, as well as in their affected children, but were less frequent and at lower levels in control mothers. Fine mapping revealed a striking difference, in which the response in the mothers of affected children was dominated by antibodies to amino acids 200–239 of the 52 kDa Ro/SSA protein ($P = 0.0002$), whereas the primary activity in control mothers was against amino acids 176–196 ($P = 0.001$). Furthermore, 8 of 9 mothers of children with CHB had antibody reactivity against amino acids 1–135 of the 52 kDa Ro/SSA protein, containing two putative zinc fingers reconstituted under reducing conditions. The authors concluded that development of CHB is strongly dependent on a specific antibody profile to 52 kDa Ro/SSA, which may be a useful tool to identify pregnant Ro/SSA-La/SSB-positive women at risk of delivering a baby with CHB. This conclusion is intriguing, but the small sample size limits generalizability.

Defining the risk of CHB based on a particular antibody profile is particularly difficult for two reasons. The first is that the maternal disease must be matched between the groups of mothers compared. For example, if the control group is mothers with SLE, as in our study done in 1993 (Buyon et al., 1993) and that of Dorner et al. (1995), it would not be surprising to find a greater frequency of anti-48 kDa La/SSB and 52 kDa Ro/SSA in the CHB-mothers. It has been previously reported that in SLE, anti-60 kDa responses predominate over anti-52 kDa response (Ben-Chetrit et al., 1990). If the control mothers have primary SS, the antibody profiles of the CHB mothers and those with healthy offspring might be equivalent as supported by the studies of Julkunen et al. (Julkunen et al., 1993a,b, 1995). In effect, these observations reinforce the findings of most studies that the serologic profile of mothers whose children have CHB closely resembles that of primary SS. One approach to defining risk would be to subset the mothers of children with CHB and compare 'SS-CHB' to 'SS-healthy' and 'SLE-CHB' to 'SLE-healthy'. However, because many mothers are asymptomatic and only identified by the birth of their affected child, an appropriate control group is difficult to assemble. A second problem is that the control mothers may have a child with CHB after having had a healthy child. In fact, data from the Research Registry reinforces this possibility. Of families with at least two children, about half had the child with CHB after a healthy child; there is one family in which the CHB child was born after 3 healthy children.

The fact that SDS-immunoblot favors recognition of denatured epitopes complicates the interpretation of antibody reactivity. It is likely that all anti-Ro/SSA responses would include reactivity with the 60 kDa Ro/SSA component if immunoprecipitation of the native protein was the assay employed (Itoh and Reichlin, 1992).

Perhaps instead of defining a high-risk profile, we should define a low-risk profile. In our experience, mothers who do not have anti-La/SSB antibodies and have anti-Ro/SSA antibodies of low titer that do not recognize either the 60 or 52 kDa component on SDS-immunoblot appear to be at lower risk (Buyon, 1993). We have evaluated sera from 124 mothers whose children have CHB. All had antibodies to Ro/SSA or La/SSB by ELISA. An isolated response to the denatured 60 kDa component on immunoblot was observed in 2 (<2%) sera, and only 2 sera (<2%) did not recognize any component of Ro/SSA or La/SSB on immunoblot (Research Registry, unpublished observation). However, this response represents only a small fraction of the anti-Ro/SSA responders in general.

A note of caution: reporting of antibody profiles is highly dependent on the assays employed. For example, Neidenbach and Sahn (1993) report an infant with cutaneous manifestations of NLS associated with maternal antibodies to La/SSB in the absence of associated antibodies to Ro/SSA. Testing was done by ELISA and immunoblot. In our experience and that of others, immunoprecipitation of the native 60 kDa Ro/SSA antigen has always been positive when anti-La/SSB antibodies are present (Buyon, 1993), and such may well be the case in this 'unique' infant.

Isacovics and Silverman (1993) have utilized limiting dilution experiments of EBV-infected peripheral blood mononuclear cells to examine the frequency of anti-Ro/SSA and anti-La/SSB antibody secreting cells in mothers whose children have NLS. These authors report that a low anti-Ro/SSA or anti-La/SSB antibody B cell precursor frequency tends to be associated with the birth of a child with NLS. Additionally, mothers of children with NLS who later developed SLE have higher anti-Ro/SSA and anti-La/SSB antibody-committed B cells than mothers who remained asymptomatic.

Maddison et al. (1995) described a novel antigen of 57 kDa recognized by 8 (38%) of 21 mothers whose children have NLS. Partial sequencing of p57 DNA demonstrated that this antigen is distinct from Ro/SSA and La/SSB. Supporting a potential pathogenic role of this antibody was its absence in the cord blood of an infant with CHB despite readily detectable circulating maternal levels. The authors proposed that this finding could be explained by selective cardiac depletion due to deposition on fetal cardiocytes. Alternatively, the antibody may not have been effectively transported across the placenta.

Although it is not known how maternal antibodies influence the development of cardiac vs. cutaneous manifestations of NLS, to date antibodies to U1RNP in the absence of reactivity to anti-Ro/SSA and/or La/SSB have never been reported in children with CHB. Sheth et al. (1995) have added two cases to eight previously reported in which anti-U1RNP antibodies and not anti-Ro/SSA-La/SSB antibodies were present in infants with cutaneous disease alone. Furthermore, Solomon et al. (1995) describe anti-U1RNP positive, anti-Ro/SSA-La/SSB negative dizygotic twins discordant for cutaneous manifestations of NLS (neither twin had cardiac disease).

The segregation of anti-U1RNP antibodies with cutaneous disease may be a useful maternal marker and should guide research efforts in sorting out cardiac vs. cutaneous susceptibility to antibody-mediated injury.

Eftekhari et al. (2000) recently reported that antibodies reactive with the serotoninergic 5-hydroxytryptamine $(5\text{-HT})_{4A}$ receptor, cloned from human adult atrium, also bind 52 kDa Ro/SSA. Moreover, affinity-purified 5-HT_4 antibodies antagonized the serotonin-induced L-type Ca channel activation in human atrial cells. Two peptides in the C terminus of 52 kDa Ro/SSA, aa365–382 and aa380–396, were identified that shared some similarity with the 5-HT_4 receptor. The former was recognized by sera from mothers of children with neonatal lupus and it was this peptide that was reported to be cross-reactive with peptide aa165–185, derived from the second extracellular loop of the 5-HT_4 receptor (Eftekhari et al., 2000). These findings are of particular importance, since over 75% of serum from mothers whose children have CHB contain antibodies to 52 kDa Ro/SSA as detected by ELISA, immunoblot, and immunoprecipitation. Given the intriguing possibility that antibodies to the 5-HT_4 receptor might represent the hitherto elusive reactivity which could directly contribute to AV block, we examined whether the 5-HT_4 receptor is a target of the immune response in these mothers (Buyon et al., 2002).

Initial experiments demonstrated mRNA expression of the 5-HT_4 receptor in the human fetal atrium. Electrophysiologic studies established that human fetal atrial cells express functional 5-HT_4 receptors. Sera from 116 mothers enrolled in the Research Registry, whose children have CHB, were evaluated. Ninety-nine (85%) of these maternal sera contained antibodies to Ro/SSA, 84% of which were reactive with the 52 kDa Ro/SSA component by immunoblot. None of the 116 sera were reactive with the peptide spanning aa165–185 of the serotoninergic receptor. Rabbit antisera, which recognized this peptide, did not react with 52 kDa Ro/SSA. Accordingly, although 5-HT_4 receptors are present and functional in the human fetal heart, maternal antibodies to the 5-HT_4 receptor are not associated with the development of CHB. These results are in agreement with those of Cavill et al. (2002). However, we are currently in the process of exchanging antisera with the Eftekhari group.

7. Identification of the Degree of Heart Block: complete AV block (third degree) vs. incomplete AV block (second degree)

At the first appearance of a fetal bradycardia it can be difficult and time-consuming to differentiate between certain types of second degree (incomplete) AV blocks and third degree (complete) AV block, but this distinction might be important, since complete AV block to date is irreversible, while incomplete AV block has been shown to be potentially reversible after dexamethasone therapy (Saleeb et al., 1999; Theander et al., 2001). The distinction is critically dependent on the analysis of the relationship between atrial and ventricular contractions during fetal echocardiography. If the block is complete (third degree), atrial and ventricular contractions are completely dissociated. If the AV block is incomplete, second degree, some atrial contractions are not followed by ventricular contractions. Problems in particular may arise if the incomplete AV block has a fixed ratio 2:1 between atrial and ventricular contractions; in fact this sequence may be difficult to ascertain echographically, with the consequence that an incomplete second degree AV block (potentially reversible) may be erroneously considered as complete (irreversible) (Theander et al., 2001). Also, blocked atrial premature contractions might be misinterpreted as second degree block.

8. Treatment and general management

8.1. Obstetric management of pregnancy at risk of developing CHB

A woman is at risk of delivering a baby affected by complete CHB if she is definitely anti-Ro/SSA positive. If the positivity is uncertain or the titer is very low, we advise to confirm the positivity with standard methods or in reference laboratories. The risk is approximately 2% (see paragraph). There are some suggestions that anti-52 kDa Ro/SSA and anti-La/SSB antibodies are more strongly associated with CHB than anti-60 kDa Ro/SSA alone, at least as tested by immunoblot (see above: Julkunen et al., 1993a,b; Buyon et al., 1993; Dorner et al., 1995; Colombo et al., 1999), but the data are incomplete. Furthermore the problem of reliability, sensitivity, and specificity of the different tests (commercial kits, home made, etc.) is even greater at this level of differentiation of the fine specificities. So, for practical purposes at present the key is a reliable positivity for anti-Ro/SSA antibodies, regardless of the methods employed. Serial echocardiograms and obstetric sonograms, performed at least every 2 wk (every week is optimal if possible) starting from the 16 wk gestation are recommended in this setting. The goal is to detect early fetal abnormalities that might precede complete AV block and that might be a target of preemptive therapy (Rosenthal et al., 1998). Prophylactic therapy with steroids is not recommended (Tseng and Buyon, 1997; Silverman and Laxer, 1997). In fact, the risk is too low to justify treatment with dexamethasone or bethametasone for all pregnant women anti-Ro/SSA positive, since this therapy has its own side effects. Other steroids do not cross the placenta, so they are not likely to have an effect on the fetus. Shinohara et al. (1999) have reported that prenatal maintenance therapy with prednisolone started before 16 wk gestation might reduce the risk of developing CHB, but this paper is heavily biased by the retrospective setting. In fact it is now recognized that the majority of women bearing children with CHB do not have recognized SLE and are often asymptomatic at the time of delivery: these women would not have been identified had the fetal abnormality not occurred (retrospective diagnosis). Furthermore the study included too few cases to see a real benefit from steroids, and there are cases of CHB in infants born to mothers who did take steroids (Waltuck and Buyon, 1994).

Overall, with regard to prophylactic therapy of the high risk mother (documentation of high titer anti-Ro/SSA and La/SSB by ELISA, anti-48 kDa La/SSB and 52 kDa Ro/SSA on immunoblot, and a previous child with NLS) we believe that initiation of prednisone, dexamethasone or plasmapheresis or intravenous immunoglobulins is not justified at the present time. Maternal prednisone (at least in low and moderate doses) early in pregnancy does not prevent the development of CHB (Waltuck and Buyon, 1994). This might be anticipated since prednisone given to the mother is not active in the fetus, and levels of anti-Ro/SSA and anti-La/SSB antibodies remain relatively constant during steroid therapy.

8.2. Risk of occurrence and preconceptional counseling of anti-Ro/SSA positive mothers

Since women with anti-Ro/SSA antibodies are relatively frequent at least in a rheumatology practice and CHB is very rare, we are faced with the following situation: frequent counseling about a rare disease. Mothers known to have autoimmune disease are at risk of delivering an affected infant, and for preconceptional counseling it would be useful to have precise figures about the risk of delivering a child with CHB. However, existing data are imprecise, since they mainly come from one retrospective study (Ramsey-Goldman et al., 1986) that indicated a risk of 5% among 47 anti-Ro/SSA positive SLE women, or from one prospective study (Lockshin et al., 1988), including only SLE patients, that found no case of CHB among 38 infants born to anti-Ro/SSA positive women (risk: 0%). Therefore, to assess the true prevalence of congenital CHB in anti-Ro/SSA positive women known to have connective tissue disease we conducted a large prospective cohort multicentric study (Brucato et al., 2001). 100 anti-Ro/SSA positive mothers were followed before getting pregnant and during the index pregnancy. Counterimmunoelectrophoresis and immunoblot were used to test for antibodies to extractable nuclear antigens. Two infants born to 100 women with anti-Ro/SSA antibodies developed CHB in utero (2%; 95% confidence interval 0.2–7%). The CHB were detected at 22 and 20 wk. No fetal death was due to CHB. One of the two CHB mothers had primary SS, while the other had UCTD. No case of CHB occurred among 53 SLE mothers: so in this prospective study CHB, the main manifestation of the entity misleadingly named 'neonatal lupus' (Julkunen et al., 1993a,b; Brucato et al., 1995a), was observed only in women with primary SS and UCTD, and not in 53 SLE mothers. This finding might be related to the low prevalence of anti-52 kDa Ro/SSA in SLE mothers, and further illustrates that this maternal–fetal syndrome appears to be closely related to primary SS and UCTD (Colombo et al., 1999; Julkunen et al., 1993a). In that particular study, we only followed mothers who had been found to be anti-Ro/SSA positive by counterimmunoelectrophoresis, a method with high specificity and rather low sensitivity, to exclude women with low or dubious titers of anti-Ro/SSA. Our results therefore refer to mothers anti-Ro/SSA positive in counterimmunoelectrophoresis, and cannot be extrapolated, for instance to those with a low-positive reactivity for anti-Ro/SSA antibodies by ELISA, for which the risk, if any, should be even lower.

8.3. In utero therapy of AV block

The substantial morbidity (~65% require lifelong pacing) and mortality (~20%) associated with CHB (Schmidt et al., 1991; Silverman, 1993; Julkunen et al., 1993a,b; Waltuck and Buyon, 1994) and the readily available technology for identification of CHB in utero have prompted the search for effective therapies. Ideally, since CHB is most often identified from 18 to 24 wk of gestation (Waltuck and Buyon, 1994; Buyon et al., 1995), intrauterine therapy should be possible. The following suggestions are experimental, based on the experience of some experts in the field, and not tested in a controlled trial. Some preliminary considerations need to be addressed. First of all, although there is no documentation regarding the reversal of third degree heart block (presumably fibrosis of conducting system) by maternal treatment with dexamethasone alone, the potential for diminishing an inflammatory fetal response attacking the cells of the conduction system and the working myocardium is plausible. It remains to be determined whether third degree block is reversible if therapy is initiated immediately upon detection (Saleeb et al., 1999). Secondly, incomplete AV block has been shown to be potentially reversible (Saleeb et al., 1999; Theander et al., 2001); moreover progression of second degree AV block to third degree AV block has been described, even after birth (Geggel et al., 1988; Brucato et al., 1995b). Thirdly, at the first appearance of a fetal bradycardia it can be extremely difficult and time-consuming to differentiate between second degree (incomplete) and third degree (complete) AV block (Theander et al., 2001). Finally, a very informative case report has been described by Rosenthal et al. (1998), who described a woman with a previous pregnancy complicated by CHB; in the next pregnancy, intensive fetal monitoring revealed at 21 wk gestation a decrease in left ventricular function, occasional premature atrial contractions, a moderate pericardial effusion, and a biphasic flow in the inferior vena cava. All these abnormalities reverted after dexamethasone 4 mg once daily, and a male newborn was delivered at 36 wk gestation, with a first degree AV block present in the electrocardiogram. This case report shows that early and treatable abnormalities may be detected, potentially averting deterioration to complete and permanent block. Overall, it seems that the presence of bradycardia in the fetus does not necessarily represent an irreversible fibrotic process, but that continued unchecked autoimmune tissue injury may cause progressive damage.

Several intrauterine regimens have been tried including dexamethasone (Carreira et al., 1993; Buyon et al., 1987; Rider et al., 1993; Copel et al., 1995), which is not metabolized by the placenta and is available to the fetus in an active form, and plasmapheresis (Buyon et al., 1987, 1988; Barclay et al., 1987). Maternal risks of dexamethasone are similar to any glucocorticoid and include infection, osteoporosis, osteonecrosis, and diabetes. In contrast, recent data suggest that dexamethasone improves maternal outcomes in postpartum-onset HELLP syndrome and reduces hypertension (Martin et al., 1997). Fetal risks include intrauterine growth restriction and oligohydramnios. In several animal studies, including mice, rats, and rabbits, fetal growth restriction was observed with higher frequency than normal (Friedman and Polifka, 1996). Tangalakis et al. (1995) have reported that prolonged use of steroids during pregnancy may significantly alter the volume and composition of fetal fluids and placental morphology in sheep. Adrenal suppression is a potential concern; however, multiple courses of antenatal dexamethasone did not show long-lasting suppressive effects on pituitary adrenal function, at least in preterm or very low birthweight infants (Ng et al., 1997). The safety of perinatal steroid use has recently come into question again, based on reports of adverse effects on growth and brain development in treated patients (Harkavy et al., 1989; Yeh et al., 1990; Van Goudoever et al., 1994; Berry et al., 1997; Jobe, 2000; Murphy et al., 2001). However, it is important to note that these studies are based on extremely low birth weight premature infants with respiratory distress syndrome and chronic lung disease, exposed to high doses of steroids, particularly dexamethasone. Such premature infants have immature brains that leave them much more susceptible to many insults, including those of their underlying unstable physiologic states requiring intensive care interventions (Harkavy et al., 1989; Yeh et al., 1990; Van Goudoever et al., 1994; Berry et al., 1997; Jobe, 2000; Murphy et al., 2001).

Therefore, possible beneficial effects need to be balanced against adverse effects, and only a randomized controlled trial will define the role of dexamethasone in the treatment of CHB. Based on these considerations, we agree with the overall schema for management proposed by Tseng and Buyon (1997). If the block is incomplete (e.g., second degree), dexamethasone 4 mg p.o. to the mother daily is recommended, with a note of caution: incomplete AV block may be very difficult to detect in utero, requiring a particular expertise (Theander et al., 2001). If the block is complete (more common clinical situation) and recent, dexamethasone is recommended as well and discontinued if no change occurs after several weeks. If the block is associated with signs of myocarditis, heart failure, or hydropic changes, dexamethasone is recommended. If the block is complete and present for more than 2–4 wk, with no effusions and no signs of hydrops, only serial echograms are done, with no therapy.

Saaleb et al. (1999) reported on a retrospective review of the data from the US-based Research Registry for Neonatal Lupus, comparing the treatment with fluorinated glucocorticoids to the natural history of untreated CHB. The cohort included 47 mothers whose sera contain anti-Ro/SSA or anti-La/SSB antibodies, and their 50 offspring with CHB, in whom at least 4 echocardiograms were performed after in utero diagnosis. In 28 pregnancies, the mothers were treated with dexamethasone 4–9 mg/day (most received 4 mg) for 4–19 wk or betamethasone 12 mg/wk for >6 wk (group A). On average, 1.6 wk passed between the detection of bradyarrhythmia and the initiation of steroids. In 22 pregnancies, fluorinated steroids were not given (group B). Mean gestational age at detection of bradyarrhythmia was 21.6 wk (group A) vs. 24.7 wk (group B), ($P = 0.01$). At the time of detection, third degree block was present in 20 fetuses in group A and 16 fetuses in group B; none were reversible despite steroids. Three fetuses in group A progressed from second degree block alternating with third degree block to permanent third degree block at birth and postnatally. In group B, one fetus with alternating second/third degree block reverted to alternating first/second degree block spontaneously, while another fetus progressed from alternating second/third to third degree block. Notably, of 3 fetuses in group A with second degree block at presentation, all reverted to first degree by birth; one remains so at the age of 4 yr, one alternates between first and second degree at 18 months, and the third is in second degree block at age 3.5 yr. However, when we updated these data, progression to a more advanced degree of block was observed after birth (Askanase et al., 2002), so these children must be closely monitored over the next 5–10 yr. Of 2 fetuses in group B with second degree block at presentation, one remained in second degree block after birth and the other progressed to third degree block after birth. Echocardiographic evaluation (within 2 days of steroid initiation, group A; within 1 wk of diagnosis of CHB, group B) revealed pericardial effusions in 13 group A vs. 4 group B ($P < 0.06$), pleural effusions in 2 group A vs. 0 group B ($P = \text{NS}$), ascites in 8 group A vs. 0 group B ($P < 0.02$), hydrops in 8 group A vs. 0 group B ($P \leqslant 0.02$), and intrauterine growth restriction in 1 group A vs. 1 group B ($P = \text{NS}$). So the group A fetuses appeared to be more severely ill than group B fetuses at the beginning of the study. Initially, 11 of 13 pericardial effusions in group A decreased after administration of steroids, however, 4 redeveloped. Three of 4 pericardial effusions in group B resolved spontaneously. Steroid therapy was most effective in the sustained resolution of pleural effusions (2/2), ascites (6/8), and hydrops (5/8). The time to resolution was extremely variable. For example, all cases of ascites initially resolved within 4 days to 11 wk. The majority of hydropic changes that resolved generally did so within 2–3 wk of steroid initiation. Two fetuses in group B developed hydrops. Oligohydramnios ensued in 8 group A and 2 group B ($P = \text{NS}$). While this latter complication is certainly a concern as a complication of maternal steroid use, it is of interest that in group A, the presence or development of oligohydramnios was significantly associated with the maternal diagnosis of SLE ($P = 0.008$). These findings suggest that maternal disease might also contribute to the development of oligohydramnios. Although fetuses in group A had more associated complications at initial presentation than those in group B, there were no significant differences between the groups with regard to the duration of pregnancy (35.7 vs. 37.1 wk), number of deaths (4 vs. 1), final degree of block, or requirement for permanent pacing (13 vs. 10). Fluorinated steroids were generally well tolerated by the mothers. One mother with SLE experienced spiking fevers towards the end of pregnancy. Infection was considered but not found and the distinction could not be made between an occult infection or a lupus flare. Varicella was diagnosed in another mother 5 wk after starting steroids. A third mother experienced ear and sinus infections 2 wk after starting steroids. A fourth mother developed a suspected bronchial pneumonia requiring antibiotics 2 wk after steroids were initiated. Glucose intolerance was not reported in any mother. The subsequent incidence of osteoporosis and/or osteonecrosis was not ascertained. Intrauterine growth restriction was noted in 5 fetuses in group A and 3 in group B. In summary, these retrospectively obtained data represent the largest experience with the extended use of maternal fluorinated glucocorticoids for the treatment of autoantibody-associated CHB. Moreover, evaluation of untreated fetuses that were serially monitored with echocardiograms provides essential information on the natural history of CHB. In the absence of such data, a critical appraisal of the efficacy of steroids would be impossible. Although the institution of steroids did not reduce the degree of block once complete AV node dissociation was documented, it remains speculative whether even third degree block could be altered if therapy was instituted immediately in all cases upon development of bradyarrhythmia. Clearly detection of AV dysfunction at a time when the block is incomplete offers the maximal chance for reversal with steroids as supported by the small numbers of fetuses with initial second degree block in this study. It is particularly encouraging that despite significant initial fetal compromise due to hydropic changes in the treated group and the possible increased risk of intrauterine growth restriction and oligohydramnios due to steroids, the mortality rates and requirement for pacing did not differ significantly between the groups. Based on these data, the PR interval and dexamethasone evaluation (PRIDE) in CHB trial was launched, as described below.

On the cardiological site, one approach has been to increase the fetal heart rate with sympathomimetics even if they do not restore coordination of AV conduction on which the heart is dependent for adequate filling. Salbutamol, a selective beta 2 adrenergic agonist, also named albuterol, may be useful particularly as a bridge to reach a more advanced gestational age. We agree that it is the preferred sympathomimetic agent. It can be given orally to the mother, e.g. at a dosage of 2 mg 6–10 times daily, according to maternal compliance. Terbutaline has only been shown to raise the fetal heart rate by 15–50%. Resolution of hydrops was reported in one case; however, the mother was simultaneously on steroids (Groves et al., 1995).

The in utero environment is preferred as long as possible because of the low resistance circulatory pathways, thereby affording minimal work to maintain cardiac output, as well as the immaturity of the lungs and other organs. However, this approach must be balanced against the heightened transfer of maternal antibodies as the pregnancy progresses, although the window of cardiac vulnerability may have passed.

9. The PRIDE trial

Many uncertainties regarding the management of pregnant woman with anti-Ro/SSA antibodies and the treatment of identified fetal heart block might be solved by an ongoing study. The PRIDE trial in CHB, funded by the NIAMS (NIH Grant 1 R01 AR 46265-01A1) is such a study. The principal investigator is Jill Buyon, from the Hospital for Joint Diseases, New York.

It actually comprises two trials in autoimmune-associated CHB. The observational trial of PRIDE is to assess if the measurement of mechanical PR interval of the fetal heart is the earliest reliable non-invasive echocardiographic marker of AV nodal dysfunction and/or myocardial injury. For this study, 100 anti-Ro/SSA positive mothers will be followed by weekly echocardiograms from 16 to 26 wk of gestation and 1 every 2 wk until 32 wk with special attention to the mechanical PR interval. Mothers of children who develop first, second or third degree block will then be offered treatment with either dexamethasone or placebo.

The interventional study was originally aimed to determine in a randomized double-blind placebo-controlled trial the effect of daily oral dexamethasone (4 mg) on the outcome of CHB. Unfortunately, despite obtaining placebo and active drug, IND approval from the FDA, and local IRB consent, it became clear that enrollment would fall short of expectations. The reason for this was that given the rarity of CHB, we could not anticipate every site in the US that would encounter a patient and have IRB approval in place when a fetus was identified with CHB. Although we sent mailings out to all US board-certified pediatric cardiologists, only 20 obtained local approval. Indeed, the cases brought to our attention wound up being from institutions in which consent had not been obtained, and given the requirement in our protocol to initiate active drug or placebo within 3 wk of identification of block, the study was not feasible. Moreover, we found that the majority of women faced with the decision to enter this randomized trial refused to be given placebo, based on either advice from their personal physicians or reading anecdotal retrospective literature. Also, there is great resistance to consent to any fetal experiments, due to a general lack of certainty of adverse effects.

10. Risk of recurrence

For prenatal counseling it is important for the mother of a patient to know the possibility of delivering a second affected child. Few prospective studies exist on this issue; the percentage seems to be between 15 and 20%, therefore substantially higher than in the first pregnancy (Brucato, 1997a,b).

In a recent nationwide study from Finland (Julkunen and Eronen, 2001a,b), the risk of recurrence of CHB was 17% (8 of 47), and data from the Research Registry for Neonatal Lupus including 105 affected mothers (Buyon et al., 1998) showed that 16% of pregnancies immediately subsequent to the birth of a child with CHB resulted in a second child with CHB. We just updated this finding, observing a 19% recurrence rate for CHB in 90 pregnancies following the birth of a child with CHB. These figures are similar to that previously reported (Waltuck and

Buyon, 1994; Brucato et al., 1995a). This risk might be considered high by some of the mothers, and in the study by Julkunen, some families have therefore reduced their planned family size.

11. Other pregnancy outcomes in women with autoimmune diseases and anti-Ro/SSA antibodies

Anti-Ro/SSA antibodies are associated with NLS but it is not clear if these antibodies are linked to other adverse pregnancy outcomes, both in SLE and non-SLE women. Most of the available data come from retrospective studies; some of them considered the anti-Ro/SSA antibodies as a possible causative factor for unexplained pregnancy loss in SLE (Hull et al., 1983; Barclay et al., 1987; Watson et al., 1986). On the other hand, Julkunen retrospectively observed that the relative risk of fetal loss was increased in patients with primary SS, but it was not associated with anti-Ro/SSA or La/SSB (Julkunen et al., 1995b). The largest retrospective study found that anti-Ro/SSA antibodies do not adversely affect pregnancy outcome in SLE patients, while they appear to be associated with recurrent pregnancy loss in non-SLE patients (Mavragani et al., 1998). Interestingly, a prospective study of pregnancy in SLE patients provided conflicting results showing that the *absence* of anti-Ro/SSA antibodies was significantly related to the occurrence of fetal loss and intrauterine growth restriction (Le Thi et al., 1994). Recently in a large multicenter cohort study, we have prospectively followed 100 anti-Ro/SSA positive women (53 SLE) during their 122 pregnancies and 107 anti-Ro/SSA negative women (58 SLE) (140 pregnancies) (Brucato et al., 2002). Anti-Ro/SSA antibodies were tested by immunoblot and counterimmunoelectrophoresis. Mean gestational age at delivery (38 vs. 37.9 wk), prevalence of pregnancy loss (9.9 vs. 18.6%), preterm birth (21.3 vs. 13.9%), cesarean sections (49.2 vs. 53.4%), premature rupture of membranes (4.9 vs. 8.1%), preeclampsia (6.6 vs. 8%), intrauterine growth retardation (0 vs. 2.3%), and newborns small for gestational age (11.5 vs. 5.8%) were similar in anti-Ro/SSA positive and negative SLE mothers; findings were similar in non-SLE women. We concluded that anti-Ro/SSA antibodies are responsible for CHB but do not affect other pregnancy outcomes, both in SLE and non-SLE women.

12. Long-term outcome

12.1. Mothers

Several studies have addressed the issue of maternal status at identification of CHB and progression toward autoimmune diseases (Julkunen et al., 1993a,b; Waltuck and Buyon, 1994; Brucato et al., 1995a; Press et al., 1996). It is now known that the mothers of affected children who at the moment of delivery are asymptomatic do not seem to have a bad prognosis, since at the most half of them will eventually develop a connective tissue disease, mild and non-life-threatening in most cases. Evolution toward primary SS is more frequent in these cases than toward SLE. Therefore, the term neonatal lupus is misleading in many cases, since it can give the false knowledge that mothers of a child with CHB will develop SLE (Brucato et al., 1995a; Press et al., 1996; Julkunen and Eronen, 2001a,b). Julkunen and Eronen (2001a,b) published an important study concerning this issue. Eighty-three mothers of children with CHB and 48 mothers of children with heart block detected after the newborn period were studied. Maternal survival was compared with survival in an age-matched population of normal Finnish women. Before the index delivery, 29 (37%) of the 78 surviving mothers of children with CHB had a self-reported clinical diagnosis of a chronic autoimmune disease, and 55 (71%) had symptoms, signs, or abnormal laboratory findings suggesting an underlying subclinical disease. Of the 23 mothers who were completely asymptomatic before the index delivery, 10 (13% of the surviving mothers) remained so after a mean follow-up of 9.6 yr (range 0–21 yr). Forty-eight (58%) of these 83 mothers developed an autoimmune disease during follow-up. The most common diagnosis was primary SS (22 definite, 11 probable), followed by SLE. The standardized mortality ratio of mothers of children with CHB was 5.1, and 3 of the 5 deaths were associated with SLE. Mothers of children with heart block detected after the newborn period had similar symptoms and signs of autoimmune diseases as the healthy controls, and their standardized mortality ratio was 1.9

Recently, Lawrence et al. (2000) raised the possibility that the long-term outcome of mothers of children with cutaneous neonatal lupus erythematosus might be worse than that of mothers of children with CHB. Twenty-four mothers were studied. Initially 10 mothers were healthy and 14 mothers had either a defined ($n = 9$) or an undifferentiated ($n = 5$) autoimmune disorder. At a mean follow-up of 7 yr, 13 (1 of whom had died) had a defined connective tissue disease, and 5 had an undifferentiated autoimmune disorder. Only 6 (25%) remained asymptomatic. By comparison, 36 (56%) of 64 mothers of children with congenital heart block were asymptomatic at follow-up, so the majority of mothers of children with cutaneous neonatal lupus erythematosus had a defined or undifferentiated autoimmune disorder at the time of the child's birth. Two problems exist with this study. First, even if the authors made every effort to avoid a selection bias, the possibility still remains. Asymptomatic mothers of CHB children are almost inevitably identified, while asymptomatic mothers of babies with skin rash may be easily overlooked if the skin rash is not typical, Second, it is well known that mothers of CHB children may subsequently deliver children affected by skin rash and vice versa (Neiman et al., 2000). In the experience of the American group, the long-term outcome of mothers of children with cutaneous neonatal lupus erythematosus is similar to that of mothers of children with CHB (Neiman et al., 2000).

12.2. Children

12.2.1. Children: long-term cardiological outcome

CHB is a severe disease. The natural history of autoimmune-associated CHB has changed recently due to greater awareness of the condition, and technical improvements in diagnostic techniques (fetal echocardiography, maternal antibody serology) and the modern era of pacemaker therapy. The most frequently encountered situation is that a child is born with permanent, complete CHB, receives a pacemaker, and does well clinically. However, it is becoming clear that a subset of patients will go on to the progressive disease of the conduction system and/or the development of a dilated cardiomyopathy. There is no documentation yet of possible reversal of third degree heart block. Mortality, usually in utero or in the first three months of life, can reach 20% even after intensive and supportive care (Schmidt et al., 1991; Vignati et al., 1999). Infants who survive the neonatal period usually have a good prognosis, but most eventually require pacing.

Our long-standing collaborative group has generated a large database of cases of autoimmune CHB through the Research Registry for Neonatal Lupus. Results of this analyses (Buyon et al., 1998; Friedman et al., 2002) have allowed us to estimate that this disease has about a 20% mortality rate (higher in fetal and neonatal presentations); 6 of these deaths occurred in utero, and 10 neonates died in the first 3 months of life. Six children died between 3 months and 3 yr of age. The cumulative probability of survival at 3 yr was 79%. None of the 67 children between 3 and 10 yr old remaining in the cohort had died at the time of the analysis. Sixty-three percent of children required pacemakers. The rate of pacemaker insertion before adulthood was 67% (52% within 9 days, 22% within 1 yr, and the rest after 1 yr of age). These findings have been confirmed by other investigators. Similar data on early mortality (24% with 7 fetal deaths, 5 neonatal deaths, and one infant death) and the association of minor structural heart disease (28%; 11 persistent patent ductus arteriosus, 6 atrial septal defect, 1 pulmonic stenosis, 1 ventricular septal defect) were reported by Gordon et al. (2001a,b) for a cohort of 64 patients with CHB. In this series, the mean gestational age at diagnosis was 26.4 wk.

Lisa Hornberger's group in Toronto (Jaeggi et al., 2002) retrospectively analyzed the single center outcome of children with isolated CHB presenting from 1965–1998, up to age 20. Cases were diagnosed from fetal life through childhood. There were a total of 102 cases, divided into 3 groups. Fetal presentation in 29 cases had a 43% mortality rate. Neonatal presentation in 33 cases had 6% mortality. There were no deaths in the 40 cases presenting in childhood, but it should be noted that 19 out of 20 tested had negative maternal antibody levels. Risk factors for death were fetal diagnosis, the presence of hydrops, gestational age at birth under 33 wk, or the development of endocardial fibroelastosis with ejection fraction ≤40%. Three neonates who had been diagnosed before birth were treated with corticosteroids. Most of the cases (88–89%) were paced by age 20. Late cardiomyopathy occurred in 5% overall, but in the antibody-positive cases it was 11%. Progression was also noted in the degree of heart block over time. Pacemaker insertions were associated with complications in 25% of cases, and there was a frequent need for pacemaker revisions.

A retrospective Finnish study (Eronen et al., 2000) has assessed the short- and long-term outcome of children with CHB: the total mortality was 16%, with almost three quarters of deaths occurring during the first year of life. Cumulative probability of survival at 10 yr of age was 82%. Moreover, a high incidence of dilated cardiomyopathy (see section 5.2.2.) and associated heart defects were found: therefore the authors suggested close echocardiographic monitoring of all the children with CHB.

It has been stated that prophylactic pace-maker implantation should always be recommended, even in asymptomatic patients, because of high incidence of unpredictable Stokes-Adams attacks and significant morbidity and mortality (Michaelsson et al., 1995). Figures on morbidity and mortality rates in published studies have to be taken with caution since in most series CHB was associated with cardiac malformations, and heart block has also been detected after birth in many cases; on the other hand, cases of CHB dead in utero might have been missed in retrospective studies.

12.2.2. Children: long-term rheumatological outcome

Finally, the possibility for a child with neonatal lupus to develop SLE or another connective tissue disease in later life seems to be extremely rare. Most of the described cases have been single reports, usually young females (McCuistion and Schoch, 1954); the risk might not be higher than in asymptomatic children of mothers with autoimmune diseases (Brucato, 1997a,b). We looked at the health outcomes of children with NLS in the Registry (Martin et al., 2002) and found no apparent increased risk of SLE, but concern was raised regarding the development of autoimmune disease (systemic or organ-specific) in early childhood. Data were obtained from children 8 yr of age or older who had manifestations of NLS (affected group) and their unaffected siblings (unaffected group). Questionnaires were sent to mothers (with anti-Ro/SSA-La/SSB antibodies) enrolled in the Registry. A control group comprised children of healthy mothers referred by the Registry enrollees. Fifty-five mothers returned questionnaires on 49 children with NL and their 45 unaffected siblings. Six children were identified with definite rheumatologic/autoimmune diseases: 2 with juvenile rheumatoid arthritis, 1 with Hashimoto's thyroiditis, 1 with psoriasis and iritis, 1 with diabetes mellitus and psoriasis, and 1 with congenital hypothyroidism and nephrotic syndrome. All had manifestations of NLS and their mothers have manifestations of autoimmune diseases: 4 SS, 1 SLE/SS, and 1 UAS. In 4 of 55 sera available and tested, the ANA was positive (2 of 33 affected children and 2 of 22 unaffected children). No child's serum contained antibodies reactive with Ro/SSA or La/SSB antigens. Immunoblot of the ANA positive sera revealed a prominent band at 65 kDa in two children (one NL affected, the other an unaffected sibling). These data suggest that children with neonatal lupus require continued follow-up, especially prior to adolescence

Key points

- Congenital heart block (CHB), defined as an AV block diagnosed *in utero,* at birth, or within the neonatal period (0–27 days after birth) is a rare disorder (1:10,000–20,000 live births) closely linked to transplacental transport of maternal antibodies anti-Ro/SSA and anti-La/SSB.
- The fetus may die in utero or a few days after birth (approximately 20%) or survive to the perinatal period and have a near normal life; in most survivors a pacemaker must be implanted.
- Skin lesions, haematological disorders, and hepatic cholestasis are transient clinical features of the syndrome.

- A spectrum and progression of conduction abnormalities may be present in infants born to mothers with anti-Ro/SSA-La/SSB antibodies.
  - Sinus bradycardia and QT interval prolongation may be observed, but this is relatively uncommon and may even be reversible.
  - An ECG should be performed on all infants born to mothers with anti-Ro/SSA-La/SSB antibodies.
- The risk of recurrence of CHB ranges from 15 to 20%.
- Most of the mothers are asymptomatic at delivery and are identified only by the birth of an affected child.
  - Their long-term outcome is generally more reassuring than previously assumed, and arthralgias and dry eyes are the commonest symptoms.
- The prevalence of CHB in newborns of prospectively followed women already known to be anti-Ro/SSA positive and with known connective tissue disease is 2% (95%; confidence interval 0.2–7%).
- A standard therapy for CHB detected in utero does not exist.
  - Serial echocardiograms and obstetric sonograms, performed at least every 2 wk starting from the 16th week of gestation, are recommended in anti-Ro/SSA positive pregnant women. Specific echocardiographic tools useful for this aim may be the mechanical PR interval and the Tei index.

and if the mother herself has an autoimmune disease. While there was no apparent increased risk of SLE, the development of some form of autoimmune disease (systemic or organ-specific) in early childhood may be of concern. During adolescence and young adulthood, individuals with neonatal lupus and their unaffected siblings do not appear to have an increased risk of developing systemic rheumatic diseases.

References

Abbot, A.E., Buyon, J.P., Friedman, S. 1998. The prevalence of cardiomyopathy observed in patients recorded in the Research Registry for Neonatal Lupus. Arthritis Rheum. 41, S262.

Askanase, A.D., Friedman, D.M., Copel, J., Dische, M.R., Dubin, A., Starc, T.J., Katholi, M.C., Buyon, J.P., 2002. Spectrum and progression of conduction abnormalities in infants born to mothers with anti-Ro/La antibodies. Lupus 11, 145.

These data have important research and clinical implications. In contrast to the AV node, permanent sinoatrial nodal involvement is not clinically apparent. Perhaps many fetuses sustain mild inflammation, but resolution is variable, as suggested by the presence of incomplete AV block. Since subsequent progression of less-advanced degrees of block can occur, an EKG should be performed on all infants born to mothers with anti-SSA/Ro-SSB/La/SSB antibodies.

Aylward, R.D. 1928. Congenital heart-block. Br. Med. J., 176, 943.

Ballard, P.L., Granberg, P., Ballard, R.A. 1975. Glucocorticoid levels in maternal and cord serum after prenatal betamethasone therapy to prevent respiratory distress syndrome. J. Clin. Invest. 56, 1548.

Bangert, J.L., Freeman, R.G., Sontheimer, R.D., et al. 1984. Subacute cutaneous lupus erythematosus and discoid lupus erythematosus. Comparative histopathologic findings. Arch. Dermatol. 120, 332.

Barclay, C.S., French, M.A.H., Ross, L.D., et al. 1987. Successful pregnancy following steroid therapy and plasma exchange in a woman with anti-Ro/SSA (SS-A) antibodies. Case report. Br. J. Obstet. Gynecol. 94, 369.

Beitins, I.Z., Bayard, F., Ances, I.G., et al. 1972. The transplacental passage of prednisone and prednisolone in pregnancy near term. J. Pediatr. 81, 936.

Ben-Chetrit, E., Fox, R.I., Tan, E.M. 1990. Dissociation of immune responses to the SS A/Ro/SSA 52 kD and 60 kD polypeptides in systemic lupus erythematosus and Sjogrens syndrome. Arthritis Rheum. 33, 349.

Benson, D.W., Silberbach, G.M., Kavanaugh-McHugh, A., et al. 1999. Mutations in the cardiac transcription factor NKX 2.5 affect diverse cardiac developmental pathways. J. Clin. Invest. 104, 1567.

Berry, M.A., Abrahamowicz, M., Usher, R.H. 1997. Factors associated with growth of extremely premature infants during initial hospitalization. Pediatrics 100, 640.

Blanford, A.T., Pearson Murphy, B.E. 1977. In vitro metabolism of prednisolone, dexamethasone, betamethasone, and cortisol by the human placenta. Am. J. Obstet. Gynecol. 127, 264.

Boutjdir, M., Chen, L., Zhang, Z.H., et al. 1997. Arrhythmogenicity of IgG and anti-52-kD SSA/Ro/SSA affinity-purified antibodies from mothers of children with congenital heart block. Circ. Res. 80, 354.

Boutjdir, M., Chen, L., Zhang, Z.H., et al. 1998. Serum and immunoglobulin G from the mother of a child with congenital heart block induce conduction abnormalities and inhibit L-type calcium channels in a rat heart model. Pediatr. Res. 44, 11.

Briggs, G.G., Freeman, R.K., Yaffe, S.J. 1994. Drugs in Pregnancy and Lactation, 4th ed., Williams and Wilkins, Baltimore.

Brucato, A. 1997a. Congenital heart block and mother's immunology (letter). Circulation 96, 2735.

Brucato, A., Franceschini, F., Buyon, J.P. 1997b. Neonatal lupus: long-term outcomes of mothers and children and recurrence rate. Clin. Exp. Rheumatol. 15, 467.

Brucato, A., Franceschini, F., Gasparini, M., et al. 1995a. Isolated congenital complete heart block: longterm outcome of mothers, maternal antibody specificity and immunogenetic background. J. Rheumatol. 22, 533.

Brucato, A., Gasparini, M., Vignati, G., et al. 1995b. Isolated congenital complete heart block: longterm outcome of children and immunogenetic study. J. Rheum. 22, 541.

Brucato, A., Buyon, J.P., Horsfall, A.C., et al. 1999. Fourth international workshop on neonatal lupus syndromes and the Ro/SSA-La/SSB system. Clin. Exp. Rheum. 117, 130.

Brucato, A., Cimaz, R., Catelli, L., et al. 2000. Anti-Ro-associated sinus bradycardia in newborns [letter]. Circulation 102, E88.

Brucato, A., Frassi, M., Franceschini, F., et al. 2001. Risk of congenital complete heart block in newborns of mothers with anti-Ro/SSA antibodies detected by counterimmunoelectrophoresis: a prospective study of 100 women. Arthritis Rheum. 44, 1832.

One hundred anti-Ro/SSA-positive mothers were followed up before they became pregnant and during the index pregnancy. Counterimmunoelectrophoresis and immunoblotting were used to test for antibodies to extractable nuclear antigens. Of the 100 women with anti-Ro/SSA antibodies, 2 had infants who developed CCHB in utero (2%).

Brucato, A., Doria, A., Frassi, M., et al. 2002. Pregnancy outcome in 100 women with autoimmune diseases and anti-Ro/SSA antibodies: a prospective controlled study. Lupus 11, 71.

Brucato, A., Jonzon, A., Friedman, D., et al. 2003. Proposal for a new definition of congenital complete atrioventricular block. Lupus 12, 427.

Buyon, J.P. 1993. Congenital complete heart block. Lupus 2, 291.

Buyon, J.P. 2003. Neonatal lupus syndrome. In: R. Lahita (Ed.), Systemic Lupus Erythematosus, 4th ed., Academic Press, San Diego.

This chapter summarizes the current knowledge in the field of neonatal lupus from the clinical, laboratory and epidemiologic perspectives, and provides a comprehensive review of the literature.

Buyon, J.P., Swersky, S., Fox, H., et al. 1987. Intrauterine therapy for presumptive fetal myocarditis with acquired heart block due to systemic lupus erythematosus: experience in a mother with a predominance of La/SSB antibodies. Arthritis Rheum. 30, 44.

Buyon, J.P., Swersky, S., Parke, A., et al. 1988. Complete congenital heart block: risk of occurrence and therapeutic approach to prevention. J. Rheum. 15, 1104.

Buyon, J.P., Ben-Chetrit, E., Karp, S., et al. 1989a. Acquired congenital heart block. Pattern of maternal antibody response to biochemically defined antigens of the Ro/La/SSB antigen system in neonatal lupus. J. Clin. Invest. 84, 627.

Buyon, J.P., Slade, S.G., Chan, E.K.L., et al. 1989b. Effective separation of the 52 SSA/Ro/SSA polypeptide from the 48 kD polypeptide by altering conditions of gel electrophoresis. J. Immunol. Methods 129, 207.

Buyon, J.P., Winchester, R.J., Slade, S.G., et al. 1993. Identification of mothers at risk for congenital heart block and other neonatal lupus syndromes in their children: comparison of ELISA and immunoblot to measure anti-Ro/SSA and anti-La/SSB antibodies. Arthritis Rheum. 36, 1263.

Buyon, J.P., Waltuck, J., Kleinman, C., et al. 1995. In utero identification and therapy of congenital heart block (CHB). Lupus 4, 116.

Buyon, J.P., Nelson, J.L., Lockshin, M.D. 1996. The effects of pregnancy on autoimmune diseases. Clin. Immunol. Immunopathol. 78, 99.

Buyon, J.P., Hiebert, R., Copel, J., et al. 1998. Autoimmune-associated congenital heart block: demographics, mortality, morbidity and recurrence rates obtained from a national neonatal lupus registry. J. Am. Coll. Cardiol. 31, 1658.

An analysis of the largest neonatal lupus patient series compiled to date (105 mothers with anti-Ro/SSA-La/SSB antibodies, and their 113 infants diagnosed with CHB between 1970 and 1997). These data substantiate that autoantibody-associated CHB is not coincident with major structural abnormalities, is most often identified in the late second trimester, carries a substantial mortality in the neonatal period and frequently requires pacing. The recurrence rate of CHB is at least 2- to 3-fold higher than the rate for a mother with anti-Ro/SSA-La/SSB antibodies who never had an affected child, supporting close echocardiographic monitoring in all subsequent pregnancies, with heightened surveillance between 18 and 24 weeks of gestation.

Buyon, J.P., Clancy, R., Di Donato, F., et al. 2002. Cardiac 5-HT(4) serotoninergic receptors, 52kD SSA/Ro/SSA and autoimmune-associated congenital heart block. J. Autoimmun. 19, 79.

Carreira, P.E., Gutierrez-Larraya, F., Gomez-Reino, J.J. 1993. Successful intrauterine therapy with dexamethasone for fetal myocarditis and heart block in a mother with systemic lupus erythematosus. J. Rheum. 20, 1204.

Carter, J.B., Blieden, L.C., Edwards, J.E. 1974. Congenital heart block: anatomic correlations and review of the literature. Arch. Pathol. 97, 51.

Cavill, D., Waterman, S., Gordon, T.P. 2002. Failure to detect antibodies to the second extracellular loop of the serotonin 5-HT4 receptor in systemic lupus erythematosus and primary Sjogren's syndrome. Lupus 11, 197.

Chameides, L., Truex, R.C., Vetter, V., et al. 1977. Association of maternal systemic lupus erythematosus with congenital complete heart block. N. Engl. J. Med. 297, 1204.

Cimaz, R., Airoldi, M.L., Careddu, P., et al. 1997. Transient neonatal bradycardia without heart block associated with anti-Ro/SSA antibodies. Lupus 6, 487.

Cimaz, R., Stramba-Badiale, M., Brucato, A., et al. 2000. QT interval prolongation in asymptomatic anti-SSA/Ro-positive infants without congenital heart block. Arthritis Rheum. 43, 1049.

Cimaz, R., Meroni, P.L., Brucato, A., et al. 2003. Concomitant disappearance of electrocardiographic abnormalities and of acquired maternal autoantibodies during the first year of life in infants who had QT interval prolongation and anti-SSA/Ro/SSA positivity without congenital heart block at birth. Arthritis Rheum. 48, 266.

Colombo, G., Brucato, A., Coluccio, E., et al. 1999. DNA typing of maternal HLA in congenital complete heart block: comparison with systemic lupus erythematosus and primary Sjogren's syndrome. Arthritis Rheum. 42, 1757.

Copel, J., Buyon, J., Kleinman, C. 1995. Successful in utero therapy of fetal heart block. Am. J. Obstet. Gynecol. 173, 1384.

Dorner, T., Chaoui, R., Feist, E., et al. 1995. Significantly increased maternal and fetal IgG autoantibody levels to 52 kD Ro/SSA (SS-A) and La/SSB (SS-B) in complete congenital heart block. J. Autoimmun. 8, 675.

Eftekhari, P., Salle, L., Lezoualc'h, F., et al. 2000. Anti-SSA/Ro52 autoantibodies blocking the cardiac 5-HT4 serotoninergic receptor could explain neonatal lupus congenital heart block. Eur. J. Immunol. 30, 2782.

Eronen, M., Siren, M.K., Ekblad, H., et al. 2000. Short- and long-term outcome of children with congenital complete heart block diagnosed in utero or as a newborn. Pediatrics 106, 86.

Frohn-Mulder, I.M., Meilof, J.F., Szatmari, A., et al. 1994. Clinical significance of maternal anti-Ro/SSA antibodies in children with isolated heart block. J. Am. Coll. Cardiol. 23, 1677.

Friedman, J.M., Polifka, J.E. 1996. The Effects of Drugs on the Fetus and Nursing Infant. Johns Hopkins University Press, Baltimore.

Friedman, D.M., Rupel, A., Glickenstein, J., et al. 2002. Congenital heart block in neonatal lupus: the pediatric cardiologist's perspective. Indian J. Pediatr. 69, 517.

Friedman, D., Buyon, J., Kim, M., et al. 2003. Fetal cardiac function assessed by Doppler myocardial performance index (Tei Index). Ultrasound Obstet. Gynecol. 21, 33.

Geggel, R.L., Tucker, L., Szer, I. 1988. Postnatal progression from second- to third-degree heart block in neonatal lupus syndrome. J. Pediatr. 113, 1049.

Gildein, H.P., Gunther, S., Mocellin, R. 1993. Complete heart block in a 9 year old girl caused by borreliosis. Br. Heart J. 70, 8.

Glickstein, J.S., Buyon, J.P., Friedman, D. 2000. Pulsed Doppler echocardiographic assessment of the fetal PR interval. Am. J. Cardiol. 86, 236.

This is the first fetal echocardiographic pulsed Doppler normative study demonstrating the PR interval in the fetus throughout gestation, a valuable tool to explore the developing fetal conduction system.

Gordon, P., Khamashta, M.A., Hughes, G.R., et al. 2001a. Increase in the heart rate-corrected QT interval in children of anti-Ro-positive mothers, with a further increase in those with siblings with congenital heart block: comment on the article by Cimaz et al. Arthritis Rheum. 44, 242.

Gordon, P., Khamashta, M., Hughes, G.R.V., et al. 2001b. Early outcome in anti-Ro/SSA antibody associated with congenital heart block. Arthritis Rheum. 44 (Suppl.), S161.

Groves, A.M., Allan, L.D., Rosenthal, E. 1995. Therapeutic trial of sympathomimetics in three cases of complete heart block in the fetus. Circulation 92, 3394.

Harkavy, K.L., Scanion, J.W., Chowdhry, P.K., et al. 1989. Dexamethasone therapy for chronic lung disease in ventilator- and oxygen-dependent infants: a controlled trial. J. Pediatr. 115, 979.

Harley, J.B., Kaine, J.L., Fox, O.F., et al. 1985. Ro(SS-A) antibody and antigen in a patient with congenital complete heart block. Arthritis Rheum. 28, 1321.

Hubscher, O., Batista, N., Rivero, S., et al. 1995. Clinical and serological identification of 2 forms of complete heart block in children. J. Rheum. 22, 1352.

Sera from 17 mothers of 18 children with CHB of unidentified cause were studied. CHB detected before the age of 3 months was highly associated with the presence of anti-Ro/SSA-La/SSB antibodies in the mothers, while CHB diagnosed later generally was not.

Hull, R.G., Harris, E.N., Morgan, S.H., Hughes, G.R. 1983. Anti-Ro antibodies and abortions in women with SLE. Lancet 2, 1138.

Isacovics, B., Silverman, E.D. 1993. Limiting dilution analysis of Epstein-Barr virus infectable B cells secreting anti-Ro/SSA and anti-La/SSB antibodies in neonatal lupus erythematosus and systemic lupus erythematosus. J. Autoimmun. 6, 481.

Itoh, Y., Reichlin, M. 1992. Autoantibodies to the Ro/SSA antigen are conformation dependent. I. Anti-60kD antibodies are mainly directed to the native protein; anti-52kD antibodies are mainly directed to the denatured protein. Autoimmunity 14, 57.

Jaeggi, E.T., Hamilton, R.M., Silverman, E.D., et al. 2002. Outcome of children with fetal, neonatal or childhood diagnosis of isolated congenital atrioventricular block. J. Am. Coll. Cardiol. 39, 130.

Jobe, A.H. 2000. Glucocorticoids in perinatal medicine misguided rockets? J. Pediatr. 137, 1.

Julkunen, H., Eronen, M. 2001a. Long-term outcome of mothers of children with isolated heart block in Finland. Arthritis Rheum. 44, 647.

Julkunen, H., Eronen, M. 2001b. The rate of recurrence of isolated congenital heart block: a population-based study. Arthritis Rheum. 44, 487.

Julkunen, H., Kurki, P., Kaaja, R., et al. 1993a. Isolated congenital heart block. Long-term outcome of mothers and characterization of the immune response to SS-A/Ro/SSA and to SS-B/La. Arthritis Rheum. 36, 1588.

A retrospective clinical study of 33 mothers, a mean of 11.2 years after the delivery of their first child with CHB. A clinical and immunologic study of 31 of these mothers, compared with 89 healthy mothers, 45 mothers with SLE, and 19 mothers with primary SS, all of whom had healthy children. The mothers of CHB children had clinical and immunologic characteristics more closely related to primary SS than to SLE or any other connective tissue disease.

Julkunen, H., Kaaja, R., Wallgren, E., et al. 1993b. Isolated congenital heart block: fetal and infant outcome and familial incidence of heart block. Obstet. Gynecol. 82, 11.

Julkunen, H., Siren, M.K., Kaaja, R., et al. 1995a. Maternal HLA antigens and antibodies to SS A/Ro/SSA and SS B/La. Comparison with systemic lupus erythematosus and primary Sjögren's syndrome. Br. J. Rheum. 34, 901.

Julkunen, H., Kaaja, R., Kurki, P., Palosuo, T., Friman, C. 1995b. Fetal outcome in women with primary Sjogren's syndrome. A retrospective case-control study. Clin. Exp. Rheumatol. 13, 65.

Kanagasegar, S., Cimaz, R., Kurien, B.T., et al. 2002. Neonatal lupus manifests as isolated neutropenia and mildly abnormal liver functions. J. Rheum. 29, 187.

Kephardt, D.C., Hood, A.F., Provost, T.T. 1987. Neonatal lupus erythematosus: new serologic findings. J. Invest. Dermatol. 77, 331.

Laemmli, U.K. 1970. Cleavage of structural proteins during the assembly of the head of bacteriophage T4. Nature 227, 680.

Laxer, R.M., Roberts, E.A., Gross, K.R., et al. 1990. Liver disease in neonatal lupus erythematosus. J. Pediatr. 116, 238.

Lawrence, S., Luy, L., Laxer, R., Krafchik, B., Silverman, E., 2000. The health of mothers of children with cutaneous neonatal lupus erythematosus differs from that of mothers of children with congenital heart block. Am. J. Med. 108, 705.

Le Thi, H.D., Wechsler, B., Piette, J.C., Bletry, O., Godeau, P. 1994. Pregnancy and its outcome in systemic lupus erythematosus. Q. J. Med. 87, 721.

Lee, L.A. 1990. Maternal autoantibodies and pregnancy-II: the neonatal lupus syndrome. In: A.L. Parke (Ed.), Bailliere's Clinical Rheumatology: Pregnancy and the Rheumatic Diseases. Bailliere Tindall, London, p. 69.

Lee, L.A. 1993. Neonatal lupus erythematosus. J. Invest. Dermatol. 100, 9S.

Lee, L.A., Reed, B.R., Harmon, C. 1983. Autoantibodies to SS-A/Ro/SSA in congenital heart block. Arthritis Rheum. 20, S24.

Lee, L.A., Reichlin, M., Ruyle, S.Z., et al. 1993. Neonatal lupus liver disease. Lupus 2, 333.

Lee, L.A., Sokol, R.J., Buyon, J.P. 2002. Hepatobiliary disease in neonatal lupus: prevalence and clinical characteristics in cases enrolled in a national registry. Pediatrics 109, E11.

Nineteen (9%) of 219 patients who had NLS and were enrolled in a national registry had probable or possible NLE hepatobiliary disease. Patients with conjugated hyperbilirubinemia with mild or no elevations of aminotransferases, occurring in the first few weeks of life and mild elevations of aminotransferases occurring at approximately 2 to 3 months of life have an excellent prognosis.

Lin, C.T., Shen, Z., Boros, P., et al. 1994. Fc receptor-mediated signal transduction. J. Clin. Immunol. 14, 1.

Lockshin, M.D., Bonfa, E., Elkon, K., et al. 1988. Neonatal lupus risk to newborns of mothers with systemic lupus erythematosus. Arthritis Rheum. 31, 697.

Machado, M.V.L., Tynan, M.J., Curry, P.V.L., et al. 1988. Fetal complete heart block. Br. Heart J. 60, 512.

Maddison, P.J., Lee, L., Reichlin, M., et al. 1995. Anti-p57: a novel association with neonatal lupus. Clin. Exp. Immunol. 99, 42.

Martin, J.N. Jr., Perry, K.G. Jr., Blake, P.G., et al. 1997. Better maternal outcomes are achieved with dexamethasone therapy for postpartum HELLP (hemolysis, elevated liver enzymes, and thrombocytopenia) syndrome. Am. J. Obstet. Gynecol. 177, 1011.

Martin, V., Lee, L.A., Askanase, A.D., et al. 2002. Long term follow-up of children with neonatal lupus and their unaffected siblings. Arthritis Rheum. 46, 2377.

These data suggest that children with neonatal lupus require continued follow-up, especially prior to adolescence and if the mother herself has an autoimmune disease. While there was no apparent increased risk of systemic lupus erythematosus, the development of some form of autoimmune disease (systemic or organ-specific) in early childhood may be of concern. During adolescence and young adulthood, individuals with neonatal lupus and their unaffected siblings do not appear to have an increased risk of developing systemic rheumatic diseases.

Mavragani, C.P., Dafni, U.G., Tzioufas, A.G., Moutsopoulus, H.M. 1998. Pregnancy outcome and anti-Ro/SSA in autoimmune diseases: a retrospective cohort study. Br. J. Rheumatol. 37, 740.

Mazel, J.A., El Sherif, N., Buyon, J., et al. 1999. Electrocardiographic abnormalities in a murine model injected with IgG from mothers of children with congenital heart block. Circulation 99, 1914.

McCue, C.M., Mantakas, M.E., Tingelstad, J.B. 1977. Congenital heart block in newborns of mothers with connective tissue disease. Circulation 56, 82.

McCuistion, C.H., Schoch, E.P. 1954. Possible discoid lupus erythematosus in a newborn infant. Report of a case with subsequent development of acute systemic lupus erythematosus in the mother. Arch. Dermatol. Syph. 70, 782.

Mehdirad, A.A., Fatkin, D., DiMarco, J.P., et al. 1999. Electrophysiologic characteristics of accessory atrioventricular connection in an inherited form of Wolff–Parkinson–White Syndrome. J. Cardiovasc. Electrophysiol. 10, 629.

Meilof, J.F., Frohn-Mulder, I.M., Stewart, P.A., et al. 1993. Maternal autoantibodies and congenital heart block: no evidence for the existence of a unique heart block-associated anti-Ro/SS-A autoantibody profile. Lupus 2, 239.

Michaelsson, M., Engle, M.A., 1972. Congenital complete heart block: an international study of the natural history. Cardiovasc. Clin. 4, 85.

Michaelsson, M., Jonzon, A., Riesenfeld, T. 1995. Isolated congenital complete atrioventricular block in adult life. A prospective study. Circulation 92, 442.

Moak, J.P., Barron, K.S., Hougen, T.J., et al. 2001. Congenital heart block: development of late-onset cardiomyopathy, a previously underappreciated sequela. J. Am. Coll. Cardiol. 37, 238.

Morquio, L. 1901. Sur une maladie infantile et familiale characterisee par des modifications permanentes du pouls, des attaques syncopales et epileptiformes et al mort subite. Arch. Med. Int. 4, 467.

Murphy, B.P., Inder, T.E., Huppi, P.S., et al. 2001. Impaired cerebral cortical gray matter growth after treatment with dexamethasone for neonatal chronic lung disease. Pediatrics 107, 217.

Neidenbach, P.J., Sahn, E.E. 1993. La/SSB (SS-B)-positive neonatal lupus erythematosus: report of a case with unusual features. J. Am. Acad. Dermatol. 29, 848.

Neiman, A.R., Lee, L.A., Weston, W.L., et al. 2000. Cutaneous manifestations of neonatal lupus without heart block: characteristics of mothers and children enrolled in a national registry. J. Pediatr. 137, 674.

Assessment of 47 mothers with anti-SSA/Ro, anti-SSB/La, and/or anti-U1-RNP antibodies and their 57 infants diagnosed with cutaneous NLE (absent heart disease) between 1981 and 1997. In 37 children, the rash resolved without sequelae; a quarter had residual sequelae including telangiectasia and dyspigmentation.

One child developed Hashimoto's thyroiditis, and 2 developed systemic-onset juvenile rheumatoid arthritis. Of 20 subsequent births, 6 (30%) children had CHB, supporting close monitoring of future pregnancies.

Ng, P.C., Wong, G.W., Lam, C.W., et al. 1997. Pituitary-adrenal response in preterm very low birth weight infants after treatment with antenatal corticosteroids. J. Clin. Endocr. Metab. 82, 3548.

Nield, L.E., Silverman, E.D., Smallhorn, J.F., et al. 2002. Endocardial fibroelastosis associated with maternal anti-Ro/SSA and anti-La/SSB antibodies in the absence of atrioventricular block. J. Am. Coll. Cardiol. 40, 796.

A retrospective review of the clinical history, echocardiography, and pathology of fetuses and children with EFE associated with CHB born to mothers positive for anti-Ro/SSA or anti-La/SSB antibodies at 5 centers. EFE occurs in the presence of autoantibody-mediated CHB despite adequate ventricular pacing. Autoantibody-associated EFE has a very high mortality rate, whether developing in fetal or postnatal life, and may be an etiologic factor in cases of fetal and neonatal "idiopathic" dilated cardiomyopathy.

Plant, R.K., Steven, R.A. 1945. Complete A–V block in a fetus. Am. Heart J. 30, 615.

Prendiville, J.S., Cabral, D.A., Poskitt, K.J., et al. 2003. Central nervous system involvement in neonatal lupus erythematosus. Pediatr. Dermatol. 20, 60.

Press, J., Uziel, Y., Laxer, R.M., Luy, L., et al. 1996. Long-term outcome of mothers of children with complete congenital heart block. Am. J. Med. 100, 328.

Follow-up of 64 mothers of children with CHB: 86% of the initially healthy mothers remained well at follow-up; 25% of the mothers with an undifferentiated autoimmune syndrome and only 2% of the initially healthy mothers developed SLE.

Priori, S.G., Barhanin, J., Hauer, R.N., et al. 1999. Genetic and molecular basis of cardiac arrhythmias: impact on clinical management parts I and II. Circulation 99, 518.

Qu, Y., Xiao, G.Q., Chen, L., et al. 2001. Autoantibodies from mothers of children with congenital heart block downregulate cardiac L-type ca channels. J. Mol. Cell. Cardiol. 33, 1153.

Ramsey-Goldman, R., Hom, D., Deng, J.S., et al. 1986. Anti-SS-A antibodies and fetal outcome in maternal systemic lupus erythematosus. Arthritis Rheum. 29, 1269.

Rider, L., Buyon, J., Rutledge, J., et al. 1993. Postnatal treatment of neonatal lupus: case report and review of the literature. J. Rheum. 20, 1208.

Reichlin, M., Brucato, A., Frank, M.B., et al. 1994. Autoantibodies to native 60 kD Ro/SSA and denaturated 52 kD Ro/SSA are concentrated in eluates from heart of a child who died with complete congenital heart block. Arthritis Rheum. 37, 1698.

Rosenthal, D., Druzin, M., Chin, C., et al. 1998. A new therapeutic approach to the fetus with congenital complete heart block: preemptive, targeted therapy with dexamethasone. Obstet Gynecol. 92, 689.

Ross, G., Sammaritano, L., Nass, R., et al. 2003. Effects of mothers' autoimmune disease during pregnancy on learning disabilities and hand preference in their children. Arch. Pediatr. Adolesc. Med. 157, 397.

Saleeb, S., Copel, J., Friedman, D., et al. 1999. Comparison of treatment with fluorinated glucocorticoids to the natural history of autoantibody-associated congenital heart block: retrospective review of the research registry for neonatal lupus. Arthritis Rheum. 42, 2335.

While prospective trials are needed, these data (from retrospective review of 50 CHB-affected pregnancies in 47 women with anti-Ro/SSA-La/SSB antibodies) suggest that fluorinated steroids should be considered for fetuses with incomplete block or hydropic changes. Serial echocardiograms are recommended to monitor fetal progress.

Salomonsson, S., Dorner, T., Theander, E., et al. 2002. A serologic marker for fetal risk of congenital heart block. Arthritis Rheum. 46, 1233.

Schmidt, K.G., Ulmer, H.E., Silverman, N.H., et al. 1991. Perinatal outcome of fetal complete atrioventricular block: a multicenter experience. J. Am. Coll. Cardiol. 17, 1360.

Schwartz, P.J., Stramba-Badiale, M., Segantini, A., et al. 1998. Prolongation of the QT interval and the sudden infant death syndrome. N. Engl. J. Med. 338, 1709.

Scott, J.S., Maddison, P.J., Taylor, P.V., et al. 1983. Connective-tissue disease, antibodies to ribonucleoprotein, and congenital heart block. N. Engl. J. Med. 309, 209.

Sheth, A.P., Esterly, N.B., Ratoosh, S.L., et al. 1995. U1RNP positive neonatal lupus erythematosus: association with anti-La/SSB antibodies? Br. J. Dermatol. 132, 520.

Shinohara, K., Miyagawa, S., Fujita, T., et al. 1999. Neonatal lupus erythematosus: results of maternal corticosteroid therapy. Obstet. Gynecol. 93, 952.

Silverman, E.D. 1993. Congenital heart block and neonatal lupus erythematosus: prevention is the goal. J. Rheumatol. 20, 1101.

Silverman, E.D., Laxer, R.M. 1997. Neonatal lupus erythematosus. Rheum. Dis. Clin. North. Am. 23, 599.

Silverman, E.D., Mamula, M.J., Hardin, J.A., et al. 1991. The importance of the immune response to the Ro/La/SSB particle in the development of complete heart block and neonatal lupus erythematosus. J. Rheumatol. 18, 120.

Silverman, E.D., Buyon, J.P., Laxer, R.M., et al. 1995. Autoantibody response to the Ro/La/SSB particle may predict outcome in neonatal lupus erythematosus. Clin. Exp. Immunol. 100, 499.

Siren, M.K., Julkunen, H., Kaaja, R. 1998. The increasing incidence of isolated CHB in Finland. J. Rheumatol. 25, 1862.

Solomon, B.A., Laude, T.A., Shalita, A.R. 1995. Neonatal lupus erythematosus: discordant disease expression of U1RNP-positive antibodies in fraternal twins—is this a subset of neonatal lupus erythematosus or a new distinct syndrome? J. Am. Acad. Dermatol. 32, 858.

Tangalakis, K., Mortiz, K., Shandley, L., et al. 1995. Effect of maternal glucocorticoid treatment on ovine fetal fluids at 0.6 gestation. Reproduct. Fertility & Dev. 7, 1595.

Theander, E., Brucato, A., Gudmundsson, S., et al. 2001. Primary Sjogren's syndrome—treatment of fetal incomplete atrioventricular block with dexamethasone. J. Rheumatol. 28, 373.

Tseng, C.E., Buyon, J.P. 1997. Neonatal lupus syndromes. Rheum. Dis. Clin. North Am. 23, 31.

Udink ten Cate, F.E., Breur, J.M., Cohen, M.I., et al. 2001. Dilated cardiomyopathy in isolated congenital complete atrioventricular block: early and long-term risk in children. J. Am. Coll. Cardiol. 37, 1129.

Van Goudoever, J.B., Wattimena, J.D., Carnielli, V.P., et al. 1994. Effect of dexamethasone on protein metabolism in infants with bronchopulmonary dysplasia. J. Pediatr. 124, 112.

Vignati, G., Brucato, A., Pisoni, M.P., et al. 1999. Clinical course of pre- and post-natal isolated congenital atrioventricular block diagnosed in utero. G. Ital. Cardiol. 29, 1478.

Waltuck, J., Buyon, J.P. 1994. Autoantibody-associated congenital heart block: Outcome in mothers and children. Ann. Int. Med. 120, 544.

Assessment of 57 anti-Ro/SSA-La/SSB-positive mothers and their 60 children with CHB: 48% of the initially healthy mothers developed autoimmune symptoms; 28% of affected children died within 1 month of birth; 4 (16%) of 25 subsequent pregnancies were complicated by CHB; and 67% of the surviving affected children required pacemakers.

Wang, D.W., Viswanathan, P.C., Balser, J.R., et al. 2002. Clinical, genetic and biophysical characterization of SCN5A mutations associated with atrioventricular conduction block. Circulation 105, 341.

Watson, R.M., Braunstein, B.L., Watson, A.J., Hochberg, M.C., Provost, T.T. 1986. Fetal wastage in women with anti-Ro/SSA antibody. J. Rheumatol. 13, 90.

Watson, R., Kang, J.E., May, M., et al. 1988. Thrombocytopenia in the neonatal lupus syndrome. Arch. Dermatol. 124, 560.

Weston, W.L., Morelli, J.G., Lee, L.A. 1999. The clinical spectrum of anti-Ro-positive cutaneous neonatal lupus erythematosus. J. Am. Acad. Dermatol. 40, 675.

Winkler, R.B., Nora, A.H., Nora, J.J. 1977. Familial congenital complete heart block and maternal systemic lupus erythematosus. Circulation 56, 1103.

Xiao, G.Q., Hu, K., Boutjdir, M. 2001. Direct inhibition of expressed cardiac l- and t-type calcium channels by IgG from mothers whose children have congenital heart block. Circulation 103, 1599.

Yater, W.M. 1929. Congenital heart block: review of the literature; report of a case with incomplete heterotaxy; the electrocardiogram in dextrocardia. Am. J. Dis. Child. 38, 112.

Yeh, T.F., Torre, J.A., Rastogi, A., Anyebuno, M.A., Pildes, R.S. 1990. Early postnatal dexamethasone therapy in premature infants with severe respiratory distress syndrome: a double-blind, controlled study. J. Pediatr. 117, 273.

Handbook of Systemic Autoimmune Diseases, Volume 1
The Heart in Systemic Autoimmune Diseases
A. Doria and P. Pauletto, editors

CHAPTER 12

Cardiac Involvement in Scleroderma

J. Gerry Coghlan[a], Christopher P. Denton*[,b]

[a]*Royal Free Hospital, London, UK*

[b]*Royal Free and University College Medical School, London, UK*

1. Introduction

Physicians caring for patients with scleroderma are struck by individual patients who develop intractable biventricular heart failure or recurrent severe pericardial effusions with haemodynamic compromise. Such patients are infrequent but right heart failure secondary to pulmonary hypertension is probably quite common and this lends further support to the impression that cardiac events are a major cause of morbidity and mortality in this population.

There is general agreement in the published literature that subclinical cardiac involvement in scleroderma is near universal, and clinical involvement, although less common, is associated with a very adverse prognosis. What remains unclear is whether overt cardiac disease is predominantly secondary to pulmonary hypertension or primary cardiac disease, the cause of primary cardiac involvement, whether the observed adverse outcome is due to cardiac disease or simply reflects the consequences of disease burden and the clinical significance of subclinical cardiac abnormalities.

Although much has been published on cardiac involvement in scleroderma, the general approach has been either a registry based search for correlations between abnormal findings and outcome or utilisation of a technique (e.g. tissue Doppler) and deducing the relevance of findings by comparison with allied situations rather than outcome. Studies have rarely addressed the underlying pathological conditions in any detail or critically evaluated the evidence supporting hypotheses of pathogenesis.

Proposed mechanisms of cardiac involvement in scleroderma include ischaemic damage, myocarditis, replacement fibrosis, systemic hypertension and pulmonary hypertension. Significant progress in our understanding and management of renal and pulmonary vascular involvement has increased the relative importance of cardiac pathology. In this chapter, we review what is known and the potential relevance of cardiac abnormalities in scleroderma and consider possible future directions for resolving the questions which remain unanswered.

2. Evidence for and prognostic impact of clinical cardiac involvement

A number of large registry studies have been published, which underline the poor prognosis associated with scleroderma and identify cardiac abnormalities as a major adverse factor (Ruangjutipopan et al., 2002; Steen and Medsger, 2000; Abbott et al., 2002; Bulpitt et al., 1993; Follansbee et al., 1993; Lee et al., 1992). More recent registries suggest that the prognosis associated with scleroderma may be much more benign (Vlachoyiannopoulos et al., 2000; Nishioka et al., 1996) and not predicted by cardiac abnormalities noted at study entry. If the more recent

* Corresponding author.
E-mail address: c.denton@rfc.ucl.ac.uk (C. Denton).

DOI: 10.1016/S1571-5078(03)01012-2

'population' based data are accurate, one must conclude that previous registries have over-estimated the significance of cardiac involvement. This would be unsurprising for two reasons. First, 'regression to the mean' (Morton and Torgerson, 2003) registries are by definition non-random samples, and by choosing any two imperfectly correlated variables (evidence of cardiac involvement and mortality) one is likely to get an extreme result, which can be improved by any intervention. Second, most registries are developed in tertiary referral centres, and referral patterns will select patients with the most difficult clinical courses. The natural consequence is that patients with abnormal cardiac findings (e.g. q waves) who are doing reasonably well will not be referred, and will thus not have the possibility of affecting either the numerator or the denominator when calculations of prognostic impact are made. One must therefore treat with caution any conclusions based on data that would not themselves have led to referral of the patients to a publishing centre. One may probably conclude that evidence of severe cardiac compromise is associated with a poor prognosis (Steen and Medsger, 2000) and is found in up to 15% of scleroderma patients attending referral centres. Whether as proposed other abnormalities such as axis deviation, ventricular hypertrophy, arrhythmias (Lee et al., 1992) have significance beyond that seen in the normal population remains a matter of conjecture.

3. Prevalence of subclinical cardiac involvement

The same caveat, by definition, must extend to assessments of subclinical cardiac involvement. If one proposes that patients with adverse clinical courses have more active disease and greater internal organ involvement, it follows that the prevalence of cardiac abnormalities will be exaggerated in patients studied at referral centres. However, findings that are near universal in any population must be evaluated since, even if this a selected population, the abnormality is either truly universal and informs us about the nature of the disease process or closely associated with the reasons for referral and thus potentially of substantial clinical importance.

Diastolic dysfunction has been found in 50–80% of patients in association with scleroderma, whether studied using echocardiography (Plazak et al., 2002; Candell-Riera et al., 1996; Di Bello et al., 1999; Armstrong et al., 1996) or nuclear medicine (Nakajima et al., 2001). The abnormalities tend to predominantly affect the longitudinal (endocardial) fibres and fit well with the histological findings of diffuse patchy fibrosis (Follansbee et al., 1993, 1990; Bulkley et al., 1976, 1978) found in over 40–70% of autopsies. No clear association with outcome has been defined, though it has been suggested that the abnormalities are likely to result from intermittent vasospastic ischaemia, and therapy directed at relieving ischaemia will improve outcome in patients with scleroderma.

Nuclear studies using older techniques suggest a high prevalence of perfusion defects (Alexander et al., 1986; Morelli et al., 1997; Lekakis et al., 1998); abnormalities whether fixed or reversible perfusion defects have been found in 50–100% of patients with scleroderma. Other studies fail to confirm these findings (Nakajima et al., 2001) or suggest that only minor abnormalities can be found (Ishida et al., 2000). Finally, more recent studies have used 24 h ambulatory monitoring to determine the heart rate variability in patients with scleroderma; these have shown reduced heart rate variability in most patients which is taken as evidence for widespread autonomic dysfunction (Wranicz et al., 2000; Morelli et al., 1996). Even allowing for methodological limitations the bulk of available data support the notion that some degree of myocardial involvement is common in scleroderma, the pathobiology of which has yet to be resolved.

4. Ischaemic heart disease

One of the most widely accepted hypotheses is that ischaemic damage underlies much of the cardiac pathology found in scleroderma. Evidence comes from histology, ECG and thallium scanning. Histology shows replacement fibrosis and contraction band necrosis (Follansbee et al., 1993; Bulkley et al., 1978, 1976), which in other situations is associated with ischaemic injury (Follansbee et al., 1985).

The data on myocardial ischaemia are much more problematic; histology shows either normal intramyocardial vessels (Bulkley et al., 1976) or occasional mild intimal or medial thickening (Follansbee et al., 1985). The presence of an excess of focal fibrosis has nevertheless been proposed as evidence of an ischaemic pathogenesis (Follansbee et al., 1990) even though in this study the hallmark abnormality of contraction band necrosis was not found to be more prevalent in the hearts of patients with scleroderma when compared to controls. More recent methodology including cell typing raises the possibility that a low-grade inflammation is the actual driver (Liangos et al., 2000). Histological features which are not readily explained by ischaemic injury are also frequent—fibrinous pericarditis, subvalvular thickening (Bulkley et al., 1976; Follansbee et al., 1990).

ECG abnormalities, in particular septal q waves, are advanced as further evidence of ischaemic damage (Follansbee et al., 1985); more importantly recent guidelines on the diagnosis of myocardial infarction accept the presence of pathological q waves as evidence of myocardial infarction (Task Force of the ESC, 2003). However, such q waves are not associated with regional wall motion abnormalities or evidence of coronary disease (Follansbee et al., 1993). One problem with interpreting ECG abnormalities is that minor ECG abnormalities are found in a large percentage of the normal population, and the prevalence rises with age. In the Framingham cohort of middle-aged women, the prevalence of abnormal ECGs was 40% (Kannel and Castelli, 1972); if one uses this population as a comparator, then only conduction defects and septal q waves appear to occur excessively in the scleroderma population. Septal 'r' waves require functioning septal conduction tissue and are thus absent in left bundle branch block without infarction (Josephson, 1993); a possible alternate explanation thus, is conducting tissue fibrosis rather than infarction.

Several publications using thallium scintigraphy have found an increased prevalence of resting (Morelli et al., 1997), exercise induced (Steen et al., 1996) or cold pressor induced (Alexander et al., 1986; Lekakis et al., 1998) perfusion defects in patients with scleroderma, and these have in some cases been associated with an adverse prognosis (Candell-Riera et al., 1996). No excess of perfusion defects has been documented when compared with other patients with Raynaud's phenomenon (Candell-Riera et al., 1996). Further, with the development of more specific techniques such as technetium scanning, stress echocardiography and stress MUGA scanning, these inducible perfusion defects have not been persistent (Nakajima et al., 2001; Ishida et al., 2000). Data from nuclear studies have been very inconsistent, some series reporting frequent large defects, others showing minor defects, and the frequency of cold pressor inducible defects varies from 0 up to 60% (Geirsson et al., 1996). Given that most data have been obtained from ungated thallium studies and that this technique is associated with a 30% false positive rate (Chung and Lahiri, 2000), it is best to regard much of the data published literature in this field with circumspection. The results of the studies examining coronary sinus blood flow are also unhelpful with one showing impaired vasodilator reserve (Nitenberg et al., 1986) and another showing the absence of vasospasm in response to cold pressor testing (Colfer et al., 1993). Thus, the ischaemic hypothesis relies heavily on the presumed mechanism of production of the damage found at autopsy. The evidence on which the case for ischaemic myocardial damage has been built is thus very tenuous.

Three potential mechanisms of ischaemic damage have been proposed: coronary arterial vasospasm, small vessel disease and occlusive coronary disease. The theoretical basis for assuming an excess of macrovascular coronary disease is derived from the observed endothelial dysfunction and fibroproliferative tendency, which have been proposed as the pathobiological model of scleroderma (Kissin and Korn, 2002), and reports of an excess of lower limb macrovascular disease in the scleroderma population. Recent studies have also identified altered large blood vessel elasticity as a general feature of scleroderma (Cheng et al., 2003a,b). Vascular lesions in the skin, kidney and lungs of patients with scleroderma show consistent features, with medial hypertrophy followed by luminal occlusion (Taylor et al., 2002). TGFB1 over-expression has been found, with evidence of upregulation of CTGF and PDGF (Schachna and Wigley, 2002). Downstream endothelin levels and adrenaline levels have also been shown to increase. These changes are thought to drive the smooth muscle and fibromuscular hypertrophy observed. Histology of the coronaries have not shown any excess of fibromuscular hypertrophy to date (Follansbee et al., 1993, 1990; Bulkley et al., 1978, 1976).

There is evidence of abnormal thickening of the large vessels in the leg (Veale et al., 1995; Youssef et al., 1993) and carotid (Cheng et al., 2003b; Ho et al., 2000), yet to date there have been no publications showing an excess of large vessel coronary disease either angiographically or on post-mortem studies. Whether or not macrovascular coronary disease is more common in patients with scleroderma is clinically significant, as this may provide a treatable cause of cardiac dysfunction. In the absence of evidence for macrovascular disease or significant pathology of the small vessels of the myocardium, vasospasm has been promoted as the cause of the observed myocardial damage (Steen et al., 1996). Unfortunately, 30 years after cardiac Raynaud was first proposed (Gupta et al., 1975) as the unifying cause of myocardial ischaemia in scleroderma, clear confirmation that this exists as a clinically important entity is lacking.

5. Myocarditis

Myositis is well known to occur in scleroderma evidenced by histological findings and electromyography. Follansbee et al. (1993) have shown an association between cardiac mortality and myositis raising the possibility that associated myocarditis is occurring in these patients. Myocarditis may well explain the frequent occurrence of exudative pericardial effusions, and could explain the endocardial lesions found on histology. The ECG evidence of conducting tissue damage could readily be the consequence of an autoimmune inflammatory process. At present, there are few published data suggesting that widespread low-grade myocarditis occurs in this population leading to diastolic dysfunction and the other cardiac abnormalities seen. We have observed an excess of troponin T release from patients with scleroderma (Mukerjee et al., 2003), and noted a weak association with outcome at 5 years. An attractive hypothesis is that low-grade intermittent myocardial inflammation causes mild myocardial damage in the first few years when the disease process is most active, leading to evidence of mild fibrosis with diastolic dysfunction in the stable phase of the disease. To prove this, one would have to screen patients using troponin testing early in the disease, and biopsy those with evidence of activity. Further, one would have to demonstrate some relationship between the intensity or duration of the inflammatory phase and the eventual degree of myocardial damage.

6. Hypertension

Surprisingly little has been published about the impact of systemic and pulmonary hypertension on the heart given the prevalence of these conditions. Renal impairment is one of the acknowledged predictors of poor prognosis in patients with scleroderma, and this effect is aggravated by evidence of cardiac involvement. Given the known impact of renal disease on coronary disease and the association with hypertension, this is somewhat surprising. Pulmonary hypertension has been suggested as occurring in up to 50% of patients with scleroderma, though a prevalence of 12% is probably closer to the mark (Mukerjee et al., 2003) (caveats about referral centre populations being accepted). Increased afterload leading to right heart failure is a well-recognised cause of death in this population, and individuals with diastolic dysfunction who improve as systemic hypertension is controlled are recognised. The question thus arises: could the cardiac mortality and diastolic dysfunction simply represent the consequences of non-cardiac disease?

In patients with scleroderma, pulmonary hypertension carries a particularly adverse prognosis, however, death is still primarily cardiac (Mukerjee et al., 2003). The fact that an adverse outcome relative to primary pulmonary hypertension is seen at relatively low pressures suggests that there is, in patients with scleroderma, an additional cardiac impairment which compromises cardiac adaptation to afterload. Studies of diastolic dysfunction include examples where systemic hypertension has been specifically excluded. Thus, one may conclude that although afterload problems are a significant cause of mortality in this population, there is an additional cardiac component to the disease process that affects outcome. It is possible to resolve the differences between population studies and referral centre studies if one accepts that the background level of cardiac involvement is insufficient by itself to alter prognosis, but can impair the response to many secondary insults which may occur in this population.

7. The future

On the basis of the presently available evidence it is reasonable to accept that a low-level cardiac involvement is seen in a significant proportion of patients with scleroderma. In the majority of patients, this does not influence prognosis, though it may impair exercise tolerance and increase overall heart rate. Additional stresses, whether pulmonary or renal, are not uncommon in patients with scleroderma, and are poorly tolerated, in part, because of underlying cardiac defects. Elucidating the nature of the cardiac involvement is important as this may throw light on the pathobiological nature of scleroderma, and since developing ways of preventing cardiac impairment may improve quality and quantity of life in patients who suffer many other stresses. If one accepts that this is an autoimmune condition then it is unlikely that a purely vascular explanation will suffice; we need to explore the nature of the process in a more sophisticated manner. It is clear that disease activity is maximal relatively early in diffuse cutaneous scleroderma, and it is now possible to identify patients with active cardiac involvement from highly sensitive analytical techniques, such as troponin testing. We need to select patients with active cardiac involvement, analyse vasoreactivity invasively, and obtain myocardial biopsies for study using modern immunofluorescent techniques. Only through studying such patients invasively can the true value and clinical usefulness of less invasive test such as nuclear imaging and gated cardiac MRI be determined and validated, and basic disease mechanisms underlying cardiac scleroderma be unequivocally elucidated.

Key points

- Subclinical cardiac involvement is frequent in systemic sclerosis, the clinical significance of which is not presently known.
- Clinically apparent cardiac involvement in systemic sclerosis is found in upto 15% of patients (those seen in referral centres) and is associated with an adverse outcome.
- The pathophysiology of cardiac involvement in systemic sclerosis is unknown. Cardiac Raynauld's phenomenon, accelerated coronary atherosclerosis, and autoimmune myocardial damage may all contribute.
- Newer investigation techniques which may help identify patients with active cardiac involvement include Troponin testing and Cardiac MRI scanning.
- Right ventricular dysfunction determines the prognosis of patients with systemic sclerosis associated pulmonary hypertension. Right ventricular failure occurs at lower pulmonary pressures in patients with systemic sclerosis when compared to patients with primary pulmonary hypertension. This suggests that subclinical cardiac involvement is significant in the presence of additional stressors.

References

Abbott, K.C., Trespalacios, F.C., Welch, P.G., Agodoa, L.Y. 2002. Scleroderma at end stage renal disease in the United States: patient characteristics and survival. J. Nephrol. 15, 236.

Alexander, E.L., Firestein, G.S., Weiss, J.L., Heuser, R.R., Leitl, G., Wagner, H.N. Jr., Brinker, J.A., Ciuffo, A.A., Becker, L.C., 1986. Reversible cold-induced abnormalities in myocardial perfusion and function in systemic sclerosis. Ann. Intern. Med. 105, 661.

Armstrong, G.P., Whalley, G.A., Doughty, R.N., Gamble, G.D., Flett, S.M., Tan, P.L., Sharpe, D.N. 1996. Left ventricular function in scleroderma. Br. J. Rheumatol. 35, 983.

Bulkley, B.H., Ridolfi, R.L., Salyer, W.R., Hutchins, G.M. 1976. Myocardial lesions of progressive systemic sclerosis. A cause of cardiac dysfunction. Circulation 53, 483.

Bulkley, B.H., Klacsmann, P.G., Hutchins, G.M. 1978. Angina pectoris, myocardial infarction and sudden cardiac death with normal coronary arteries: a clinicopathologic study of 9 patients with progressive systemic sclerosis. Am. Heart J. 95, 563.

An early series recognizing that cardiac involvement was an important cause of death in systemic sclerosis but was not always associated with structural pathology.

Bulpitt, K.J., Clements, P.J., Lachenbruch, P.A., Paulus, H.E., Peter, J.B., Agopian, M.S., Singer, J.Z., Steen, V.D., Clegg, D.O., Ziminski, C.M. 1993. Early undifferentiated connective tissue disease: III. Outcome and prognostic indicators in early scleroderma (systemic sclerosis). Ann. Intern. Med. 118, 602.

Candell-Riera, J., Armadans-Gil, L., Simeon, C.P., Castell-Conesa, J., Fonollosa-Pla, V., Garcia-del-Castillo, H., Vaque-Rafart, J., Vilardell, M., Soler-Soler, J. 1996. Comprehensive noninvasive assessment of cardiac involvement in limited systemic sclerosis. Arthritis Rheum. 39, 1138.

Cheng, K.S., Tiwari, A., Boutin, A., Denton, C.P., Black, C.M., Morris, R., Seifalian, A.M., Hamilton, G. 2003a. Differentiation of primary and secondary Raynaud's disease by carotid arterial stiffness. Eur. J. Vasc. Endovasc. Surg. 25, 336.

Cheng, K.S., Tiwari, A., Boutin, A., Denton, C.P., Black, C.M., Morris, R., Hamilton, G., Seifalian, A.M. 2003b. Carotid and femoral arterial wall mechanics in scleroderma. Rheumatology, 42, 1299.

Chung, G., Lahiri, A. 2000. Myocardial perfusion imaging in modern cardiology. Br. J. Cardiol. 7, 619.

Colfer, H.T., Das, S.K., Dabich, L., Randall, O.S., Pitt, B. 1993. Effect of cold stress on coronary sinus blood flow in patients with scleroderma. J. Assoc. Acad. Minor. Phys. 4, 62.

Di Bello, V., Ferri, C., Giorgi, D., Bianchi, M., Bertini, A., Martini, A., Storino, F.A., Paterni, M., Pasero, G., Giusti, C. 1999. Ultrasonic videodensitometric analysis in scleroderma heart disease. Coron. Artery Dis. 10, 103.

Follansbee, W.P., Curtiss, E.I., Rahko, P.S., Medsger, T.A. Jr., Lavine, S.J., Owens, G.R., Steen, V.D. 1985. The electrocardiogram in systemic sclerosis (scleroderma). Study of 102 consecutive cases with functional correlations and review of the literature. Am. J. Med. 79, 183.

Follansbee, W.P., Miller, T.R., Curtiss, E.I., Orie, J.E., Bernstein, R.L., Kiernan, J.M., Medsger, T.A. Jr. 1990. A controlled clinicopathologic study of myocardial fibrosis in systemic sclerosis (scleroderma). J. Rheumatol. 17, 656.
Seminal paper describing cardiac involvement with fibrosis in systemic sclerosis that establishes a substantial prevalence of subclinical disease.

Follansbee, W., Zerbe, T., Medsger, T. 1993. Cardiac and skeletal muscle disease in systemic sclerosis (scleroderma): a high risk association. Am. Heart J. 125, 194.

Geirsson, A., Danielsen, R., Petursson, E. 1996. Left ventricular myocardial perfusion and function in systemic sclerosis before and after diltiazem treatment. Scand. J. Rheumatol. 25, 317.

Gupta, M.P., Zoneraich, S., Zeitlin, W., Zoneraich, O., D'Angelo, W. 1975. Scleroderma heart disease with slow flow velocity in coronary arteries. Chest 67, 116.

Ho, M., Veale, D., Eastmond, C., Eastmond, C., Nuki, G., Belch, J. 2000. Macrovascular disease and systemic sclerosis. Ann. Rheum. Dis. 59, 39.

Ishida, R., Murata, Y., Sawada, Y., Nishioka, K., Shibuya, H. 2000. Thallium-201 myocardial SPECT in patients with collagen disease. Nucl. Med. Commun. 21, 729.

Josephson, M. 1993. Intraventricular Conduction Disturbances. Clinical Cardiac Electrophysiology, 2nd ed., Lea and Febiger, Philadelphia, PA, p. 117.

Kannel, W.B., Castelli, W.P. 1972. The Framingham study of coronary disease in women. Med. Times 100, 173.

Kissin, E., Korn, J.H. 2002. Poptosis and myofibroblasts in the pathogenesis of systemic sclerosis. Curr. Rheumatol. Rep. 4, 129.

Lee, P., Langevitz, P., Alderdice, C.A., Aubrey, M., Baer, P.A., Baron, M., Buskila, D., Dutz, J.P., Khostanteen, I., Piper, S. 1992. Mortality in systemic sclerosis (scleroderma). Q. J. Med. 82, 139.

Lekakis, J., Mavrikakis, M., Emmanuel, M., Prassopoulos, V., Papazoglou, S., Papamichael, C., Moulopoulou, D., Kostamis, P., Stamatelopoulos, S., Moulopoulos, S. 1998. Cold-induced coronary Raynaud's phenomenon in patients with systemic sclerosis. Clin. Exp. Rheumatol. 16, 135.

Liangos, O., Neure, L., Kuhl, U., Pauschinger, M., Sieper, J., Distler, A., Schwimmbeck, P.L., Braun, J. 2000. The possible role of myocardial biopsy in systemic sclerosis. Rheumatology (Oxford) 39, 674.

Morelli, S., Piccirillo, G., Fimognari, F., Sgreccia, A., Ferrante, L., Morabito, G., DeMarzio, P., Valesini, G., Marigliano, V. 1996. Twenty-four hour heart period variability in systemic sclerosis. J. Rheumatol. 23, 643.
This paper confirms that there is likely to be altered cardiac electrophysiology in many patients with systemic sclerosis although the clinical and therapeutic implications remain uncertain.

Morelli, S., Sgreccia, A., De Marzio, P., Perrone, C., Ferrante, L., Gurgo, A.M., Gurgo diCastelmenardo, A.M., Aguglia, G., De Vincentiis, G., Scopinaro, F., Calvieri, S. 1997. Noninvasive assessment of myocardial involvement in patients with systemic sclerosis: role of signal averaged electrocardiography. J. Rheumatol. 24, 2358.

Morton, V., Torgerson, D. 2003. Effect of regression to the mean on decision making in health care. Br. Med. J. 326, 1083.

Mukerjee, D., St. George, D., Coleiro, B., Denton, C.P., Devar, J., Black, C.M. and Coghlan, J.G., 2003. Prevalence and outcome in systemic sclerosis associated pulmonary arterial hypertension (SScPAH): application of a registry approach. Annals Rheum Disease. Ann Rheum Dis. 62: 1088–93.

Nakajima, K., Taki, J., Kawano, M., Higuchi, T., Sato, S., Nishijima, C., Takehara, K., Tonami, N. 2001. Diastolic dysfunction in patients with systemic sclerosis detected by gated myocardial perfusion SPECT: an early sign of cardiac involvement. J. Nucl. Med. 42, 183.

Nishioka, K., Katayama, I., Kondo, H., Shinkai, H., Ueki, H., Tamaki, K., Takehara, K., Tajima, S., Maeda, M., Hayashi, S., Kodama, H., Miyachi, Y., Mizutani, H., Fujisaku, A., Sasaki, T., Shimizu, M., Kaburagi, J. 1996. Epidemiological analysis of prognosis of 496 Japanese patients with progressive systemic sclerosis (SSc). Scleroderma Research Committee Japan. J. Dermatol. 23, 677.

Nitenberg, A., Foult, J.M., Kahan, A., Perennec, J., Devaux, J.Y., Menkes, C.J., Amor, B. 1986. Reduced coronary flow and resistance reserve in primary scleroderma myocardial disease. Am. Heart J. 112, 309.

Plazak, W., Zabinska-Plazak, E., Wojas-Pelc, A., Podolec, P., Olszowska, M., Tracz, W., Bogdaszewska-Czabanowska, J. 2002. Heart structure and function in systemic sclerosis. Eur. J. Dermatol. 12, 257.

Ruangjutipopan, S., Kasitanon, N., Louthrenoo, W., Sukitawut, W., Wichainun, R. 2002. Causes of death and poor survival prognostic factors in Thai patients with systemic sclerosis. J. Med. Assoc. Thai. 85, 1204.

Schachna, L., Wigley, F.M. 2002. Targeting mediators of vascular injury in scleroderma. Curr. Opin. Rheumatol. 14, 686.

Steen, V.D., Medsger, T.A. Jr. 2000. Severe organ involvement in systemic sclerosis with diffuse scleroderma. Arthritis Rheum. 43, 2437.

Steen, V.D., Follansbee, W.P., Conte, C.G., Medsger, T.A. Jr. 1996. Thallium perfusion defects predict subsequent cardiac dysfunction in patients with systemic sclerosis. Arthritis Rheum. 39, 677.

Task Force of the ESC, 2003. Management of acute myocardial infarction in patients presenting with ST-segment elevation. Eur. Heart J. 24, 28.

Taylor, M.H., McFadden, J.A., Bolster, M.B., Silver, R.M. 2002. Ulnar artery involvement in systemic sclerosis (scleroderma). J. Rheumatol. 29, 102.

Veale, D.J., Collidge, T.A., Belch, J.J. 1995. Increased prevalence of symptomatic macrovascular disease in systemic sclerosis. Ann. Rheum. Dis. 54, 853.

Vlachoyiannopoulos, P.G., Dafni, U.G., Pakas, I., Spyropoulou-Vlachou, M., Stavropoulos-Giokas, C., Moutsopoulos, H.M. 2000. Systemic scleroderma in Greece: low mortality and strong linkage with HLA-DRB1*1104 allele. Ann. Rheum. Dis. 59, 359.

Wranicz, J.K., Strzonda, M., Zieliska, M., Cygankiewicz, I., Ruta, J., Dziankowska-Bartkowiak, B., Sysa-Jedrzejowska, A. 2000. Evaluation of early cardiovascular involvement in patients with systemic sclerosis. Przegl. Lek. 57, 389.

Youssef, P., Englert, H., Bertouch, J. 1993. Large vessel occlusive disease associated with CREST syndrome and scleroderma. Ann. Rheum. Dis. 52, 464.
The first report of increased macrovascular disease in systemic sclerosis. Occult left ventricular cardiac involvement may first present at times of cardiovascular stress related to the disease (e.g. hypertensive renal crisis) or related to high volume fluid loads associated therapy or as a result of cardiotoxic drugs.

Handbook of Systemic Autoimmune Diseases, Volume 1
The Heart in Systemic Autoimmune Diseases
A. Doria and P. Pauletto, editors

CHAPTER 13

Cardiac Involvement in Autoimmune Myositis and Overlap Syndromes

Ingrid E. Lundberg

Rheumatology Unit, Department of Medicine at Karolinska Hospital, Karolinska Institutet, SE-171 76 Stockholm, Sweden

1. Introduction

This chapter will be focused on the chronic idiopathic inflammatory myopathies with reference to cardiac involvement. The overlap syndromes is a less well-defined group, in this chapter only cardiac involvement in one condition which is sometimes referred to as an overlap syndrome, the mixed connective tissue disease (MCTD) will be addressed.

Chronic idiopathic inflammatory muscle disorders, myositis, encompass a group of muscle disorders which are characterized clinically by weakness and fatigue of skeletal muscle and by autoimmune phenomena such as infiltration of T-lymphocytes and macrophages in skeletal muscle tissue and by the presence of autoantibodies (Plotz et al., 1995). Based on some different clinical features and different histopathological findings in muscle tissue three major subgroups of myositis have been identified; dermatomyositis, polymyositis and inclusion body myositis (Dalakas, 1991; Arahata and Engel, 1984; Engel and Arahata, 1986). The clinical manifestations of the idiopathic inflammatory myopathies are not limited to symptoms from skeletal muscles but other organs are frequently involved such as the skin in dermatomyositis, and also lungs, heart, joints with arthralgias and arthritis and the gastrointestinal tract with esophagus dysmotility.

Epidemiological data of idopathic inflammatory myopathies in general are relatively limited and older studies are hampered by the use of different definitions of myositis. After 1975 the criteria proposed by Bohan and Peter (1975a,b) are the most often used for diagnosis of polymyositis and dermatomyositis. Older studies could include more heterogenous populations of muscle disorders and are more difficult to draw conclusions from. These problems also relate to epidemiology data of cardiac manifestations in myositis. The criteria which were proposed by Bohan and Peter were based on clinical observations leading to the diagnosis of polymyositis and dermatomyositis. Later a third subset of myositis was identified, inclusion body myositis (Yunis and Samaha, 1971), with some distinct clinical and histopathological features from polymyositis and dermatomyositis and defined in the criteria suggested by Griggs et al. (1995). In older studies inclusion body myositis patients were not distinguished from polymyositis patients, which makes it difficult to make a distinction between cardiac manifestations in polymyositis and inclusion body myositis in older studies. Recently, a revision of the Bohan and Peter criteria for classification of idiopathic inflammatory myopathies was suggested in which results of magnetic resonance imaging, presence of myositis-specific autoantibodies, more specific histopathologic changes in muscle tissue and the criteria for inclusion body myositis are included (Targoff et al., 1997).

The idiopathic inflammatory myopathies as a whole group are rare disorders and reports of incidence and prevalence are few. The incidence of hospital-diagnosed polymyositis and dermatomyositis according to the Bohan and Peter criteria was

E-mail address: ingrid.lundberg@medks.ki.se (I.E. Lundberg).

DOI: 10.1016/S1571-5078(03)01013-4

determined to be 5.5 per million population (Oddis et al., 1990). An annual incidence rate between 2.2 and 7.6 per million population was reported in an Israeli study, a county-based Swedish study and an Australian population-based study (Benbassat et al., 1980; Weitoft, 1997; Patrick et al., 1999). The different incidence numbers could depend on varying inclusion criteria as well as varying case retrieval strategies used in these studies which makes comparisons difficult, but ethnic or geographical differences cannot be excluded.

Prevalence data of polymyositis and dermatomyositis are more scarce and vary from 5 per 100,000 population in Japan to 11 per 100,000 in a county-based survey from Sweden (Ahlstrom et al., 1993). The relative prevalence of dermatomyositis in relation to polymyositis varies between different studies. Recently, an interesting report suggested a latitude gradient with an increasing relative prevalence of dermatomyositis along the geographical latitude in Europe (Hengstman et al., 2000). There is a female predominance with a female to male ratio of 2:1 among patients with polymyositis and dermatomyositis in most epidemiology studies although this was most pronounced during childbearing age (Oddis et al., 1990; Medsger et al., 1970; Benbassat et al., 1980).

Population-based epidemiological data on IBM are scarce. An incidence of 2.2–4.9 per million population was reported from two European studies (Lindberg et al., 1994; Badrising et al., 2000). In a recently published nation-wide study the prevalence of IBM was reported to be 4.9 patients per million inhabitants in the Netherlands (Badrising et al., 2000). When adjusted for age distribution the prevalence was 16 per million inhabitants over 50 years of age. The relative prevalence of inclusion body myositis of all inflammatory myopathies was reported to vary between 16 and 28% in series from large neuromuscular centres (Lotz et al., 1989; Mhiri and Gherardi, 1990). The male to female ratio for inclusion body myositis was 2:1.

Mixed connective tissue disease is even more a rare condition than the myositis. MCTD is clinically characterized by the combined features of other defined autoimmune disorders, namely, systemic lupus erythematosus (SLE), systemic sclerosis (SSc), rheumatoid arthritis and polymyositis (Sharp et al., 1972). The most typical clinical symptoms are Raynaud's phenomenon, puffy hands, arthritis and myositis. A hallmark of patients with MCTD is the presence of anti-ribonucleoprotein (RNP) antibodies in high titers (Sharp et al., 1972).

2. Epidemiology/prevalence of heart involvement in myositis/MCTD

2.1. Prevalence of cardiac involvement in myositis

Although the heart is a muscle, clinical manifestations of cardiac involvement are seldom evident and the real frequency of heart involvement in myositis is uncertain. Cardiac involvement in polymyositis or dermatomyositis was first reported by Oppenheim (1899). Until the 1970s cardiac involvement was considered to be a rare manifestation of the inflammatory myopathies. Since 1975 cardiac involvement has been recognized as a manifestation in polymyositis and dermatomyositis but the published reports of heart involvement in patients with myositis are still limited. There are very few, if any, controlled studies including unselected well-defined patient populations with population-based controls in which cardiac manifestations in myositis patients have been investigated. The limitations of available reports make it difficult to draw conclusions about the prevalence of different types of cardiac manifestations, pathogenesis and prognosis of heart disease in myositis patients. Moreover, in most reports the number of patients in each study is too low to analyse whether there are differences between cardiac involvement in the three subsets of myositis. Furthermore, epidemiology data concerning cardiac manifestations in inclusion body myositis is largely missing. Most of the patients involved in the different studies are adult, although there are a few reports which include children which will also be mentioned briefly in this overview.

The frequency of heart involvement, between 6 and 75%, is still uncertain due to lack of epidemiological studies in which heart involvement has been addressed. The frequency varies depending on patient selection, definition of heart involvement, whether clinical manifest or subclinical cardiac involvement is considered, and the methods used to detect cardiac involvement (Gottdiener et al., 1978; Gonzales-Lopez et al., 1996). Most of the published reports have been conducted as cross-sectional studies of cardiac involvement in patients from one clinical cohort; the number of patients in each study is limited. The types of heart involvement that have been reported in patients with idiopathic inflammatory myopahties are several; conduction abnormalities, congestive heart failure, myocarditis, myocardial fibrosis, left ventricular dysfunction, enhanced left ventricular function, mitral valve prolaps, coronary artery disease, small vessel disease and atherosclerosis (Gottdiener et al., 1978; Denbow et al., 1979; Haupt and Hutchins, 1982; Stern et al., 1984). Clinically manifest heart problems are relatively infrequent in most reports varying in frequency between less than 10 and 25% of patients with myositis (Bohan et al., 1977; Gottdiener et al., 1978; Denbow et al., 1979; Henriksson and Sandstedt, 1982; Haupt and Hutchins, 1982; Hochberg et al., 1986; Gonzales-Lopez et al., 1996). In a small Finnish study including 16 cases of polymyositis and dermatomyositis, 69% of the patients had features of cardiac involvement, most of them were clinically apparent heart problems such as congestive heart failure in four and coronary heart disease in six patients (Oka and Raasakka, 1978). No control population was included in this study which makes it difficult to draw conclusions about the underlying reasons for the cardiac problems in this cohort, but a high frequency of traditional risk factors for cardiac disease which are not disease related cannot be excluded.

The prevalence of cardiac involvement in children with myositis is not known. There are a few case reports of myocardial infarction and pericarditis, and in one autopsy study two of the children had autopsy signs of congestive heart failure (Haupt and Hutchins, 1982). In a recently published evaluation in which all cases with juvenile dermatomyositis at the Department of Hospital for Sick Children were screened with electrocardiograms (ECG), and most also with echocardiogram, no case with clinically significant cardiac disease was detected (Ramanan and Feldman, 2002).

2.2. MCTD—prevalence of cardiac involvement

The frequency of cardiac involvement in patients with MCTD varies from 11 to 85% depending upon patient selection and definitions of cardiac involvement as well as upon methods used to detect cardiac manifestations (Lundberg and Hedfors, 1991; Alpert et al., 1983). In the study by Alpert et al. (1983), in which a high prevalence of cardiac manifestations was reported, all patients were subject to investigations of cardiac involvement regardless of symptoms. The most frequently detected cardiac manifestations were pericarditis (29%), and mitral valve prolapse (26%). Of those who underwent cardiac catheterization pulmonary hypertension was recorded in 65%. Intima hyperplasia of coronary arteries was also common.

3. Etiology and pathogenesis

The etiology of idiopathic inflammatory myopathies is not known in detail although recent data suggest that both environmental and genetic factors such as HLA-DR type and cytokine polymorphisms are important risk factors (Shamim et al., 2000; Pachman et al., 2000). Risk factors to develop cardiac manifestations have only been investigated in a few studies and there are no epidemiological studies in which genetic background and environmental exposures have been addressed. In one study only increasing age was an independent risk factor to develop cardiac involvement in patients with poly- and dermatomyositis (Taylor et al., 1993). In that study there was no association between disease activity assessed as serum levels of creatine phosphokinase (CPK) or history of treatment with immunosuppressives and the presence of heart symptoms.

There is ample evidence to support immune-mediated mechanisms in polymyositis and dermatomyositits and it is likely that both the humoral and cell-mediated immune response have important roles in the development of these disorders. The role of the immune system in disease mechanisms of inclusion body myositis is more controversial. The inflammatory infiltrates in the skeletal muscle are predominated by T-cells and macrophages with some differences between the subsets of myositis (Arahata and Engel, 1984; Engel and Arahata, 1986). In polymyositis and IBM there is a predominance of CD8 + T-cells and macrophages localized to the endomysium typically surrounding and invading non-necrotic muscle fibers (Arahata and Engel, 1984; Engel and Arahata, 1986). In dermatomyositis, the inflammatory cells are predominantly localized to the perivascular areas and mainly composed of CD4 + T-cells and macrophages and to some extent B-cells. In recent years it has been possible to characterize inflammatory molecules which are produced in muscle tissue of myositis patients and interestingly, the molecular pattern is very similar between the subsets of myositis and is predominated by pro-inflammatory cytokines mainly interleukin—(IL) 1 alpha and IL-1beta and tumor necrosis factor alpha and by chemokines such as macrophage inflammatory protein (MIP)-1 alpha (Lundberg et al., 1997; Adams et al., 1997). Cytokines are not only produced by infiltrating inflammatory cells but also by endothelial cells in blood vessels in the muscle tissue and some cytokines seem to be produced by the muscle fibers (Lundberg et al., 1997, de Bleecker et al., 1999). Increased expression of IL-1 alpha, was preferentially expressed in the endothelial cells of microvessels in the muscle tissue and was observed in muscle tissue independently of detectable inflammatory infiltrates. Moreover, the IL-1 alpha expression seemed to correlate better with the clinical symptoms than the presence of inflammatory infiltrates. This observation could indicate that IL-1 alpha has a role in the mechanisms which cause muscle weakness (Nyberg et al., 2000; Englund et al., 2002). Whether IL-1 could affect cardiac muscle in patients with myositis is not known. Increased serum levels of IL-1β, TNF-α and soluble TNF-receptors compared to healthy controls have been observed in patients with polymyositis and dermatomyositis (Shimuzu et al., 2000). Increased serum levels of TNF-α as well as increased expression of TNF-α in myocardial biopsies were demonstrated in patients with idiopathic dilated cardiomyopathy who had a high degree of tissue inflammation (Sigush et al., 2000). From experimental models it has been demonstrated that over-expression of TNF-α leads to systolic dysfunction and ventricular dilatation suggesting that TNF-α might have a systemic role and could affect heart muscle function (Bryant et al., 1998). Whether this also applies to patients with chronic inflammatory diseases is not known.

3.1. Pathogenesis and cardiac involvement—myositis

The mechanisms which lead to cardiac involvement in myositis have not been clarified in detail, although autopsy studies and occasional case reports with myocardial biopsies have given some information about the underlying mechanisms. The most often observed histopathological changes in the heart are myocarditis with or without fibrosis and coronary artery disease. Percicarditis was rarely reported.

3.1.1. Myocarditis

As the myocardium is a muscle which is pathologically similar to skeletal muscle, it is not surprising to find myocarditis with infiltration of lymphocytes and macrophages in a similar fashion as could be observed in the skeletal muscles in these conditions (Hill and Barrows, 1968; Denbow et al., 1979; Haupt and Hutchins, 1982). The myocarditis could lead to impaired left ventricular dysfunction compatible with restrictive cardiomyopathy but could also be clinically silent as reported by Denbow et al., 1979. The most consistently reported histopathological changes of myocarditis include diffuse interstitial and perivascular mononuclear cell infiltrates of lymphocytes, contraction band necrosis, degeneration of cardiac myocytes, interstitial edema, variation in myocyte size and patchy fibrosis (Gottdiener et al., 1978; Oka and Raasakka, 1978; Denbow et al., 1979; Haupt and Hutchins, 1982). There are also reports of fibrosis of the myocardium, in some cases there was a coexistence of fibrosis and infiltration of inflammatory cells which may indicate a relapsing course of the myocarditis (Hill and Barrows, 1968; Haupt and Hutchins, 1982). However, there are no published reports of which inflammatory molecules are produced in the myocardium of patients with myositis and that could have a potential role in causing the myocardial manifestations.

The most often reported cardiac manifestations in poly- and dermatomyositis are subclinical arrhythmias and conduction disturbances, in particular left anterior hemiblock and right bundle-branch block (Stern et al., 1984). One possible pathophysiologic mechanism that could lead to such disturbances could be inflammation and fibrosis in the conducting system. Histopathological changes similar to those in the myocardium were noticed in the conducting system including lymphocytic infiltration, fibrosis of the sinoatrial node and contraction band necrosis which correlated with the electrocardiographic finding of left bundle branch block in one case (Haupt and Hutchins, 1982). Focal myocardial fibrosis with a patchy distribution and fibrosis of the conduction system was observed in 25% of the cases in one autopsy study (Haupt and Hutchins, 1982). Myocardial fibrosis including the conducting system was observed at autopsy in a few young cases with polymyositis who developed bardycardia–tachycardia syndrome and evidence of complete heart block and had a fatal outcome (Lynch, 1971; Lightfoot et al., 1977; Anders et al., 1999). It has been suggested that the predisposition of the anterior division of the left bundle branch and the right bundle branch could be explained by their particular vulnerability due to anatomic reasons because of their greater lengths and narrower width as compared to the posterior fascicle (Lightfoot et al., 1977).

3.1.2. Coronary heart disease

The most often reported cardiac problems in patients with poly- and dermatomyositis, impaired left ventricular function and arrhythmias, could also be secondary to vascular changes in the heart. Vascular alterations in coronary arteries have also been reported such as vasculitis, intima proliferation, media sclerosis and microvessel disease of the heart with vasospasm angina (Oka and Raasakka, 1978; Haupt and Hutchins, 1982). In one autopsy study 44% of the patients had coronary atherosclerosis (Haupt and Hutchins, 1982), but this was less frequently observed in other studies (Denbow et al., 1979; Stern et al., 1984). Acute myocardial infarction secondary to obstructive coronary artery disease, two of whom had a myocardial infarction shortly after the diagnosis of polymyositis was reported in a study (Oka and Raasakka, 1978).

Small vessel disease characterized by the narrowing of vessel lumen by smooth muscle hyperplasia with little or no intimal proliferation was also observed (Denbow et al., 1979). This small vessel disease may cause clinical symptoms like arrhythmia and angina pectoris. Small vessel disease could be accompanied by vasospastic disease with clinically manifest Raynaud's phenomenon and spasm angina and suggests similar pathogenic mechanisms with an impaired regulation of vascular tone (Riemekasten et al., 1999). Recently a young woman with dermatomyositis and episodes of acute chest pain and myocardial infarctions had a small vessel disease of the heart demonstrated by myocardial biopsy, and vasospastic angina which improved after treatment with high doses of calcium channel blockers (Riemekasten et al., 1999). In another study two patients had signs of myocardial infarcts without the evidence of atherosclerosis, one of these had Raynaud's phenomenon suggesting vasospastic disease (Haupt and Hutchins, 1982). The pathophysiology behind Raynaud's phenomenon is multifactorial but recently it has been demonstrated that repeated attacks of vasospasm may cause ischaemic reperfusion injury to the endothelium which may result in rarefications of capillaries, ischaemia and perivascular fibrosis (Riemekasten et al., 1999). Raynaud's phenomenon is present in patients with polymyositis and dermatomyositis (Haupt and Hutchins, 1982) and is particularly common in a subset of myositis patients with the so-called anti-synthetase syndrome (Love et al., 1991). Vasospasm with or without coinciding small vessel disease could thus have a role in the pathophysiology of cardiovascular manifestations of both poly- and dermatomyositis.

3.1.3. Pericarditis

Pericarditis is an unusual cardiac manifestation in patients with inflammatory myopathies reported with a frequency of about 10% (Hochberg et al., 1986; Gonzales-Lopez et al., 1996). Signs of pericarditis on echocardiography were recorded in 8–12% (Taylor et al., 1993; Gonzales-Lopez et al., 1996).

3.1.4. Cardiac performance

The effects of hemodynamic function of the heart in patients with myositis have been investigated by echocardiography and both enhanced and decreased left ventricular function have been reported. In a study by Gottdiener et al. (1978) cardiac performance, estimated as ejection phase index of left ventricular function assessed by echocardiography, was enhanced compared with a control group. Hyperdynamic left ventricular contraction was also found in a few other studies in 12–15% of myositis patients (Taylor et al., 1993; Gonzales-Lopez et al., 1996). The mechanisms behind the enhanced ventricular function remain unclear. More recently left ventricular diastolic dysfunction (LVDD) was reported in 42% of newly diagnosed poly- and dermatomyositis patients in a study in which the highly sensitive and specific color Doppler flow was used to evaluate cardiac abnormalities (Gonzales-Lopez et al., 1996). In these patients LVDD was not associated with clinical symptoms. LVDD has been reported in other diseases such as diabetes mellitus and amyloidosis and is considered to be a predictor of poor outcome (Gonzales-Lopez et al., 1996). The frequency of LVDD in the general population was in this paper estimated to be approximately 30%. The pathophysiologic mechanisms which may cause LVDD are several, and include increased chamber stiffness due to fibrosis but may also reflect disturbances in calcium regulation (Gonzales-Lopez et al., 1996).

3.1.5. Valvular abnormalities

The most frequently reported valvular abnormality is mitral valve prolapse although the frequency is uncertain and varies between 8% which equals the frequency in the normal population and as high as 65% in a study using echocardiography (Gottdiener et al., 1978; Taylor et al., 1993). The striking discrepancy in frequency between these two reports could probably be explained both by differences in patient selection and by the different sensitivity and specificity by the echocardiographic methods used to detect mitral valve prolapse. The M-mode echocardiography used by Gottdiener et al. (1978) has a lower specificity and could overestimate the frequency of mitral valve prolapse in patients with myositis (Taylor et al., 1993). In one autopsy study there were no anomalies in the tricuspid, pulmonar or aortic valves but 1/16 patients had a 'mild floppy change of the mitral valve' and four had calcific mitral annulus fibrosis (Haupt and Hutchins, 1982).

3.2. Pathogenesis and cardiac involvement—MCTD

The pathophysiologic mechanisms behind the cardiac involvement in MCTD are partly shared with myositis and myocarditis has been reported in occasional patients with MCTD (Whitlow et al., 1980). However, there are some distinct differences compared to myositis; firstly, pericarditis seems to be a more common manifestation in patients with MCTD and secondly, the most prominent cardiac problem in patients with MCTD is pulmonary hypertension (Alpert et al., 1983; Negoro et al., 1987). From autopsy studies it was demonstrated that the pulmonary hypertension was associated with intimal proliferation of small pulmonary arteries and arterioles and smooth muscle hypertrophy with only sporadic lymphocytic infiltration in the lungs (Alpert et al., 1983). A similar finding of intimal proliferation was observed in the epicardial and intramural coronary arteries. It was hypothesized that pulmonary hypertension in MCTD was related to proliferative vascular abnormalities involving small pulmonary vessels.

4. Clinical manifestations

4.1. Clinically manifest heart involvement—myositis

Clinically manifest heart involvement was rare in most published reports of heart problems in cohorts with myositis patients (Agrawal et al., 1989). Palpitations and shortness of breath was reported in 15% in one study (Gonzales-Lopez et al., 1996). But in two other studies clinically manifest heart problems were recorded in 62% of the patients either as congestive heart failure or coronary heart disease in one study (Oka and Raasakka, 1978) or as subjective symptoms such as dyspnea on exertion, palpitations, ortopnea, nonanginal chest pain or angina pectoris (Taylor et al., 1993).

4.1.1. Congestive heart failure

One of the most frequently reported clinically manifest cardiac problem in patients with myositis is congestive heart failure and in some of these patients the heart involvement may have a fatal outcome (Oka and Raasakka, 1978; Stern et al., 1984). The frequency of congestive heart failure varies between 3 and 45% (Bohan et al., 1977; Denbow et al., 1979; Oka and Raasakka, 1978). Congestive heart failure was observed both at the time of myositis diagnosis or developed after the onset despite immunosuppressive treatment. The onset of heart failure secondary to cardiomyopathy or myocarditis usually occurs with active skeletal muscle involvement, but it may develop despite inflammatory low active skeletal muscle disease or even when in remission.

4.1.2. Coronary heart disease

Coronary heart disease with angina pectoris is another clinically evident cardiac manifestation which has been reported in patients with inflammatory myopathies. Coronary heart disease with angina pectoris was reported after myositis diagnosis in 5/16 patients and myocardial infarction in 2/16 after the onset of myositis (Oka and Raasakka, 1978). There was recently a case report of vasospastic angina (Prinzmetal's angina) that accompanied small vessel disease of the heart in a case with dermatomyositis and Raynaud's phenomenon.

4.1.3. Pericarditis

Pericarditis was rarely reported in adult patients with poly- and dermatomyositis. In a case report by Yale et al. (1993), two cases with pericarditis were identified from a cohort including 350 polymyositis and dermatomyositis cases at the Mayo Clinic. One of these presented with a pericardial tamponade.

4.1.4. Subclinical heart involvement

Subclinical cardiac involvement is much more common and the frequency varies depending on the methods used. Abnormalities on ECG are frequently observed, in 32.5–72% (DeWere and Bradley, 1975; Taylor et al., 1993; Stern et al., 1984; Gottdiener et al., 1978; Denbow et al., 1979; Gonzales-Lopez et al., 1996). These ECG abnormalities include atrial and ventricular arrhythmias, conduction abnormalities including bundle branch block, A–V blocks, ventricular premature beats, high-grade heart block, prolongation of PR-intervals, left atrial abnormality, abnormal Q-waves as well as non-specific ST-T wave changes. In a large study including 77 patients with poly- and dermatomyositis in adults and children, in which standard populations were referred to as control populations, conduction abnormalities were observed in 32% which was significantly more frequent compared to the control populations (Stern et al., 1984). The most frequently observed conduction abnormalities were left anterior hemiblock and right bundle-branch block occurring in 13 and 9% of the patients, respectively. Three patients required permanent pacemakers. A high frequency of bundle branch blocks and A–V blocks were also reported from uncontrolled studies of myositis patients and in single case reports in some cases with fatal outcome (Lynch, 1971; Gottdiener et al., 1978; Denbow et al., 1979; Haupt and Hutchins, 1982; Taylor et al., 1993; Gonzales-Lopez et al., 1996; Anders et al., 1999).

4.1.5. Heart involvement in juvenile cases with myositis

As mentioned in Section 2 clinically significant cardiac involvement in children appears to be a rare manifestation. Congestive heart failure has been reported in two cases with juvenile dermatomyositis from an autopsy study (Haupt and Hutchins, 1982). Congestive heart failure in children was observed both at the time of myositis diagnosis or developed after onset (Oka and Raasakka, 1978). There are a few case reports of pericarditis and of myocardial infarction.

4.1.6. Mortality in cardiovascular death

Cardiac involvement as a cause of death in polymyositis was reported in 10–20% (Bohan et al., 1977; Hochberg et al., 1986). This figure is uncertain as large epidemiological studies in which causes of death were investigated in patients with inflammatory myopathies are very few (Bohan et al., 1977; Hochberg et al., 1986; Schwarz et al., 1992). There are a few studies to support an over risk of cardiovascular death in patients with poly- and dermatomyositis. In a follow-up study of patients with polymyositis and dermatomysitis by DeWere and Bradley (1975), with an average follow-up time of 6 years, a nearly four times increased overall mortality was recorded for myositis patients compared to the expected in the population. A sixteen times increased death rate from myocardial infarction was reported in this myositis population (males, 9 times and females, 32 times). In a computer-assisted analysis including 153 patients, cardiovascular disease was one of the leading causes of death, observed in 9.5%, together with malignancy in 23.8% and sepsis in 19% (Bohan et al., 1977). In one autopsy study the direct cause of death was cardiovascular in 3 out of 16 cases; acute congestive heart failure in one, arrhythmia with congestive heart failure in one, and dissecting aorta aneurysm in one patient (Haupt and Hutchins, 1982).

4.1.7. Association with myositis subgroups

Whether there is a difference in cardiac involvement between polymyositis and dermatomyositis is uncertain as the number of patients in each subgroup in published studies is usually too low to allow subgroup analysis. In a study by Bohan et al. (1977) cardiopulmonary manifestations were most frequently seen in patients with polymyositis and overlap syndromes and less often with dermatomyositis. In another study no difference was found in the rate of cardiac abnormalities between polymyositis and dermatomyositis (Gonzales-Lopez et al., 1996).

4.2. Clinically manifest cardiac involvement—MCTD

The same clinical heart manifestations as were reported in patients with myositis may also occur in patient with MCTD although their relative frequency may vary. There are reports of myocarditis, mitral valve prolapse, conduction disturbances including complete heart block, pericarditis and abnormal left ventricular diastolic filling pattern (Alpert et al., 1983). In MCTD the most frequently observed cardiac manifestations are pericarditis and mitral valve prolapse. Using echocardiography to detect cardiac abnormalities right ventricular enlargement was more common than left ventricular enlargement. The most significant clinical cardiovascular problem in MCTD is pulmonary hypertension which is associated with a poor prognosis.

5. Diagnostic investigations

5.1. Radiological

With conventional *chest X-ray* cardiomegaly, assessed as cardiothoracic ratio (>0.50), has been observed in patients with poly- and dermatomyositis in up to 15% (Taylor et al., 1993; Denbow et al., 1979; Buchpiguel et al., 1996). Chest X-ray has a low sensitivity to detect cardiac involvement but has a more important role to detect lung involvement.

More recently isotope imaging techniques have been used to evaluate cardiac involvement. *Technetium 99m-pyrophosphate scintigraphy* permits detection of left ventricular global and regional wall abnormalities and both decreased function and hyperkinetic left ventricular contraction systolic function can be detected. In a study 15% of myositis patients had abnormal radionuclide ventriculography, which was much less than abnormal ECG (in 85%) and abnormal echocardiography which was observed in 42% (Taylor et al., 1993). The abnormalities determined by radionuclide ventriculography were mild motion abnormalities with normal ejection fractions (Taylor et al., 1993). In another study technetium 99m-pyrophosphate scintigraphy and gallium-67 scintigraphy were compared in skeletal and cardiac muscle. A similar uptake of the two isotopes was observed in skeletal muscle but in the cardiac muscle the uptake of technetium 99m-pyrophosphate was much more common than cardiac gallium-67 uptake, observed in 57 and 15% of patients with poly- and dermatomyositis, respectively, suggesting that the technetium 99m-pyrophosphate scintigraphy is much more sensitive to cardiac changes than gallium-67 scintigraphy. The results were compared with electrocardiography, which was abnormal in 40% of the patients. No control group was included in any of the two reported studies which used technetium 99m-pyrophosphate to determine cardiac involvement which makes it difficult to draw conclusion from the results, and the clinical usefulness of this technique needs to be determined.

Gadolinium diethylenetriaminepentaacetic enhanced magnetic resonance imaging (Gd-DTPA-MRI) has been used to distinguish active myocardial inflammation from myocardial damage in humans with myocarditis with viral infections, sarcoidosis and in ischemic myocardial damage as well as in animal models (Friedrich et al., 1998; Ohata et al., 2002). Enhanced transmural contrast with Gd-DTPA-MRI was observed in the left ventricle of the heart of a patient with polymyositis and congestive heart failure in a recently published case report (Ohata et al., 2002). An endomyocardial biopsy from the left ventricle confirmed myocardial inflammation with inflammatory infiltrates and interstitial fibrosis. Gd-DTPA-MRI could be a helpful technique to detect myocardial inflammation but its sensitivity and specificity in patients with inflammatory myopathies needs to be determined.

5.2. Functional

Electrocardiography (ECG) is the basic method to detect arrhythmias, conduction defects and ST-T changes and should be included in the evaluation of all patients with inflammatory myopathies, as ECG changes are frequent and may demand treatment (Stern et al., 1984).

Echocardiography with different techniques have been used to detect myocardial and valvular lesions as well as left ventricular function and pericardial effusions. The frequency of echocardiographic abnormalities in patients with poly- and dermatomyositis varies between 14 and 62% (Gottdiener et al., 1978; Agrawal et al., 1989; Taylor et al., 1993; Gonzales-Lopez et al., 1996). The most frequently observed abnormalities were LVDD in 42% in one study, hyperdynamic heart in various frequencies (Gottdiener et al., 1978; Gonzales-Lopez et al., 1996) and mitral valve prolapse in 0–65% of the patients. As discussed above the large variations in frequency of cardiac abnormalities in myositis patients may be due to several factors such as patient selection and different techniques. A controlled study is needed to clarify the cardiac involvement in myositis patients.

Phonocardiography has rarely been used to determine cardiac involvement in patients with myositis. In one study 33% of the patients had single or multiple systolic clicks (Gottdiener et al., 1978). Phonocardiography does not seem to be a useful method to detect cardiac involvement in myositis patients.

Endomyocardial biopsies have been used in some cases to confirm myocardial inflammation in patients with poly- or dermatomyositis (Ohata et al., 2002; Riemekasten et al., 1999).

5.3. Biochemistry/serology/immunology

5.3.1. Biochemistry—serum enzymes

Creatine kinases (CK) are enzymes in muscle cells which may be released into the blood stream upon damage of myocytes. CK consists of three isoenzymes designated MM, MB and BB. Adult skeletal muscle contains mainly CK-MM, cardiac muscle CK-MB and smooth muscle CK-BB (Yazici and Kagen, 2002). During inflammation in skeletal muscle or when there is a damage of muscle fibres regeneration of muscle fibres takes place. In regenerating muscle fibres the subunit CK-B is upregulated, which may lead to increased release of CK-MB and CK-BB into the circulation. This often results in an increase in CK-MB/total CK ratio by more than 3%, which is a threshold that is commonly used to determine myocardial damage. In a longitudinal study including 13 myositis patients there was a significant correlation between the total CK and CKMB (Kiely et al., 2000). None of these cases had evidence of myocardial involvement. Thus these enzymes cannot be reliably used to detect myocardial damage in patients with inflammatory myopathies.

The cardiac isoforms of troponins are claimed to have the highest specificity of available serum markers for myocardial damage during (Erlacher et al., 2001). Troponins are part of the contractile system of skeletal and cardiac muscle, they are associated with the thin actin filaments and regulate its contractile response after calcium release (Messner et al., 2000). The troponin complex consists of three subunits: troponin C, troponin T and troponin I. Troponin T and I each exists in three isoforms; two different skeletal muscle isoforms (slow-twitch and fast-twitch) and one cardiac isoform, whereas troponin C has only two isoforms (Messner et al., 2000). Each isoform is regulated by a separate gene. The cardiac isoform troponin I (cTnI) has a high specificity for cardiac muscle and is the most reliable marker for the detection of myocardial damage (Messner et al., 2000). Although serum levels of cTnI were increased in occasional individuals with polymyositis without the evidence of myocardial involvement it was still regarded as a specific marker to distinguish between striated and myocardial damage (Kiely et al., 2000; Erlacher et al., 2001). In contrast the cardiac isoform troponin C (cTnC) is also expressed in adult skeletal muscle and increased serum levels of the cardiac isoform troponin T (cTnT) were demonstrated in patients with end-stage renal failure and in patients with Duchenne muscular dystrophy, polymyositis or dermatomyositis without clinical evidence of myocardial damage (Messner et al., 2000; Erlacher et al., 2001). Notably, messenger RNA expression of both cTnT and cTnI were detected in skeletal muscle biopsies from patients with Duchenne muscular dystrophy and some other myopathies (Messner et al., 2000). However, on protein level cardiac troponin I was not detected in human skeletal muscle during development or regenerative muscle disease process in patients with polymyositis or Duchenne muscle dystrophy (Bodor et al., 1995). The skeletal isoform of TnI (sTnI) correlated significantly with CK levels in patients with myositis without cardiac involvement (Kiely et al., 2000). Of the different isoforms of troponin only increased serum levels of cTn1 are useful to detect cardiac involvement in patients with inflammatory myopathies.

5.3.2. Serology/Immunology

Antinuclear antibodies (ANAs) were positive in 50–80% of patients with inflammatory myopathies (Targoff, 2002). Antibodies to extractable nuclear antigens were found in 28% in a study by Taylor et al. (1993). Another group of autoantibodies, the so-called myositis specific autoantibodies, MSAs, are associated with certain clinical phenotypes, which have been used to subclassify myositis patients (Love et al., 1991). The most frequently observed MSA is the anti-Jo-1 antibody, which can be detected in approximately 20% of the myositis patients. The anti-Jo-1 antibody is directed to histidyl tRNA-synthetases, and there are other so-called anti-synthetase autoantibodies which are specific for myositis, but with a low frequency. These anti-synthetase auto-antibodies are associated with characteristic clinical features including myositis, presence of interstitial lung disease (ILD), arthritis, Raynaud's phenomenon and skin changes on the hands so-called mechanic's hands, often referred to as the synthetase syndrome (Love et al., 1991). These autoantibodies are often associated with an unfavorable prognosis. The anti-Mi-2 autoantibodies are often associated with dermatomyositis with Gottron's papules and heliotrope rash (Targoff, 2002). A third set of MSAs, autoantibodies to signal recognition particle (SRP), was in some studies reported to be associated with cardiac involvement and a severe prognosis but this could not be confirmed in other studies (Targoff, 2002). Presence of anti-RNP antibodies in high titers is a hallmark of MCTD and is also included in the criteria of this disorder (Alarcón-Segovia and Cardiel, 1989). Anti-RNP antibodies are not specific to MCTD but may also be found in patients with polymyositis, dermatomyositis, SLE and Sjögren's syndrome but often in lower titers.

6. Differential diagnosis

Fatigue is a common symptom in patients with poly- or dermatomyositis. There could be several mechanisms that cause fatigue, one of them being cardiac involvement with congestive heart failure, another cause could be pulmonary hypertension. Lung involvement, which is a frequent manifestation in polymyositis and dermatomyositis, could also cause fatigue or dyspnea and has to be considered in these patients. The prevalence of lung involvement varies between 5 and 65% depending on patient selection and types of investigations used. One common lung manifestation in inflammatory myopathies is ILD an organ involvement which is a prognostic negative factor.

7. Treatment of cardiac manifestation

7.1. Myositis

The effects of corticosteroid treatment and other immunosuppressives, which constitute the basis for the treatment in polymyositis and dermatomyositis, on cardiac manifestations in patients with poly- or myositis are conflicting. In one study congestive heart failure improved during corticosteroid treatment in some individuals but progressed in others (Oka and Raasakka, 1978; Stern et al., 1984). In a longitudinal study conduction abnormalities progressed and new disturbances developed despite corticosteroid treatment and despite remission of the polymyositis (Stern et al., 1984). In the autopsy study by Denbow et al. (1979) the occurrence of myocarditis appeared to be independent of steroid therapy. There are several reports of development of cardiac involvement during follow up such as conduction abnormalities including complete heart block independent of signs of active disease in skeletal muscle activity (Reid and Mordoch, 1979; Kehoe et al., 1981). There are also a few studies to support a risk of development of cardiac involvement with congestive heart failure in treatment-resistant active polymyositis. In one case fatal congestive heart failure with myocardial fibrosis developed in a treatment-resistant active polymyositis (Anders et al., 1999).

Besides immunosuppressive therapy, patients with congestive heart failure have been treated with traditional heart medication. Vasospastic angina (Prinzmetal's angina) should be considered in patients with poly- and dermatomyositis in particular those who have Raynaud's phenomenon (Riemekasten et al., 1999). Vasospastic angina could be provoked by acetylcholine and successfully treated with high doses of calcium channel blockers (Riemekasten et al., 1999). There are a few reports of patients with atrioventricular block who have been treated with pacemaker, in some with successful outcome, but in others the outcome has still been fatal (Oka and Raasakka, 1978; Stern et al., 1984; Afzal et al., 1999). Recently there was a report of a successful heart transplant for dilated cardiomyopathy in a woman with polymyositis, with a 14-month postoperative observation period (Afzal et al., 1999).

7.1.1. Prognosis heart involvement

Cardiac involvement was the most important clinical factor associated with poor prognosis in a few studies (Hochberg et al., 1986; Oka and Raasakka, 1978). On the contrary, in another study patients with myocarditis had a significantly longer disease duration of polymyositis compared to those without myocarditis (Denbow et al., 1979). The correlation of cardiac manifestations in polymyositis with overall severity of the disease is also controversial. No correlation was observed between the presence of conduction abnormalities on ECG and disease activity (CK levels or skeletal muscle inflammation), disease severity (function) or corticosteroid dosages in one of the studies (Stern et al., 1984; Taylor et al., 1993; Gonzales-Lopez et al., 1996).

7.2. Treatment of cardiac manifestations in MCTD

Most of the clinical manifestations in patients with MCTD are benign and can be treated symptomatically or with corticosteroids and immunosuppressives over a limited period of time. Patients with pulmonary hypertension are usually refractory to immunosuppressive treatment and have a poor prognosis. There are a few reports of favorable pulmonary hemodynamic effects in patients with MCTD and pulmonary hypertension. In one such case a positive sustained effect was reported after treatment with nasal oxygen 2 l/min in combination with high doses of diltiazem, 300 mg/day (Shinohara et al., 1994). In another report of a young woman with a rapidly progressive pulmonary hypertension a positive effect was observed after treatment with high doses of corticosteroids, nitric oxide ventilation for 6 days and plasma exchange (Lahaye et al., 1999). There are also reports of favorable long-term effects after treatment with cyclophosphamide (Dahl et al., 1992; Hammann et al., 1999)

8. Summary

Clinically manifest heart problem is relatively uncommon in patients with poly- and dermatomyositis but cardiovascular manifestations constitute a major cause of death. This could indicate that significant cardiac involvement in patients with myositis is underestimated or that cardiac involvement is a late complication of the inflammatory muscle disease or a consequence of the treatment. The clinically manifest cardiac problems most frequently reported are congestive heart failure, conduction abnormalities that may lead to complete heart block and coronary artery disease. In contrast, subclinical manifestations are frequently reported and are predominated by conduction abnormalities and arrhythmias detected by ECG. Pericarditis, which is often recorded in other connective tissue diseases, is not a common cardiac manifestation in patients with myositis, neither subclinically nor clinically. Most of the available reports of cardiac involvement in patients with myositis lack control populations, which makes it difficult to draw conclusions from these reports but there is at least evidence to support a significantly increased frequency of bundle branch blocks in a study with controls. Whether cardiac manifestation is a significant clinical problem in patients with inclusion body myositis is unclear and needs to be determined. Furthermore, the limited data available so far does not allow to make a distinction as to whether there is a difference between polymyositis and dermatomyositis. There are several reports to support that not only adults but also children with juvenile dermatomyositis may develop cardiac involvement although the frequency seems to be low.

Both autopsy studies and case reports with myocardial biopsies suggest that the underlying pathophysiologic mechanisms which may cause cardiac manifestations could involve both the myocardium with myocarditis and the blood vessels, both the coronary arteries and the small vessels of the myocardium. The histopathology of the myocarditis resembles the inflammation in the skeletal muscle with inflammatory infiltrates localized to the endomysium and to the perivascular areas and with degeneration of cardiac myocytes. It is still uncertain whether the myocardial inflammation is part of poly- and dermatomyositis disease or develops as a consequence of the disease or its treatment. The histopathologic similarities with the skeletal muscle inflammation suggest that myocarditis is a part of the chronic poly- and dermatomyositis disease. However, the infiltrating cells have not been carefully phenotyped and there are no reports in which the inflammatory molecules such as cytokines or chemokines have been characterized in the heart tissue. Furthermore, subclinical or even clinically manifest cardiac involvement may be present at the time of diagnosis of poly- or dermatomyositis, but may also develop during immunosuppressive treatment and despite the remission of the skeletal muscle symptoms. This suggests that there are different mechanisms, which cause the myocardiac involvement and the weakness and fatigue of the skeletal muscle. To address the question of whether the cardiac involvement of myositis is a part of the myositis disease or a consequence of treatment and to gain more knowledge about the pathophysiologic mechanisms that could cause cardiac problems in patients with myositis a prospective study with the evaluation of cardiac involvement at disease onset and follow up during the course of the disease in a controlled fashion would be needed. As the inflammatory myopathies are rare disorders such an approach would have to be done in an international multi-center study to enroll an adequate number of patients to be able to get answers to these important questions.

Key points

- Based on the knowledge that there is a risk to develop cardiac involvement an ECG and an echocardiography should be included in the diagnostic evaluation of patients with inflammatory myopathies.
- During follow up it should be kept in mind that significant myocardial involvement such as congestive heart failure and conduction abnormalities may develop during immunosuppressive therapy and despite remission of the skeletal muscle symptoms.
- Determination of serum levels of most cardiac enzymes are usually not helpful to identify cardiac involvement in patients with inflammatory myopathies as these enzymes could also be produced in the inflamed skeletal.
- The cardiac enzyme with the highest specificity to detect cardiac muscle damage is cardiac troponin I but the sensitivity to detect significant cardiac involvement in patients with myositis is not known.
- Long-term follow-up multi-center studies with well-defined patients with inflammatory myopathies and control individuals are needed to achieve information about the frequency and prognosis of clinically significant cardiac involvement in these patients.
- In patients with MCTD pulmonary hypertension is not uncommon. Treatment with calcium blockers and/or immunosuppressives could be beneficial although most patients with MCTD and pulmonary hypertension are refractory to the therapy that is available today.

References

Adams, E.M., Kirkley, J., Eidelman, G., et al. 1997. The predominance of beta (cc) chemokine transcripts in idiopathic inflammatory muscle diseases. Proc. Assoc. Am. Phys. 109, 275.

Afzal, A., Higgins, R.S.D., Philbin, E.F. 1999. Heart transplant for dilated cardiomyopathy associated with polymyositis. Heart 82, e4.

This is the first report of successful heart transplant in a patient with polymyositis.

Agrawal, C.S., Behari, M., Shrivastava, S., et al. 1989. The heart in polymyositis–dermatomyositis. J. Neurol. 236, 249.

Ahlstrom, G., Gunnarsson, L.G., Leissner, P., et al. 1993. Epidemiology of neuromuscular diseases, including the post-polio sequelae, in a Swedish county. Neuroepidemiology 12, 262.

Alarcón-Segovia, D., Cardiel, M.H. 1989. Comparison between three diagnostic criteria for mixed connective tissue disease. Study of 593 patients. J. Rheumatol. 16, 328.

Alpert, M.A., Goldberg, S.H., Singsen, B.H., et al. 1983. Cardiovascular manifestations of mixed connective tissue disease in adults. Circulation 68, 1182.

This is a carefully conducted study of cardiovascular manifestations in a relatively large number of patients with MCTD.

Anders, H.-J., Wanders, A., Rihl, M., et al. 1999. Myocardial fibrosis in polymyositis. J. Rheumatol. 26, 1840.

Arahata, K., Engel, A.G. 1984. Monoclonal antibody analysis of mononuclear cells in myopathies. I. Quantitation of subsets according to diagnosis and sites of accumulation and demonstration and counts of muscle fibers invaded by T-cells. Ann. Neurol. 16, 193.

Badrising, U.A., Maat-Schieman, M., van Duinen, S.G., et al. 2000. Epidemiology of inclusion body myositis in the Netherlands: a nationwide study. Neurology 55, 1385.

Benbassat, J., Geffel, D., Zlotnick, A. 1980. Epidemiology of polymyositis–dermatomyositis in Israel, 1960–76. Isr. J. Med. Sci. 16, 197.

de Bleecker, J.L., Meire, V.I., Declercq, W., et al. 1999. Immunolocalization of tumor necrosis factor-alpha and its receptors in inflammatory myopathies. Neuromuscul Disord. 9, 239.

Bodor, G.S., Porterfield, D., Voss, E.M., et al. 1995. Cardiac troponin-I is not expressed in fetal healthy or diseased adult human skeletal muscle tissue. Clin. Chem. 41, 1710.

Bohan, A., Peter, J.B. 1975a. Polymyositis and dermatomyositis (first of two parts). N. Engl. J. Med. 292, 344.

Bohan, A., Peter, J.B. 1975b. Polymyositis and dermatomyositis (second of two parts). N. Engl. J. Med. 292, 403.

Bohan, A., Peter, J.B., Bowman, R.L., et al. 1977. Computer-assisted analysis of 153 patients with polymyositis and dermatomyositis. Medicine (Baltimore) 56, 255.

Bryant, D., Becker, L., Richardson, J., et al. 1998. Cardiac failure in transgenic mice with myocardial expression of tumor necrosis factor-alpha. Circulation 97, 1375.

Buchpiguel, C.A., Roizemblatt, S., Pastor, E.H., et al. 1996. Cardiac and skeletal muscle scintigraphy in dermato- and polymyositis: clinical implementations. Eur. J. Nucl. Med. 23, 199.

Dahl, M., Chalmers, A., Wade, J., et al. 1992. Ten year survival of a patient with advanced pulmonary hypertension and mixed connective tissue disease treated with immunnosuppressive therapy. J. Rheumatol. 19, 1807.

Dalakas, M.C. 1991. Polymyositis, dermatomyositis and inclusion-body myositis. N. Engl. J. Med. 325, 1487.

Denbow, C.E., Lie, J.T., Tancredi, R.G., et al. 1979. Cardiac involvement in polymyositis. Arthritis Rheum. 22, 1088.

DeWere, R., Bradley, W.G. 1975. Polymyositis: its presentation, morbidity and mortality. Brain 98, 637.

Engel, A.G., Arahata, K. 1986. Mononuclear cells in myopathies: quantitation of functionally distinct subsets, recognition of antigen-specific cell-mediated cytotoxicity in some diseases, and implications for the pathogenesis of the different inflammatory myopathies. Hum. Pathol. 17, 704.

Englund, P., Nennesmo, I., Klareskog, L., et al. 2002. Interleukin-1α expression in capillaries and major histocompatibility complex class I expression in type II muscle fibers from polymyosit and dermatomyositis patients. Arthritis Rheum. 46, 1044.

Erlacher, P., Lercher, A., Falkensammer, J., et al. 2001. Cardiac troponin and β-type myosin heavy chain concentrations in patients with polymyositis or dermatomyositis. Clin. Chim. Acta 306, 27.

Friedrich, M.G., Strohm, O., Schulz-Menger, J., et al. 1998. Contrast media-enhanced magnetic resonance imaging visualize myocardial changes in the course of viral myocarditis. Circulation 97, 1802.

Gonzales-Lopez, L., Gamez-Nava, J.I., Sanchez, L., et al. 1996. Cardiac manifestations in dermato-polymyositis. Clin. Exp. Rheumatol. 14, 373.

Gottdiener, J.S., Sherber, H.S., Hawley, R.J., et al. 1978. Cardiac manifestations in polymyositis. Am. J. Cardiol. 41, 1141.

Griggs, R.C., Askanas, V., DiMauro, S., et al. 1995. Inclusion body myositis and myopathies. Ann. Neurol. 38, 705.

Hammann, C., Genton, C.Y., Delabays, A., et al. 1999. Myocarditis of mixed connective tissue disease; favourable outcome after intravenous pulsed cyclophosphamide. Clin. Rheumatol. 18, 85.

Haupt, H.M., Hutchins, G.M. 1982. The heart and cardiac conduction system in polymyositis–dermatomyositis: a clinicopathologic study of 16 autopsied patients. Am. J. Cardiol. 50, 998.

Hengstman, G.J., van Venrooij, W.J., Vencovsky, J., et al. 2000. The relative prevalence of dermatomyositis and polymyositis in Europe exhibits a latitudinal gradient. Ann. Rheum. Dis. 59, 141.

Henriksson, K.G., Sandstedt, P. 1982. Polymyositis—treatment and prognosis. A study of 107 patients. Acta Neurol. Scand. 65, 280.

Hill, D.L., Barrows, H.S. 1968. Identical skeletal and cardiac muscle involvement in a case of fatal polymyositis. Arch. Neurol. 19, 545.

Hochberg, M.C., Feldman, D., Stevens, M.B. 1986. Adult onset polymyositis/dermatomyositis: an analysis of clinical and laboratory features and survival in 76 patients with a review of the literature. Sem. Arthritis Rheum. 15, 168.

Kehoe, R., Bauernfeind, R., Tommasco, C., et al. 1981. Cardiac conduction defects in polymyositis. Ann. Intern. Med. 94, 41.

Kiely, P.D., Bruckner, F.E., Nisbet, J.A., et al. 2000. Serum skeletal troponin I in inflammatory muscle disease: relation to creatine kinase, CKMB and cardiac troponin I. Ann. Rheum. Dis. 59, 750.

Lahaye, I.E., Rogiers, P.E., Nagler, J.M., et al. 1999. Vanishing pulmonary hypertension in mixed connective tissue disease. Clin. Rheumatol. 18, 45.

Lightfoot, P.R., Bharati, S., Lev, M. 1977. Chronic dermatomyositis with intermittent trifascicular block. Chest 71, 3.

Lindberg, C., Persson, L.I., Bjorkander, J., et al. 1994. Inclusion body myositis: clinical, morphological, physiological and laboratory findings in 18 cases. Acta Neurol. Scand. 89, 121.

Lotz, B.P., Engel, A.G., Nishino, H., et al. 1989. Inclusion body myositis. Observations in 40 patients. Brain 112, 727.

Love, L.A., Leff, R.L., Fraser, D.D., et al. 1991. A new approach to the classification of idiopathic inflammatory myopathy: myositis-specific autoantibodies define useful homogeneous patient groups. Medicine (Baltimore) 70, 360.

Lundberg, I., Hedfors, E. 1991. Clinical course of patients with anti-RNP antibodies. A prospective study of 32 patients. J. Rheumatol. 18, 1511.

Lundberg, I., Ulfgren, A.K., Nyberg, P., et al. 1997. Cytokine production in muscle tissue of patients with idiopathic inflammatory myopathies. Arthritis Rheum. 40, 865.

Lynch, P.G. 1971. Cardiac involvement in chronic polymyositis. Br. Heart J. 33, 416.

Medsger, T.A. Jr., Dawson, W.N. Jr., Masi, A.T. 1970. The epidemiology of polymyositis. Am. J. Med. 48, 715.

Messner, N., Baum, H., Fischer, P., et al. 2000. Expression of messenger RNA of the cardiac isoforms of troponin and T and I in myopathic skeletal muscle. Am. J. Clin. Pathol. 114, 544.

Mhiri, C., Gherardi, R. 1990. Inclusion body myositis in French patients. A clinicopathological evaluation. Neuropathol. Appl. Neurobiol. 16, 333.

Negoro, N., Kanayama, Y., Yasadu, M., et al. 1987. Nuclear ribonucleoprotein immune complexes in pericardial fluid of a patient with mixed connective tissue disease. Arthritis Rheum. 30, 97.

Nyberg, P., Wikman, A.L., Nennesmo, I., et al. 2000. Increased expression of interleukin 1alpha and mhc class i in muscle tissue of patients with chronic, inactive polymyositis and dermatomyositis. J. Rheumatol. 27, 940.

Oddis, C.V., Conte, C.G., Steen, V.D., et al. 1990. Incidence of polymyositis–dermatomyositis: a 20-year study of hospital diagnosed cases in Allegheny County, PA 1963–1982. J. Rheumatol. 17, 1329.

Ohata, S., Shimada, T., Shimizu, H., et al. 2002. Myocarditis associated with polymyositis diagnosed by gadolinium-DTPA enhanced magnetic resonance imaging. J. Rheumatol. 29, 861.

Oka, M., Raasakka, T. 1978. Cardiac involvement in polymyositis. Scand. J. Rheumatol. 7, 203.

Oppenheim, H. 1899. Zur Dermatomyositis. Berl. Klin. Wochenschrift 36, 805.

Pachman, L.M., Liotta-Davis, M.R., Hong, D.K., et al. 2000. TNFalpha-308A allele in juvenile dermatomyositis: association with increased production of tumor necrosis factor alpha, disease duration, and pathologic calcifications. Arthritis Rheum. 43, 2368.

Patrick, M., Buchbinder, R., Jolley, D., et al. 1999. Incidence of inflammatory myopathies in Victoria, Australia, and evidence of spatial clustering. J. Rheumatol. 26, 1094.

Plotz, P.H., Rider, L.G., Targoff, I.N., et al. 1995. Myositis immunologic contributions to understanding cause, pathogenesis and therapy. Ann. Intern. Med. 122, 715.

Ramanan, A.V., Feldman, B.M. 2002. Clinical outcome in juvenile dermetomyositis. Curr. Opin. Rheum. 14, 658.
This is a recent update on clinical manifestations and out-come in patients with juvenile dermatomyositis.

Reid, J., Mordoch, R. 1979. Polymyositis and complete heart block. Br. Heart J. 41, 628.

Riemekasten, G., Opitz, C., Audring, H., et al. 1999. Beware of the heart, the multiple picture of cardiac involvement in myositis. Rheumatology 38, 1153.

Schwarz, M.I. 1992. Pulmonary and cardiac manifestations of polymyositis–dermatomyositis. J. Thorac. Imag. 7, 46.

Shamim, E.A., Rider, L.G., Miller, F.W. 2000. Update on the genetics of the idiopathic inflammatory myopathies. Curr. Opin. Rheumatol. 12, 482.

Sharp, G.S., Irvin, W.S., Tan, E.M., et al. 1972. Mixed connective tissue disease. An apparently distinct rheumatic disease syndrome with a specific antibody to extractable nuclear antigen. Am. J. Med. 52, 148.

Shimuzu, T., Tomita, Y., Son, K., et al. 2000. Elevation of serum soluble tumour necrosis factor receptors in patients with polymyositis and dermatomyositis. Clin. Rheum. 19, 352.

Shinohara, S., Murata, I., Yamada, H., et al. 1994. Combined effects of diltiazem and oxygen in pulmonary hypertension of mixed connective tissue disease. J. Rheumatol. 21, 1763.

Sigush, H.H., Lehmann, M.H., Schnittler, U., et al. 2000. Tumor necrosis factor—a expression in idiopathic dilated cardiomatyopathy: correlation to myocardial inflammatory activity. Cytokine 12, 1261.

Stern, R., Godbold, J.H., Chess, Q., et al. 1984. ECG abnormalities in polymyositis. Arch. Intern. Med. 144, 2185.
This is thoroughly performed study of electrocardiographic manifestations of a large group of patients with polymyositis and dermatomyositis.

Targoff, I.N. 2002. Laboratory testing in the diagnosis and management of idiopathic inflammatory myopathies. Rheum. Dis. Clin. North Am. 28, 859.
This is a very comprehensive and recent update on autoantibodies and relation to clinical manifestations in patients with inflammatory myopathies.

Targoff, I.N., Miller, F.W., Medsger, T.A. Jr., et al. 1997. Classification criteria for the idiopathic inflammatory myopathies. Curr. Opin. Rheumatol. 9, 527.

Taylor, A.J., Wortham, D.C., Burge, J.R., et al. 1993. The heart in polymyositis: a prospective evaluation of 26 patients. Clin. Cardiol. 16, 802.

Weitoft, T. 1997. Occurrence of polymyositis in the county of Gavleborg, Sweden. Scand. J. Rheumatol. 26, 104.

Whitlow, P.L., Gilliam, J.N., Chubick, A., et al. 1980. Myocarditis in mixed connective tissue disease. Arthritis Rheum. 23, 7808.

Yale, S.H., Adlakha, A., Stanton, S.M. 1993. Dermatomyositis with pericardial tamponade and polymyositis with pericardial effusion. Am. Heart J. 126, 997.

Yunis, E.J., Samaha, F.J. 1971. Inclusion body myositis. Lab. Invest. 25, 240.

Yazici, Y., Kagen, L.J. 2002. Cardiac involvement in myositis. Curr. Opin. Rheumatol. 14, 663.

Handbook of Systemic Autoimmune Diseases, Volume 1
The Heart in Systemic Autoimmune Diseases
A. Doria and P. Pauletto, editors

CHAPTER 14

Cardiac Involvement in the Antiphospholipid Syndrome

Doruk Erkan*[,a], Mary J. Roman[b], Felicia Tenedios[a], Michael D. Lockshin[a]

[a]*Department of Rheumatology, Hospital for Special Surgery, Weill Medical College of Cornell University, 535 East 70th Street, New York, NY 10021, USA*

[b]*Division of Cardiology, Weill Medical College of Cornell University, New York, NY, USA*

1. Introduction

The antiphospholipid syndrome (APS) is characterized by thrombosis (either arterial or venous) and/or pregnancy morbidity in the presence of circulating antiphospholipid antibodies (aPL), most commonly anticardiolipin antibodies (aCL) or positive lupus-anticoagulant test (LAC) (Table 1) (Wilson et al., 1999). The prevalence of aPL is 2–5% in the general population and increases with age. Several large-scale studies report the prevalence of LAC and aCL in systemic lupus erythematosus (SLE) patients between 15–34 and 12–30%, respectively (Petri, 2000a). In the absence of an underlying connective tissue disorder (CTD), this syndrome is the 'primary' APS, whereas 'secondary' APS occurs in patients with other CTDs, most often SLE.

The presence of aPL in the absence of symptoms does not indicate APS; asymptomatic aPL-positive patients exist. These asymptomatic patients are generally identified as part of an autoimmune disease serologic evaluation, most commonly SLE, or during evaluation for an elevated activated partial thromboplastin time, e.g. during presurgical screening. A subgroup of APS patients is diagnosed solely after pregnancy morbidity without vascular events. APS-related vascular events can range from superficial thrombosis to life-threatening multiple organ system thromboses developing over a short period (catastrophic APS). Thus, APS represents a spectrum; patients should not be evaluated and managed as a single disease entity (Table 2).

APS can result in both venous and arterial non-inflammatory thromboses anywhere within the vascular tree. APS patients may present with deep venous thrombosis, pulmonary embolism, transient ischemic attack, stroke, occlusive ocular disease, mesenteric ischemia, renal artery and vein thrombosis, superficial arterial thrombosis, or coronary artery disease (angina, myocardial infarction, or sudden death).

Cardiac manifestations of the APS range from asymptomatic valvular lesions to life-threatening myocardial infarction (Table 3) (Levine et al., 2002), although the association of some of these manifestations with aPL is still under debate. The most commonly reported cardiac manifestation of aPL is heart valve abnormalities; thickening of the valve leaflets is the most common (Cervera, 2000). These manifestations can occur in asymptomatic (no history of vascular or pregnancy events) aPL-positive patients as well as in primary and secondary APS patients.

Despite numerous prevalence studies on the cardiac manifestations of aPL (impeded by variable definitions of positive aPL), the pathogenesis and

* Corresponding author.
E-mail address: derkan@pol.net (D. Erkan).

DOI: 10.1016/S1571-5078(03)01014-6

Table 1
Summary of the Sapporo Classification Criteria for the APS (Wilson et al., 1999)

Clinical criteria
Vascular thrombosis
Arterial, venous, or small vessel thrombosis, in any organ or tissue
Pregnancy morbidity
One or more unexplained deaths of morphologically normal fetus at or beyond the 10th week of gestation or
One or more premature births of a morphologically normal neonate at or before the 34th week of gestation because of severe preeclampsia or eclampsia, or severe placental insufficiency or
Three or more unexplained consecutive spontaneous abortions before the 10th week of gestation
Laboratory criteria
aCL of IgG and/or IgM isotype in blood, present in medium or high titer, on two or more occasions, at least 6 weeks apart and/or
Lupus anticoagulant present in the plasma on two or more occasions at least 6 weeks apart

Definite APS is considered to be present if at least one of the clinical and one of the laboratory criteria are met.

the optimal management are unknown. This chapter will discuss each of the aPL-related cardiac manifestations (Table 3) in the following order: prevalence; pathogenesis; clinical presentation; diagnostic investigations and differential diagnosis; and treatment.

Table 2
The spectrum of APS

Asymptomatic aPL-positive patients
Medium-to-high titer IgG/M aCL and/or positive LAC test
Low titer aCL or isolated IgA aCL
APS patients with only pregnancy morbidity
Patients who fulfill the Sapporo Criteria
Patients who do not fulfill the Sapporo criteria (i.e. single early pregnancy loss with positive aPL)
APS patients with vascular thrombosis with or without pregnancy morbidity
Patients with venous events
Patients with arterial events
Patients with catastrophic APS

aPL: antiphospholipid antibodies; aCL: anticardiolipin antibodies; LAC: lupus-anticoagulant.

Table 3
Cardiac manifestations of the APS

Valve abnormalities
Vegetations
Valve thickening
Valvular dysfunction
Thrombotic and atherosclerotic coronary occlusion
Ventricular hypertrophy and dysfunction
Intracardiac thrombus

2. Prevalence

2.1. Valve abnormalities

Heart valve abnormalities (vegetations and/or thickening) are the most commonly reported cardiac manifestation of aPL. Hojnik et al. (1996) reviewed echocardiographic studies of primary APS patients; the four largest transthoracic echocardiography (TTE) studies (totaling 168 primary APS patients) reported a 32–38% prevalence of valve lesions compared to 0–5% among control subjects. Valvular lesions most frequently involved left-sided valves, with the mitral valve more commonly affected than the aortic valve. Using transesophageal echocardiography (TEE), which is generally more sensitive for detection of valvular lesions than TTE, Turiel et al. (2000) demonstrated valve abnormalities in 33/40 (82%) of primary APS patients. This study also suggested that aCL titer >40 GPL is a risk factor for thromboembolic events; embolic events were identified in 25% of patients. Mitral valve thickening was the most common abnormality (63%), which was associated with aortic valve thickening in 32% and tricuspid valve thickening in 8%. Mitral valve thickening also correlated with aCL titer. Another TEE study found valvular abnormalities in 22 of 29 primary APS patients (76%) (Espinola-Zavaleta et al., 1999).

Echocardiographic studies disagree as to whether patients with SLE are more or less likely than primary APS patients to have valve disease and whether SLE patients with and without aPL differ in prevalences of valvular disease. Nesher et al. (1997) demonstrated in a meta-analysis of 13 studies that 48% of aPL-positive SLE patients had valve lesions compared with 21% of aPL-negative SLE patients. Valvular lesions were found in 36% of primary APS patients. These abnormalities included valve thickening, vegetation, regurgitation, and stenosis. Nihoyannopoulos et al. (1990) demonstrated that 50% of SLE patients with very high-titer aCL (defined as aCL >100 ELISA units) have valvular disease compared to 37% of SLE patients with high-titer aCL (defined as aCL 9-100 ELISA units) and 14% of SLE patients without aPL. In a series of 132 SLE patients Khamashta et al. (1990) reported that among aPL-positive SLE patients, 16% had valvular vegetations and 38% had mitral regurgitation (vs. 1.2 and 12%, respectively, of aPL-negative SLE patients). In contrast, Roldan et al. (1992) found comparable prevalences of valvular abnormalities in SLE patients with (77%) and without (72%) aPL.

Clinically significant valvulopathy appears to be uncommon in aPL-positive patients. Significant valvular disease leading to congestive heart failure occurred in 5% of primary APS and SLE patients in a meta-analysis (Nesher et al., 1997). Galve et al. (1988) demonstrated that SLE patients with hemodynamically significant valvular disease were significantly older and had longer disease duration compared to SLE patients with valvular lesions and minimal or no regurgitation.

Of 39 primary APS patients followed for 10 years at the Hospital for Special Surgery, 13% eventually required cardiac valve replacement and 5% were permanently incapacitated because of cardiac disease. Nine of the 22 (41%) patients with available echocardiograms, primarily TTEs, had valve thickening and/or vegetations; the mitral valve was affected in 4 patients (one had mild regurgitation), the aortic valve was involved in 2 patients (one had mild and one had moderate regurgitation), and both valves were involved in 3 patients (all three had mild aortic regurgitation, one had mild mitral regurgitation, one had moderate mitral regurgitation, and one had mild mitral stenosis) (Erkan et al., 2000).

In summary, valvular abnormalities occur with increased frequency in primary APS. The presence of aPL in SLE may increase the likelihood of valvular abnormalities, particularly in the setting of high antibody titers. Despite the high prevalence of echocardiographic (and autopsy) evidence of valvular involvement, clinically important valvular heart disease is uncommon. Differences in the existing literature with regard to these issues likely relate to small sample sizes, methodologic differences (definitions of valvular disease, TTE vs. TEE, inclusion of control population), and selection bias (method of ascertainment, referral center).

2.2. Thrombotic/atherosclerotic coronary occlusion

Both preclinical (carotid plaque) and clinical (myocardial infarction) atherosclerotic disease are more prevalent in SLE patients than in the general population (Manzi et al., 1999; Lockshin et al., 2001a; Petri, 2000b; Roman et al., 2001). However, whether primary APS or the presence of aCL in SLE predisposes to atherosclerosis is uncertain.

The prevalence of myocardial infarction in primary APS patients is relatively low. Asherson et al. (1989) reported 70 primary APS patients in whom 5 had myocardial infarction and Font et al. (1991) found a history of myocardial infarction in 1 of 23 primary APS patients. Our recent cross-sectional analysis of 77 primary and secondary APS patients yielded only 1 patient with a history of myocardial infarction (Erkan et al., 2002a). In the Hopkins Lupus Cohort study, the incidence of myocardial infarction was 3.3% in the aPL-positive and 5.9% in aPL-negative SLE patients ($p = 0.06$), and the presence of carotid plaque by ultrasonography was equally prevalent in the two groups (Lockshin et al., 2003). Although the incidence of myocardial infarction in SLE patients aged 35–44 years old was estimated to be 50-fold greater in the Pittsburgh Lupus Registry than in historical age-matched controls, data regarding the relation of aCL to myocardial infarction in this population are not available (Manzi et al., 1997).

Among 42 patients with aPL in the absence of SLE, Ames et al. (2002) found that IgG aCL titer related independently to carotid intimal-medial thickness (IMT), which may be a measure of diffuse atherosclerosis; although plaque, an unequivocal manifestation of atherosclerosis, was measured in this study, no mention is made of its relation to aPL.

The prevalence of aCL in patients presenting with myocardial infarction is between 5 and 15% (Cuadrado and Hughes, 2001) and increases to 21% before the age of 45 (Hamsten et al., 1986); however, the association is controversial. Hamsten et al. (1986) and Bili et al. (2000) found aCL to be an independent risk factor for recurrent cardiac events, among survivors of myocardial infarction. In contrast, Sletnes et al. (1992) found no association between aCL and myocardial infarction and reported that aCL was not a risk factor for mortality or recurrent myocardial infarction in patients who survived acute myocardial infarction. Likewise De Caterina et al. (1990) did not detect differences in aCL levels between unselected patients with angiographic evidence of coronary artery disease and healthy controls. Thus routine aPL screening for myocardial infarction patients is not recommended, however, testing should be considered in young patients with coronary artery disease or myocardial infarction in the absence of other obvious atherosclerosis risk factors.

2.3. *Ventricular hypertrophy and dysfunction*

Left ventricular hypertrophy and systolic and/or diastolic dysfunction may occur in association with hypertension, valvular heart disease, atherosclerotic coronary artery disease, myocarditis, and SLE, especially with active disease (Roman et al., 2001). Very limited data regarding these ventricular abnormalities and no data regarding the prevalence of left ventricular hypertrophy (not attributable to hemodynamically significant valvular disease) are available in APS. The prevalence of systolic and diastolic dysfunction has only been examined in very small studies. In a prospective study of 18 primary APS patients without clinically evident cardiac disease, Courday et al. (1995) showed prolonged iso-volumetic relaxation time, abnormal left ventricular early filling pattern, and decreased myocardial-lengthening rate compared to age- and sex-matched healthy controls. Comparing 10 primary APS patients with age- and sex-matched healthy controls, Hasnie et al. (1995) showed an association between primary APS and impaired diastolic filling as evidenced by decreased peak early filling velocity (52 ± 10 cm/s in primary APS patients vs. 67 ± 12 cm/s in normal controls, $p < 0.01$). Leung et al. (1990) demonstrated an association between isolated myocardial dysfunction (global or segmental) and aPL ($p < 0.05$) in SLE patients. In this study, 4 of 5 SLE patients with isolated left ventricular dysfunction (two patients had congestive heart failure and two were asymptomatic) had positive aPL. Thus, given the very small number of patients studied, the extent to which aPL independently impacts left ventricular size and function in the absence of other confounding processes and whether such an impact is of clinical relevance remains uncertain.

2.4. *Intracardiac thrombi*

Several case reports have documented intracardiac thrombus formation in patients with primary APS, usually identified in the evaluation of source of embolus (Erkan et al., 2002b). Thrombus may be difficult to differentiate from intracardiac tumors such as myxoma, although magnetic resonance imaging (MRI) may be useful in making the distinction (vide infra).

3. Pathogenesis

The pathogenic mechanisms of APS-related thrombosis and thus aPL-related cardiac manifestations are poorly understood. Whether aPL promotes thrombosis by affecting endothelial cells, platelets, or the coagulation system is not yet clear. Multiple mechanisms and risk factors for thrombosis are likely to exist. Proposed mechanisms regarding endothelial cells include: endothelial cell damage or activation by aPL; coexisting anti-endothelial antibodies contributing to thrombosis; and aPL-induced increased monocyte adhesion to endothelial cells. Alternatively, activation of platelets followed by the binding of aPL to platelet membrane phospholipid-bound proteins may initiate platelet adhesion and thrombosis. The possibility of an interaction between the coagulation cascade and aPL has been investigated intensively. These antibodies may inhibit certain reactions in the coagulation cascade catalyzed by phospholipids such as inhibition of the activation of the protein C and protein S systems. Furthermore, there are studies indicating that complement activation may be necessary for the induction of clinical complications caused by aPL (Lockshin, 2001b).

3.1. Valve abnormalities

aPL may stimulate thrombin formation on endothelium. Deposits of immunoglobulins (consisting of aCL) and complement (but not serum albumin) are found in the subendothelial connective tissue of the deformed valves of APS patients. The aCL isotype is mainly IgG, which appears as a continuous ribbon-like layer along the surface of the leaflets and cusps. Complement (C1q, C3c, C4) deposits are similar in form and location, but are more granular, suggesting immune complexes. Control valves from aPL-negative patients and control tissue specimens from an APS patient do not demonstrate such staining (Ziporen et al., 1996). Histopathology of the valves demonstrates superficial or intravalvular fibrin deposits and subsequent re-organization: vascular proliferation, fibroblast influx, fibrosis and calcification. This results in valve thickening, fusion and rigidity causing disrupted function.

Inflammation may be present but is not a prominent feature of this valvular lesion (Garcia-Torres et al., 1996; Espinola-Zavaleta et al., 1999). Amital et al. (1999) suggested that the deposition of aPL in heart valves initiates an inflammatory process. Support for this hypothesis came from Afek et al. (1999) who demonstrated that markers of endothelial cell activation are up-regulated in valves of APS patients.

In summary, immunoglobulin and complement deposition can be demonstrated in heart valves, however, it is unclear whether antibody deposition results in valvular lesions or preexisting valve lesions stimulate antibody deposition.

3.2. Thrombotic/atherosclerotic coronary occlusion

aPL may contribute to atherosclerosis via cross-reactivity with oxidized low-density lipoproteins (LDL), endothelial cell activation, and other means. The possible role of infection in inducing both APS and atherosclerosis is an exciting research area, the treatment implications of which are not yet known. Furthermore, medications (such as corticosteroids) used to treat aPL associated CTDs and other related comorbid conditions (such as hypertension or hyperlipidemia) may contribute to the development of atherosclerotic coronary disease.

Antioxidized-LDL is found to be a marker of atherosclerosis (Witztum, 1994) and predictive of myocardial infarction in the general population (Puurunen et al., 1994). Plasma fibrinogen and homocysteine (Ames et al., 2002) are also independent predictors of increased carotid IMT, a potential indirect measure of atherosclerosis. High plasma homocysteine is a known risk factor for thrombosis independent of aPL (Lee and Frenkel, 2003), and elevated plasma homocysteine may be implicated in the thrombotic tendency of primary APS.

In addition to epicardial coronary artery occlusions, myocardial infarction can occur in APS patients with normal coronary arteries, possibly due to microvascular thrombosis (Lagana et al., 2001).

3.3. Ventricular hypertrophy and dysfunction

The pathogenesis of ventricular hypertrophy and dysfunction (in the absence of valvular or coronary artery disease) is unclear and may not be independently related to the presence of aPL. Myocardial thrombotic microangiopathy (thrombosis of myocardial microcirculation) has been demonstrated in both catastrophic APS and in primary APS patients who presented with myocardial infarction and normal angiography (Asherson et al., 1998; Kattwinkel et al., 1992). It may be speculated that microvascular thrombosis can also result in myocardial hypertrophy and dysfunction (Leung et al., 1990). In addition, chronic pulmonary embolism can also result in right ventricular failure.

3.4. Intracardiac thrombi

Thrombosis on the endocardial surface results in intracardiac thrombus formation, however, as discussed above, the mechanism is unclear.

4. Clinical manifestations

4.1. Valve abnormalities

Valve abnormalities in patients with APS are similar to those of SLE: thickening of leaflets, and irregular nodular excrescences on the closure lines or undersurfaces of the mitral and aortic valves. They can vary from minimal thickening to severe valve distortion and dysfunction requiring surgical replacement (Ziporen et al., 1996). These lesions generally have minor hemodynamic significance and are clinically silent. However, in some patients they can produce regurgitation, more frequently associated with valvular thickening. Mitral regurgitation is the most common aPL-associated hemodynamic abnormality (Cervera, 2000; Espinola-Zavaleta et al., 1999). Involvement of the tricuspid or pulmonary valve is rare. Severe valvular regurgitation can result in congestive heart failure symptoms such as fatigue, dyspnea, or orthopnea.

Arterial thromboembolism is more common in patients with than without valve disease. Stroke, transient ischemic attack, or amaurosis fugax may be caused by emboli. Several studies have also reported a strong association between valve lesions and brain infarcts (Cervera et al., 1991; Galve et al., 1992; Garcia-Torres et al., 1996).

4.2. Thrombotic/atherosclerotic coronary occlusion

Patients can present with a wide spectrum of clinical problems ranging from asymptomatic atherosclerotic lesions to sudden death. Acute thrombosis can result in myocardial infarction with or without left ventricular dysfunction, valvular regurgitation, or congestive heart failure. Chest pain is the major presentation of coronary artery occlusion, and the left anterior descending artery is commonly involved in primary APS patients (Espinosa et al., 2002).

4.3. Ventricular hypertrophy and dysfunction

In the absence of systolic or diastolic dysfunction, left ventricular hypertrophy is usually asymptomatic. Both systolic and diastolic dysfunction may cause exertional dyspnea and other signs of congestive heart failure.

4.4. Intracardiac thrombi

Thrombi may occur in any of the four chambers of the heart. Patients can present with fever, chest pain, murmur, or embolic phenomena. It has been reported that patients with aCL titer >40 GPL may be at a 2-fold increased risk of occurrence of further thromboembolic events and death (Levine et al., 1997).

5. Diagnostic investigations and differential diagnosis

5.1. Valve abnormalities

Doppler echocardiography is the most important diagnostic tool in the detection of cardiac valve abnormalities. Valvular vegetations and thickening are the two important morphological patterns. Libman–Sacks lesions in aPL-negative SLE patients and vegetations in APS are similar with respect to localization and echocardiographic appearance of lesions (Brenner et al., 1991).

Fourteen percent of patients with infective endocarditis may have aPL (Kupferwasser et al., 1999). However, SLE patients may also present with pseudoinfective endocarditis (fever, cardiac murmurs, vegetations, splinter hemorrhages, increased SLE activity, and negative blood cultures), which can be very difficult to differentiate from infective endocarditis. High white blood cell count, high C-reactive protein, and low titers of aPL should point toward the diagnosis of infective endocarditis.

Rheumatic heart disease (RHD)-related valvular diseases should also be considered in the differential diagnosis. In aPL lesions, valve thickening is generally diffuse and if localized thickening is present, it involves the mid-portion or base of the leaflet. Chordae tendinae involvement is rare. In RHD patients, the mitral valve leaflet tips are thickened with subvalvular (chordal) involvement developing over time. Both aortic and mitral rheumatic disease may involve commissural fusion resulting in valvular stenosis.

5.2. *Thrombotic/atherosclerotic coronary occlusion*

Chest pain caused by angina may be diagnosed by stress testing, either exercise or pharmacologic. In general, an imaging modality should be added to the stress electrocardiogram in women to enhance the predictive accuracy of the study. Stress testing detects the presence of flow-limiting lesions of the epicardial vessels but may also be abnormal in the setting of diffuse microvascular disease and/or hypertension. Electrocardiography and serologic markers are used for the initial diagnosis of acute myocardial infarction.

5.3. *Ventricular hypertrophy and dysfunction*

Left ventricular mass and systolic performance can be reliably measured using standard echocardiographic techniques. Doppler echocardiography is required to assess diastolic function. Standard parameters measured to assess the presence of impaired diastolic filling and/or elevated left atrial pressure include the ratio of peak early (E) and late or atrial (A) filling velocities, deceleration time of the E wave, isovolumic relaxation time, pattern of pulmonary venous inflow, and tissue Doppler imaging.

5.4. *Intracardiac thrombi*

The ability of TTE to detect intracardiac thrombi may be limited in the setting of poor acoustic windows, as occurs in the presence of chronic obstructive lung disease or obesity. In these patients, TEE should be performed if clinical suspicion is high.

Clinicians should also be aware of the usefulness and major advantages of cardiac MRI for the differentiation of cardiac masses, especially when echocardiography is inconclusive. MRI can differentiate between tumor and thrombus, a major advantage over echocardiography (Seelos et al., 1992). Tumors are hyperintense on spin echo (SE) T2-weighted images. Furthermore, on gradient-recalled echo images (GRE), a clot has lower signal intensity compared to the myocardium, while tumor has intermediate signal intensity. If gadolinium (superparamagnetic contrast media) is administered, tumor enhances, but thrombus does not. These signal characteristics are quite useful for differentiating between the tumor and clot. MRI also helps to define the age of clot, which is very important to determine the most appropriate treatment. On SE images, fresh clot shows high intensity, whereas an old clot has low signal intensity (Erkan et al., 2002b). Furthermore, myxomas are usually solitary, not calcified, and attach near the fossa ovalis of the interatrial septum (Espinosa et al., 2002).

6. Treatment

6.1. *Valve abnormalities*

Though they may have different pathogeneses and treatment implications, valvulitis, valve deformity/-failure, and valve vegetations are not clearly distinguished in most publications, impeding interpretation in some treatment studies. Standard measures should be used in patients with congestive heart failure; however, the management of asymptomatic patients is under debate.

Espinola-Zavaleta et al. (1999) performed a 1-year TEE follow-up study on 13 primary APS patients receiving anticoagulant or antiplatelet therapy, most treated with low-dose aspirin (100 mg/day) and/or warfarin (international normalized ratio, INR > 3). Valve lesions persisted unchanged in 6 patients (46%); new lesions appeared in the remaining 7 (54%). The investigators concluded that oral anticoagulant or antithrombotic therapy does not contribute to the disappearance of vegetations. Skyrme-Jones et al. (1995) described a single primary APS patient in whom echocardiographic follow-up demonstrated the resolution of mitral vegetations after warfarin treatment.

Nesher et al. (1997) reported improvement in valve thickness and hemodynamics of four APS patients in association with corticosteroid treatment. Four patients with subacute onset of congestive heart failure secondary to severe mitral regurgitation, with leaflets thickened 3- to 6-fold, who had not responded to treatment with diuretics, afterload reduction, and anticoagulation, received 40–60 mg/day prednisone for a period of 6–12 months. All improved; the regurgitant jet area decreased from 7.5 ± 0.8 to $1.6 \pm 1.2\ \text{cm}^2$. Although other contributory factors (pregnancy, hypertension) also changed, rapid decrease in leaflet thickness (from 14.3 ± 4 to 8.5 ± 3 mm) suggests that corticosteroid therapy reduced valvular regurgitation. However, Shahian et al. (1995) found no effect of corticosteroid treatment on chronic mitral regurgitation in one patient with primary APS, and Hojnik et al. (1996) stated, without presenting primary data, that steroid therapy is ineffective in the treatment of valvular disease. It is important to note that corticosteroids may result in scarring and deformity by accelerating the healing process (Galve et al., 1992). Thus it is unclear whether corticosteroids should be used for the treatment of aPL-related valvular diseases.

No systematic study on immunosuppressive or anti-inflammatory treatment of aPL-related valvular disease exists. In patients with SLE and recurrent systemic embolism, surgical excision of uninfected valvular vegetations may not prevent recurrence (Roldan et al., 1992).

We surveyed clinical APS experts participated in the Sapporo (Japan 1998) and Tours (France 2000) APS Meeting Advisory Board regarding treatment of asymptomatic (no history of vascular or pregnancy events) aPL-positive patients with valve disease (Erkan et al., 2002c). Thirteen of 17 experts preferred low-dose aspirin alone, 2 chose no treatment, 1 warfarin, and 1 low-dose aspirin plus low-dose corticosteroid. There is no published consensus regarding treatment of *symptomatic* patients.

6.2. Thrombotic/atherosclerotic coronary occlusion

For persons who have suffered a thrombotic coronary occlusion, anticoagulation is usually prescribed. Ruiz-Irastorza et al. (2002) recommends a target INR of 3.5. Measurement of plasma homocysteine and fibrinogen may help define aPL subjects at high vascular risk. In the Hopkins Lupus Cohort, hydroxychloroquine was shown to have an additional protective effect, likely multifactorial, including benefit on lupus activity, hyperlipidemia, anti-platelet and 'desludging' effects, and a reduction in aPL titers (Petri, 2000c). In older stroke patients with low-titer aPL, aspirin may be as effective as low-dose warfarin in preventing recurrence (Brey and Levine, 2002), as well as possibly preventing primary thrombosis in women identified with APS-associated pregnancy complications (Erkan et al., 2001).

Statin treatment is associated with regression of atherosclerotic lesions and with a reduction in cardiovascular complications. Statins may also influence anti-β_2GPI-induced proadhesive and proinflammatory endothelial phenotype (Meroni et al., 2001a, b). Thus, statins are an additional tool for treatment but currently untested for APS patients as an adjunctive treatment.

6.3. Ventricular hypertrophy and dysfunction

No published studies have addressed treatment of these possible manifestations of cardiac disease. In general, standard pharmacologic approaches should be used, i.e. treatment of hypertension and heart failure regimens demonstrated to control symptoms and prolong life. It remains to be established whether antiplatelet, anticoagulant or other treatment can prevent or improve dysfunction in patients with primary APS.

6.4. Intracardiac thrombi

Timely detection of thrombosis is crucial in the management of APS. Individual physicians, primarily in case reports, have treated intracardiac thrombi with aggressive anticoagulation and/or surgical excision. Substantial data favoring either approach do not exist. O'Neill et al. (1995) used anticoagulation as the initial treatment of three APS patients with left-sided thrombi complicated by systemic embolization; all thrombi resolved completely in 6 weeks to 3 months. These authors proposed that initial treatment of an intracardiac lesion should be a trial of systemic anticoagulation before surgical intervention. Heightened surgical risk in these patients (vide infra) strongly supports an initial non-surgical approach.

6.5. Cardiovascular surgery in APS patients

Patients with positive aPL may be prone to excessive postoperative morbidity and mortality after cardiovascular surgical procedures. In one retrospective report, 16 of 19 patients with a positive ELISA for IgG aCL suffered major postoperative complications,

Table 4
Experience with postoperative thrombosis prophylaxis after cardiovascular surgeries in antiphospholipid antibody positive patients (APL) and in patients meeting the Sapporo criteria for APS

Author	Dx	Surgery	Postop. regimen and timing (day)		Postop. thrombosis
Sheikh et al.	–[a]	CABG	–	–	Yes
Sheikh et al.	APS	MVR	Heparin/warfarin	1/1	No
Matsuyama et al.	APS	AVR	Warfarin	1	No
Yoshida et al.	APS	MVP	Heparin/warfarin	NR	No
Yoshida et al.	APS	CABG/MVP	Heparin/warfarin	NR	No
East et al.	APS	CABG/MVR	Warfarin	NR	No
East et al..	APS	MVR	Warfarin	NR	No
Hogan et al.	APL	AVR	Aspirin	NR	No
Ducart et al.	APL	CABG	NR	NR	No
Myers et al.	APL	AVR/MVR	Warfarin	NR	No
Erkan et al.	APS	MVR	Heparin/warfarin	1/3	No
Erkan et al.	APS	MVR/AVR	Heparin/warfarin	1/1	No

Dx: diagnosis; Postop: post-operative; CABG: coronary artery by-pass grafting; MVR: mitral valve replacement; AVR: aortic valve replacement; MVP: mitral valve prolapse; NR: not reported.
[a] APS was diagnosed after the surgery.

and 12 died of complications related to surgical interventions (Ciocca et al., 1995).

However, there are numerous reports of uncomplicated cardiac valve replacements in APS patients (Sheikh et al., 1997; Matsuyama et al., 1999; Yoshida et al., 2000; East et al., 2000). Hogan et al. (2000) recently reviewed the intraoperative management of cardiac valvular surgeries in APS patients. Intraoperative heparin monitoring during cardiopulmonary bypass surgery can be challenging because APS patients may have elevated baseline activated coagulation time (ACT) level (Hogan et al., 2000; Ducart et al., 1997). Suggested methods for monitoring include: doubling the baseline ACT level (Sheikh et al., 1997); obtaining heparin concentrations by protamine titration rather than following ACT levels (Hogan et al., 2000; Ducart et al., 1997); and performing heparin-ACT titration curves preoperatively to determine patient-specific target ACT levels (East et al., 2000). Heparin, followed by warfarin, is generally used to prevent postoperative thrombotic complications; however, there is no consensus on the timing of the initiation of anticoagulation, especially warfarin. Reported cases of cardiovascular surgeries, anticoagulation regimens, and outcomes are shown in Table 4.

When an APS patient undergoes a surgical procedure, serious perioperative complications (recurrent thrombosis, catastrophic exacerbation, or bleeding) may occur despite prophylaxis. Thus,

Table 5
Recommendations for the perioperative medical management of the APS patients (Erkan et al., 2002a–d)

Preoperative assessment
- Prolonged activated partial thromboplastin time (aPTT) and/or slightly prolonged prothrombin time (PT) when known to be due to APS are *not*contraindications for surgical procedures
- Platelet count greater than 100×10^9 l due to APS requires no specific therapy; thrombocytopenia does not protect against thrombosis
- Surgical and interventional procedures should be the last option in the management of APS patients

Perioperative considerations
- Minimize intravascular manipulation for access and monitoring
- Set pneumatic blood pressure cuffs to inflate infrequently to minimize stasis in the distal vascular bed
- Avoid tourniquets
- Maintain high suspicion that any deviation from a normal course may reflect arterial or venous thrombosis

Perioperative anticoagulation
- Keep periods without anticoagulation to an absolute minimum
- Employ pharmacological and physical anti-thrombosis interventions vigorously and start immediately before the operation, continuing until the patient is fully ambulating
- Be aware that APS patients can develop recurrent thrombosis despite appropriate prophylaxis
- Be aware that current conventional doses of anti-thrombotic regimens can result in 'under-anticoagulation'; APS patients may benefit from an aggressive approach with higher doses than standard doses
- Manage APS patients whose only clinical manifestation is pregnancy morbidity as if they had vascular thrombosis

perioperative strategies should be clearly identified before any surgical procedure, pharmacological and physical anti-thrombosis interventions vigorously employed, periods without anticoagulation kept to an absolute minimum, and any deviation from a normal course be considered a potential disease-related event. Strategies that may guide physicians in their preoperative, intraoperative, and postoperative management of APS patients are summarized in Table 5 (Erkan et al., 2002d).

6.6. 10th International Antiphospholipid Antibodies Meeting Therapy Committee Consensus Report on the Cardiac Manifestations of the Antiphospholipid Syndrome

The 10th International Congress on aPL was held in Taormina, Sicily, Italy between September 29 and October 3, 2002. In a precongress meeting, diagnosis and treatment guidelines were evaluated by physicians who have special expertise in APS. The Cardiac Committee's treatment recommendations are shown in Table 6 (Lockshin et al., 2003).

Table 6
10th International aPL Meeting Therapy Committee Consensus Report on the Cardiac Manifestations of the APS (Lockshin et al., 2003)

Valve abnormalities

Anticoagulation for *symptomatic* patients with valvulopathy

Prophylactic antiplatelet therapy may be appropriate for hemodynamically stable *asymptomatic* (no history of vascular or pregnancy) patients (recommended by 13/17 experts in an independent review)

Committee members disagreed whether corticosteroid therapy is helpful

Distinguishing among valvulitis, valve deformity, and vegetations is important, as treatment implications may differ

Thrombotic and atherosclerotic (coronary) vascular occlusion

Aggressive treatment of all risk factors for atherosclerosis (hypertension, hypercholesterolemia, smoking) and liberal use of folic acid, B vitamins, and cholesterol-lowering drugs (preferably statins)

Hydroxychloroquine for cardiac protection in APS patients may be considered

Warfarin anticoagulation for those who have suffered non-atherosclerotic thrombosis, but developing data may support the use of antiplatelet agents instead

Ventricular dysfunction

No recommendations on this aspect of cardiac disease

Intracardiac thrombi

Intensive warfarin anticoagulation, and consultation with cardiac surgeons when appropriate

Key points

- Cardiac manifestations of the APS range from asymptomatic valvular lesions to life-threatening myocardial infarction.
- The most commonly reported cardiac manifestation is heart valve abnormalities; thickening of the valve leaflets is the most common, however, clinically significant valvulopathy appears to be uncommon.
- The prevalence of myocardial infarction in primary APS patients is relatively low.
- The extent to which aPL independently impacts left ventricular size and function in the absence of other confounding processes and whether such an impact is of clinical relevance remains uncertain.
- A recent committee consensus report for the treatment recommendations of cardiac disease in APS may guide physicians for the management of aPL-related cardiac manifestations.
- When an APS patient undergoes a surgical procedure, serious perioperative complications (recurrent thrombosis, catastrophic exacerbation, or bleeding) may occur despite prophylaxis.

References

Afek, A., Shoenfeld, Y., Manor, R., Goldberg, I., Ziporen, L., George, J., Polak-Charcon, S., Amigo, M.C., Garcia-Torres, R., Segal, R., Kopolovic, J. 1999. Increased endothelial cell expression of alpha3beta1 integrin in cardiac valvulopathy in the primary (Hughes) and secondary antiphospholipid syndrome. Lupus 8, 502.

Ames, P.R.J., Margarita, A., Delgado Alves, J., Tommasino, C., Iannaccone, L., Brancaccio, V. 2002. Anticardiolipin antibody titer and plasma homocysteine level independently predict intima media thickness of carotid arteries in subjects with idiopathic antiphospholipid antibodies. Lupus 11, 208.

Amital, H., Langevitz, P., Levy, Y., Afek, A., Goldberg, I., Pras, M., Livneh, A., Shoenfeld, Y. 1999. Valvular deposition of antiphospholipid antibodies in the antiphospholipid syndrome: a clue to the origin of the disease. Clin. Exp. Rheumatol. 17, 99.

Asherson, R.A., Khamashta, M.A., Ordi-Ros, J., Derksen, R.H., Machin, S.J., Barquinero, J., Outt, H.H., Harris, E.N., Vilardell-Torres, M., Hughes, G.R. 1989. The 'primary' antiphospholipid syndrome: major clinical and serological features. Medicine (Baltimore) 68, 366.

Asherson, R.A., Cervera, R., Piette, J.C., Font, J., Lie, J.T., Burcoglu, A., Lim, K., Munoz-Rodriguez, F.J., Levy, R.A., Boue, F., Rossert, J., Ingelmo, M. 1998. Catastrophic antiphospholipid syndrome. Clinical and laboratory features of 50 patients. Medicine (Baltimore) 77, 195.

Bili, A., Moss, A.J., Francis, C.W., Zareba, W., Watelet, L.F., Sanz, I. 2000. Antiphospholipid antibodies and recurrent coronary events—a prospective study of 1150 patients. Circulation 102, 1258.

This study demonstrated that anticardiolipin antibodies are independent risk factors for recurrent cardiac events in patients with myocardial infarction.

Brenner, B., Blumenfeld, Z., Markiewicz, W., Reisner, S.A. 1991. Cardiac involvement in patients with primary antiphospholipid syndrome. J. Am. Coll. Cardiol. 18, 931.

Brey, R., Levine, S.R. 2002. APL and the brain: treatment. Lupus 11, 2002 (Abstract).

Cervera, R., Khamashta, M.A., Font, J., Reyes, P.A., Vianna, J.L., Lopez-Soto, A., Amigo, M.C., Asherson, R.A., Azqueta, M., Pare, C. 1991. High prevalence of significant heart valve lesions in patients with the primary antiphospholipid syndrome. Lupus 1, 43.

Cervera, R. 2000. Recent advances in antiphospholipid antibody-related valvulopathies. J. Autoimmun. 15, 123.

A summary of echocardiographic findings, pathogenesis, and clinical manifestations of antiphospholipid antibody-related valvulopathies.

Ciocca, R.G., Choi, J., Graham, A.M. 1995. Antiphospholipid antibodies lead to increased risk in cardiovascular surgery. Am. J. Surg. 170, 198.

Coudray, N., de Zuttere, D., Bletry, O., Piette, J.C., Wechsler, B., Godeau, P., Pourny, J.C., Lecarpentier, Y., Chemla, D. 1995. M mode and doppler echocardiographic assessment of left ventricular diastolic function in primary antiphospholipid syndrome. Br. Heart J. 74, 531.

Cuadrado, M.J., Hughes, G.R.V. 2001. Hughes (antiphospholipid) syndrome. Clinical features. Rheum. Dis. Clin. North Am. 27, 507.

De Caterina, R., d'Ascanio, A., Mazzone, A., Gazzetti, P., Bernini, W., Neri, R., Bombardieri, S. 1990. Prevalence of anticardiolipin antibodies in coronary artery disease. Am. J. Cardiol. 65, 922.

Ducart, A.R., Collard, E.L., Osselaer, J.C., Broka, S.M., Eucher, P.M., Joucken, K.L. 1997. Management of anticoagulation during cardiopulmonary bypass in a patient with a circulating lupus anticoagulant. J. Cardiothorac. Vasc. Anesth. 11, 878.

East, C.J., Clements, F., Mathew, J., Slaughter, T.F. 2000. Antiphospholipid syndrome and cardiac surgery: management of anticoagulation in two patients. Anesth. Analg. 90, 1098.

Erkan, D., Yazici, Y., Sobel, R., Lockshin, M. 2000. Primary antiphospholipid syndrome: functional outcome after 10 years. J. Rheumatol. 27, 2817.

Erkan, D., Merrill, J.T., Yazici, Y., Sammaritano, L., Buyon, J.P., Lockshin, M.D. 2001. High thrombosis rate after fetal loss in antiphospholipid syndrome. Effective prophylaxis with aspirin. Arthritis Rheum. 44, 1466.

Erkan, D., Yazici, Y., Peterson, M., Sammaritano, L., Lockshin, M.D. 2002a. A cross-sectional study of clinical thrombotic risk factors and preventive treatments in antiphospholipid syndrome. Rheumatology 41, 924.

Erkan, D., Erel, H., Yazici, Y., Prince, M.R. 2002b. The role of cardiac magnetic resonance imaging in antiphospholipid syndrome. J. Rheumatol. 29, 2658.

Erkan, D., Sammaritano, L., Lockshin, M.D. 2002c. Management of the difficult aspects of antiphospholipid syndrome. In: R.A. Asherson, R. Cervera, J.C. Piette, Y. Shoenfeld (Eds.), Antiphospholipid Syndrome II. Elsevier, Amsterdam, p. 353.

Erkan, D., Leibowitz, E., Berman, J., Lockshin, M.D. 2002d. Perioperative medical management of antiphospholipid syndrome: Hospital for Special Surgery experience, review of the literature and recommendations. J. Rheumatol. 29, 843.

When an Antiphospholipid Syndrome (APS) patient undergoes a surgical procedure, serious perioperative complications may occur despite prophylaxis. This paper summarizes strategies that may guide physicians in their preoperative, intraoperative, and postoperative management of APS patients.

Espinola-Zavaleta, N., Vargas-Barron, J., Colmenares-Galvis, T., Cruz-Cruz, F., Romero-Cardenas, A., Keirns, C., Amigo, M.C. 1999. Echocardiographic evaluation of patients with primary antiphospholipid syndrome. Am. Heart J. 137, 973.

Espinosa, G., Cervera, R., Font, J., Garcia-Carrasco, M., Battagliotti, C., Ingelmo, M. 2002. Cardiac and pulmonary manifestations in the antiphospholipid syndrome. In: R.A. Asherson, R. Cervera, J.C. Piette, Y. Shoenfeld (Eds.), Antiphospholipid Syndrome II—Autoimmune Thrombosis. Elsevier, Amsterdam, p. 169.

Font, J., Lopez-Soto, A., Cervera, R., Balasch, J., Pallares, L., Navarro, M., Bosch, X., Ingelmo, M. 1991. The 'primary' antiphospholipid syndrome: antiphospholipid antibody pattern and clinical features of a series of 23 patients. Autoimmunity 9, 69.

Galve, E., Candell-Riera, J., Pigrau, C., Permanyer-Miralda, G., Garcia-Del-Castillo, H., Soler-Soler, J. 1988. Prevalence, morphologic types, and evolution of cardiac valvular disease in systemic lupus erythematosus. N. Engl. J. Med. 319, 817.

Galve, E., Ordi, J., Barquinero, J., Evangelista, A., Vilardell, M., Soler-Soler, J. 1992. Valvular heart disease in the primary antiphospholipid syndrome. Ann. Intern. Med. 116, 293.

Garcia-Torres, R., Amigo, M.C., de la Rosa, A., Moron, A., Reyes, P.A. 1996. Valvular heart disease in primary antiphospholipid syndrome (PAPS): clinical and morphological findings. Lupus 5, 56.

Hamsten, A., Norberg, R., Bjorkholm, M., de Faire, U., Holm, G. 1986. Antibodies to cardiolipin in young survivors of myocardial infarction: an association with recurrent cardiovascular events. Lancet 1 (8473), 113.

Hasnie, A.M., Stoddard, M.F., Gleason, C.B., Wagner, S.G., Longaker, R.A., Pierangeli, S., Harris, E.N. 1995. Diastolic dysfunction is a feature of the antiphospholipid syndrome. Am. Heart J. 129, 1009.

Hogan, W.J., McBane, R.D., Santrach, P.J., Plumhoff, E.A., Oliver, W.C. Jr, Schaff, H.V., Rodeheffer, R.J., Edwards, W.D., Duffy, J., Nichols, W.L. 2000. Antiphospholipid syndrome and perioperative hemostatic management of cardiac valvular surgery. Mayo Clin. Proc. 75, 971.

Hojnik, M., George, J., Ziporen, L., Shoenfeld, Y. 1996. Heart valve involvement (Libman–Sacks endocarditis) in the antiphospholipid syndrome. Circulation 93, 1579.

Kattwinkel, N., Villanueva, A.G., Labib, S.B., Aretz, H.T., Walek, J.W., Burns, D.L., Klenz, J.T. 1992. Myocardial infarction caused by cardiac microvasculopathy in a patient with the primary antiphospholipid syndrome. Ann. Intern. Med. 116 (12 Pt 1), 974.

Khamashta, M.A., Cervera, R., Asherson, R.A., Font, J., Gil, A., Coltart, D.J., Vazquez, J.J., Pare, C., Ingelmo, M., Oliver, J. 1990. Association of antibodies against phospholipids with heart valve disease in systemic lupus erythematosus. Lancet 335 (8705), 1541.

Kupferwasser, L.I., Hafner, G., Mohr-Kahaly, S., Erbel, R., Meyer, J., Darius, H. 1999. The presence of infection-related antiphospholipid antibodies in infective endocarditis determines a major risk factor for embolic events. J. Am. Coll. Cardiol. 33, 1365.

Lagana, B., Baratta, L., Tubani, L., Golluscio, V., Delfino, M., Rossi Fanelli, F. 2001. Myocardial infarction with normal coronary arteries in a patient with primary antiphospholipid syndrome—case report and literature review. Angiology 52, 785.

Lee, R., Frenkel, E.P. 2003. Hyperhomocysteinemia and thrombosis. Hematol. Oncol. Clin. North Am. 17, 85.

Leung, W.H., Wong, K.L., Lau, C.P., Wong, C.K., Liu, H.W. 1990. Association between antiphospholipid antibodies and cardiac abnormalities in patients with systemic lupus erythematosus. Am. J. Med. 89, 411.

Levine, J.S., Branch, D.W., Rauch, J. 2002. The antiphospholipid syndrome. N. Engl. J. Med. 346, 752.

Levine, S.R., Salowich-Palm, L., Sawaya, K.L., Perry, M., Spencer, H.J., Winkler, H.J., Alam, Z., Carey, J.L. 1997. IgG anticardiolipin antibody titer >40 GPL and the risk of subsequent thrombo-occlusive events and death. A prospective cohort study. Stroke 28, 1660.

Lockshin, M.D., Salmon, J.E., Roman, M.J. 2001a. Atherosclerosis and lupus: a work in progress. Arthritis Rheum. 44, 2215–2217.

Lockshin, M.D. 2001b. Antiphopholipid antibody syndrome. In: S. Ruddy, E.D. Harris, C.B. Sledge (Eds.), Kelley's Textbook of Rheumatology. Saunders Company, Philadelphia, p. 1145.

Lockshin, M.D., Tenedios, F., Petri, M., McCarty, G., Forastiero, R., Krilis, S., Tincani, A., Erkan, D., Khamashta, M.A., Shoenfeld, Y. 2003. Cardiac disease in antiphospholipid syndrome: recommendations for treatment. Committee consensus report. Lupus 12, 518.

The 10th International Congress on antiphospholipid antibodies was held in Taormina, Sicily, Italy between September 29 and October 3, 2002. A Cardiac Committee reviewed cardiac involvement in the Antiphospholipid Syndrome and published treatment recommendations.

Manzi, S., Meilahn, E.N., Rairie, J.E., Conte, C.G., Medsger, T.A. Jr, Jansen-McWilliams, L., D'Agostino, R.B., Kuller, L.H. 1997. Age-specific incidence rates of myocardial infarction and angina in women with systemic lupus erythematosus: comparison with the Framingham Study. Am. J. Epidemiol. 145, 408.

Manzi, S., Selzer, F., Sutton-Tyrrell, K., Fitzgerald, S.G., Rairie, J.E., Tracy, R.P., Kuller, L.H. 1999. Prevalence and risk factors of carotid plaque in women with systemic lupus erythematosus. Arthritis. Rheum. 42, 51.

Matsuyama, K., Ueda, Y., Ogino, H., Sugita, T., Matsubayashi, K., Nomoto, T., Yoshimura, S., Yoshioka, T. 1999. Aortic valve replacement for aortic regurgitation in a patient with primary antiphospholipid syndrome. Jpn. Circ. J. 63, 725.

Meroni, P.L., Raschi, E., Testoni, C., Tincani, A., Balestrieri, G. 2001a. Antiphospholipid antibodies and the endothelium. Rheum. Dis. Clin. 27, 587.

Meroni, P.L., Raschi, E., Testoni, C. 2001b. Statins prevent endothelial cell activation induced by antiphospholipid (anti-beta2-glycoprotein I) antibodies: effect on the proadhesive and proinflammatory phenotype. Arthritis Rheum. 44, 2870.

Nesher, G., Ilany, J., Rosenmann, D. Abraham, A.S. 1997. Valvular dysfunction in antiphospholipid syndrome: prevalence, clinical features, and treatment. Sem. Arthritis Rheum. 27, 27 .

The pathogenesis, prevalence (including a meta-analysis), clinical presentation, and treatment options of Antiphospholipid Syndrome-related valvular dysfunction were discussed.

Nihoyannopoulos, P., Gomez, P., Joshi, M., Loizou, S., Walport, M.J., Oakley, C.M. 1990. Cardiac abnormalities in systemic lupus erythematosus. Association with raised anticardiolipin antibodies. Circulation 82, 369.

O'Neill, D., Magaldi, J., Dobkins, D., Greco, T. 1995. Dissolution of intracardiac mass lesions in the primary antiphospholipid syndrome. Arch. Intern. Med. 155, 325–327.

Petri, M. 2000a. Epidemiology of the antiphospholipid antibody syndrome. J. Autoimmun. 15, 145.

Petri, M. 2000b. Hopkins Lupus Cohort. 1999 update. Rheum. Dis. Clin. North Am. 26, 199.

Petri, M. 2000c. Detection of coronary artery disease and the role of traditional risk factors in the Hopkins Lupus Cohort. Lupus 9, 170.

Puurunen, M., Manttari, M., Manninen, V., Tenkanen, L., Alfthan, G., Ehnholm, C., Vaarala, O., Aho, K., Palosuo, T. 1994. Antibody against oxidized low-density lipoprotein predicting myocardial infarction. Arch. Intern. Med. 154, 2605.

Roldan, C.A., Shively, B.K., Lau, C.C., Gurule, F.T., Smith, E.A., Crawford, M.H. 1992. Systemic lupus erythematosus valve disease by transesophageal echocardiography and the role of antiphospholipid antibodies. J. Am. Coll. Cardiol. 20, 1127.

Roman, M.J., Salmon, J.E., Sobel, R., Lockshin, M.D., Sammaritano, L., Schwartz, J.E., Devereux, R.B. 2001. Prevalence and relation to risk factors of carotid atherosclerosis and left ventricular hypertrophy in systemic lupus erythematosus and antiphospholipid antibody syndrome. Am. J. Cardiol. 87, 663.

Ruiz-Irastorza, G., Khamashta, M.A., Hunt, B.J., Escudero, A., Cuadrado, M.J., Hughes, G.R. 2002. Bleeding and recurrent thrombosis in definite antiphospholipid syndrome. Arch. Intern. Med. 162, 1164.

Seelos, K., Caputo, G.R., Carrol, C.L., Hricak, H., Higgins, C.B. 1992. Cine gradient refocused (GRE) echo imaging of intravascular masses: differentiation between tumor and non-tumorous thrombus. J. Comput. Assist. Tomogr. 16, 169.

Shahian, D.M., Labib, S.B., Schneebaum, A.B. 1995. Etiology and management of chronic valve disease in antiphospholipid antibody syndrome and systemic lupus erythematosus. J. Card. Surg. 10, 133.

Sheikh, F., Lechowicz, A., Setlur, R., Rauch, A., Dunn, H. 1997. Recognition and management of patients with antiphospholipid antibody syndrome undergoing cardiac surgery. Cardiothorac. Vasc. Anesth. 11, 764.

Skyrme-Jones, R.A., Wardrop, C.A., Wiles, C.M., Fraser, A.G. 1995. Transesophageal echocardiographic demonstration of resolution of mitral vegetations after warfarin in a patient with the primary antiphospholipid syndrome. J. Am. Soc. Echocardiogr. 8, 251.

Sletnes, K.E., Smith, P., Abdelnoor, M., Arnesen, H., Wisloff, F. 1992. Antiphospholipid antibodies after myocardial infarction and their relation to mortality, reinfarction, and non-haemorrhagic stroke. Lancet 339 (8791), 451–453.

Turiel, M., Muzzupappa, S., Gottardi, B., Crema, C., Sarzi-Puttini, P., Rossi, E. 2000. Evaluation of cardiac abnormalities and embolic sources in primary antiphospholipid syndrome by transesophageal echocardiography. Lupus 9, 406.

Wilson, W.A., Gharavi, A.E., Koike, T., Lockshin, M.D., Branch, D.W., Piette, J.C., Brey, R., Derksen, R., Harris, E.N., Hughes, G.R., Triplett, D.A., Khamashta, M.A. 1999. International consensus statement on preliminary classification criteria for definite antiphospholipid syndrome: report of an international workshop. Arthritis Rheum. 42, 1309.

The first published international consensus statement on the preliminary classification criteria for definite antiphospholipid syndrome.

Witztum, J.L. 1994. The oxidation hypothesis of atherosclerosis. Lancet 344 (8925), 793.

Yoshida, M., Sasako, Y., Kobayashi, J., Minatoya, K., Bando, K., Kitamura, S. 2000. Mitral valve plasty in systemic lupus erythematosus in the setting of antiphospholipid syndrome. Jpn. J. Thorac. Cardiovasc. Surg. 48, 391.

Ziporen, L., Goldberg, I., Arad, M. 1996. Libman–Sacks endocarditis in the antiphospholipid syndrome: immunopathologic findings in deformed heart valves. Lupus 5, 196.

Handbook of Systemic Autoimmune Diseases, Volume 1
The Heart in Systemic Autoimmune Diseases
A. Doria and P. Pauletto, editors

CHAPTER 15

Cardiac Involvement in Systemic Vasculitis

Christian Pagnoux[a], Luigi Boiardi[b], Carlo Salvarani[b], Loïc Guillevin[*,a]

[a]*Department of Internal Medicine, Hôpital Cochin, 27, rue du Faubourg Saint-Jacques, Paris F-75014, France*

[b]*Division of Rheumatology, Department of Internal Medicine, Arcispedale S. Maria Nuova, V.le Umberto 1°N 50, 42100 Reggio Emilia, Italy*

1. Introduction

Systemic vasculitides are a heterogeneous group of diseases characterized by inflammation of vessels, which results in their obstruction, with ensuing extensive tissue ischemia and infarction, and/or aneurysm formation. Their classification varies according to the type of vessels affected, running from aorta to capillaries to veins, with different end-organs targeted. The heart can be involved, with varying frequency depending on the type of vasculitis. Even though cardiac manifestations are rarely predominant, they can be life threatening and, as such, require therapeutic adaptation. After briefly reviewing the definitions, classification and pathogenic mechanisms of vasculitides, we describe the cardiac manifestations that can occur in each vasculitis and their corresponding therapies. The potential involvement of the aorta, its proximal branches and of pulmonary arteries in some vasculitides is also addressed, but peripheral vascular manifestations are not within the scope of this chapter.

2. Definition and classification of vasculitides

Vasculitides are defined based upon their histological features. Three main lesions can commonly be observed: fibrinoid necrosis of vessel walls, perivascular inflammatory infiltrates, and subsequent fibrotic scar replacement (Fig. 1). Vasculitic lesions usually have a segmental distribution pattern, with a predilection for arterial bifurcations. Fibrinoid necrosis occurs very early and predominates in the internal layer of the artery media, concomitantly with inflammatory lymphocyte, plasma cell, histiocyte, and some neutrophil infiltration of or around the vessel walls. Segmental necrosis in medium-sized vessels may give rise to microaneurysms. These lesions usually progress to fibrosis, and thrombosis can occur, resulting in tissue ischemia and damage. As some vasculitides have an activity pattern of successive flares, different histological stages may be seen in a single specimen. Giant cell arteritis (GCA) and Takayasu's arteritis, in which there are no (or only mild) fibrinoid necrosis and which affect large-sized vessels, should be distinguished from necrotizing angiitis. Thus, the presence of fibrinoid necrosis in a temporal artery should be interpreted as a sign of small or medium-sized vessel arteritis with temporal artery involvement, with exclusion of the diagnosis

*Corresponding author.
E-mail addresses: loic.guillevin@cch.ap-hop-paris.fr (L. Guillevin), salvarani.carlo@asmn.re.it (C. Salvarani).

DOI: 10.1016/S1571-5078(03)01015-8

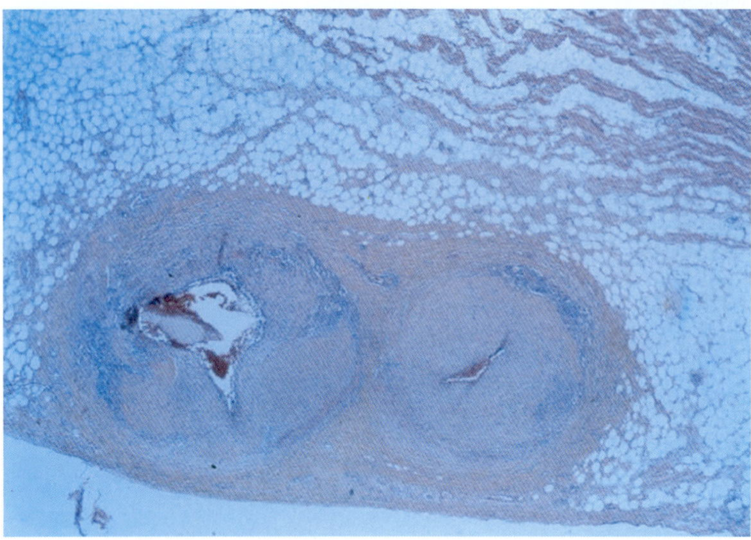

Figure 1. Histology of small vessel vasculitis in an endomyocardial biopsy: characteristic arterial wall-thickening associated with inflammatory infiltrates, fibrotic scar replacement, stenosis and endoluminal thrombosis.

of GCA (Chomette et al., 1983; Généreau et al., 1999; Saveuse et al., 1988). On the other hand, granulomatous inflammation is one of the characteristic features of Wegener's granulomatosis (WG) and Churg–Strauss syndrome (CSS).

Primary vasculitides can be classified according to the 1990 American College of Rheumatology classification criteria (Arend et al., 1990; Bloch et al., 1990; Calabrese et al., 1990; Fries et al., 1990; Hunder et al., 1990a,b; Leavitt et al., 1990; Lightfoot et al., 1990; Masi et al., 1990; Mills et al., 1990) or to the more accurate and complete Nomenclature of Systemic Vasculitides, established at the Chapel Hill Consensus Conference (Jennette et al., 1994) (Table 1). This latter classification distinguishes large, medium-sized and small vessel vasculitides, and also recognizes some overlap syndromes, with some, but not predominant, involvement of small vessels in polyarteritis nodosa (PAN) and medium-sized vessels in microscopic polyangiitis (MPA), CSS and WG (ANCA Workshop, Birmingham, UK, 1998, unpublished revised version of the nomenclature).

Diagnosis of vasculitis theoretically requires histological proof. However, as tissue easily accessible to biopsy may show only non-specific inflammation or even be normal, diagnosis sometimes has to rely on the combination of clinical findings, and results of biological, immunological and radiological investigations. Anti-neutrophil cytoplasmic autoantibodies (ANCA, cf. Pathogenesis of vasculitides) and angiography are useful tools to help make the diagnosis of necrotizing vasculitides. Angiographic findings, such as multiple, 1–5 mm diameter aneurysms or irregular vessel narrowing are present in approximately 80% of PAN patients (D'Izarn et al., 1976; Guillevin et al., 1995a). Even though suggestive, such findings are not absolutely specific, since arterial aneurysms may also be seen in thrombotic thrombocytopenic purpura, mycotic aneurysms, fibromuscular dysplasia, atrial myxoma, malignant arterial hypertension and in few patients with small vessel vasculitides (Ha et al., 2000; Jee et al., 2000; Miller, 2000). Indeed, to date, no diagnostic criteria for vasculitides have been established.

Some vasculitides are secondary manifestations or complications of other systemic diseases (McLaren et al., 2002), e.g. systemic lupus erythematosus (36–56% of the patients) (D'Cruz, 1998; Drenkard et al., 1997; Golan, 2002), rheumatoid arthritis (up to 22% of the patients) (Bely and Apathy, 1996; Goronzy and Weyand, 1994; Vollertsen and Conn, 1990), Cogan's syndrome (15%) (Vollertsen et al., 1986), Behçet's disease or Buerger's disease in which vascular involvement is the main feature. Vasculitis may also

Table 1
Names and definitions of vasculitides adopted by the Chapel Hill Consensus Conference on the Nomenclature of Systemic Vasculitis

Large vessel vasculitis	
Giant cell (temporal) arteritis	Granulomatous arteritis of the aorta and its major branches, with a predilection for the extracranial branches of the carotid artery. *Often involves the temporal artery. Usually occurs in patients older than 50 and is often associated with polymyalgia rheumatica.*
Takayasu's arteritis	Granulomatous inflammation of the aorta and its major branches. *Usually occurs in patients younger than 50.*
Medium-sized vessel vasculitis	
Polyarteritis nodosa	Necrotizing inflammation of medium-sized or small arteries without glomerulonephritis or vasculitis in arterioles, capillaries, or venules.
Kawasaki disease	Arteritis involving large, medium-sized, and small arteries, and associated with mucocutaneous lymph node syndrome. *Coronary arteries are often involved. Aorta and veins may be involved. Usually occurs in children.*
Small vessel vasculitis	
Wegener's granulomatosis[a]	Granulomatous inflammation involving the respiratory tract, and necrotizing vasculitis affecting small to medium-sized vessels (e.g. capillaries, venules, arterioles, and arteries). *Necrotizing glomerulonephritis is common.*
Churg–Strauss syndrome[a]	Eosinophil-rich and granulomatous inflammation involving the respiratory tract, and necrotizing vasculitis affecting small to medium-sized vessels, and associated with asthma and eosinophilia.
Microscopic polyangiitis[a]	Necrotizing vasculitis, with few or no immune deposits, affecting small vessels (i.e. capillaries, venules, or arterioles). *Necrotizing arteritis involving small and medium-sized arteries may be present. Necrotizing glomerulonephritis is very common. Pulmonary capillaritis often occurs.*
Henoch-Schönlein purpura	Vasculitis with IgA-dominant immune deposits, affecting small vessels (i.e. capillaries, venules, or arterioles). *Typically involves skin, gut, and glomeruli, and is associated with arthralgias or arthritis.*
Essential cryoglobulinemic vasculitis	Vasculitis, with cryoglobulin immune deposits, affecting small vessels (i.e. capillaries, venules, or arterioles), and associated with cryoglobulins in serum. *Skin and glomeruli are often involved.*
Cutaneous leukocytoclastic angiitis	Isolated leukocytoclastic angiitis without systemic vasculitis or glomerulonephritis.

Jennette et al. Arthritis Rheum. 1994, with permission. Large vessel refers to the aorta and the largest branches directed toward major body regions (e.g. to the extremities and the head and neck); medium-sized vessel refers to the main visceral arteries (e.g. renal, hepatic, coronary, and mesenteric arteries); small vessel refers to venules, capillaries, arterioles, and the intraparenchymal distal arterial radicals that connect with arterioles. Some small and large vessel vasculitides may involve medium-sized arteries, but large and medium-sized vessel vasculitides do not involve vessels smaller than arteries. Essential components are represented by normal type; italicized type represents usual, but not essential, components.

[a] Strongly associated with antineutrophil cytoplasmic autoantibodies.

occur in a setting of infection (e.g. hepatitis B virus (HBV), hepatitis C virus (HCV), human immunodeficiency virus (HIV) or cytomegalovirus) (Guillevin et al., 1997; Lortholary et al., 1999), cancer, malignant hemopathy or drug hypersensitivity (Calabrese et al., 1990; Garcia-Porrua et al., 2001). In the late 1980s, HBV was responsible for one-third of the PAN cases (Guillevin et al., 1993). HBV-related PAN now represents less than 10% of all PAN cases (Guillevin et al., 2001; Guillevin and Lhote, 1997), while HCV is responsible for more than 80% of mixed cryoglobulinemia (Rieu et al., 2002). Identification of these latter secondary vasculitic syndromes is important because of their better outcomes when a specific (and effective) treatment of the underlying cause is prescribed, and because the use of immunosuppressants may even be deleterious in virus-related vasculitides.

3. Pathogenesis of vasculitides

Several pathogenic pathways have been implicated in the development of these diseases, with the main mechanisms differing according to the type of vasculitis. These mechanisms are only partly understood and some are probably still unknown. Small vessel vasculitides (WG, CSS, MPA) are strongly associated with the presence of ANCA, whereas immune complexes may be responsible for Henoch-Schönlein purpura, cryoglobulinemic vasculitis and PAN.

3.1. Immune complexes

Deposition of circulating immune complexes in the vessel walls seems relevant in some vasculitides, like PAN, cryoglobulinemia, and necrotizing vasculitis occurring in rheumatoid arthritis. In the presence of an excess amount of antigen, immune complexes would form, and be deposited in vessel walls, where they facilitate the activation of the complement components and the attraction of neutrophils, which together can cause local damage to the endothelium. The identification of vascular deposits in Henoch-Schönlein purpura, and the detection of HBV-derived antigens and their corresponding antibodies in the vessels of patients with HBV-related vasculitis (Gower et al., 1978) support this concept of immune-complex involvement in their pathogeneses.

3.2. Anti-neutrophil cytoplasmic antibodies

First detected in a small cohort of patients with pauci-immune glomerulonephritis (Davies et al., 1982), antibodies specific to antigens in the cytoplasm of ethanol-fixed neutrophils have been shown to be strongly associated with three major small vessel vasculitides: WG, MPA, and CSS (Falk and Jennette, 1988; Van der Woude et al., 1985). ANCA are specific to peptides contained in neutrophil granules and monocyte lysosomes. Indirect immunofluorescence assays give a homogeneous, cytoplasmic (C-ANCA), perinuclear pattern (P-ANCA), or diffuse label pattern. Antigens recognized and identified by antigen-specific enzyme-linked immunosorbent assays (ELISA), are proteinase 3 (PR3) for C-ANCA, myeloperoxidase (MPO) for 90% of the P-ANCA, and elastase, cathepsin G, lactoferrin and lysozyme in the remaining cases (Ledford, 1997; Specks et al., 1993). Tumor necrosis factor-alpha (TNFα), as an inflammatory mediator, stimulates neutrophils, thereby inducing the translocation of the PR3 to the cytoplasmic membrane, where ANCA may bind to it. Such interactions would contribute directly to vascular damage. Indeed, high numbers of circulating endothelial cells, with a necrotic phenotype, have been observed in patients with active ANCA-associated vasculitides. Their numbers were significantly less abundant in vasculitis patients in remission or those with ANCA-negative vasculitides (Woywodt et al., 2003). This association is further supported by the development of necrotizing glomerulonephritis in recombinase-activating gene-2-deficient (Rag2($-/-$)) mice, but also in wild-type C57BL/6J mice, after injection of purified anti-MPO IgG (Heeringa et al., 1998; Xiao et al., 2002). C-ANCA are detected in 60–90% of cases of systemic WG, and in 50–75% of those with localized forms of WG (Kallenberg et al., 1992). Antibody titers seem to fluctuate with the disease activity, but must not be used as a tool to initiate or modify therapy, since this relationship is not constant (Girard et al., 2001; Tervaert et al., 1990). P-ANCA are more often associated with pauci-immune glomerulonephritis

(80% of the patients), MPA (50–75%) or CSS (47%) (Ewert et al., 1991; Guillevin et al., 1999a; Hagen et al., 1998). However, ANCA have also been detected in some non-vasculitic pathologies, such as inflammatory bowel and autoimmune liver diseases, rheumatoid arthritis, tuberculosis (Flores-Suarez et al., 2003) and drug reactions (Guillevin et al., 1995a; Halbwachs-Mecarelli et al., 1992; Specks et al., 1993).

3.3. Cytokines and adhesion molecules

Many cytokines are present at sites of inflammation and their circulating levels are high in patients with vasculitis (Sundy et al., 2000; Tesar et al., 1998). Some of them may be responsible for clinical symptoms (fever and weight loss induced by interleukin-1 (IL-1), TNFα and IL-6), some may favor fibrosis and thrombosis (transforming growth factor-beta (TGFβ)), while others may act as chemoattractants for polymorphonuclear leukocytes, or have inflammatory capacities (interferon-gamma (IFNγ)). Adhesion molecules are involved in the interactions between these activated leukocytes and endothelial cells (Sundy and Haynes, 2000). In addition, high levels of soluble endothelial receptors for neutrophils (intercellular adhesion molecule-1 (ICAM-1), E-selectin and vascular cell adhesion molecule-1 (VCAM-1)) have been detected in patients with active WG, MPA (Ara et al., 2001; Becvar et al., 1997; Mrowka and Sieberth, 1994, 1995; Ohta et al., 2001; Pall et al., 1994; Stegeman et al., 1994), Takayasu's arteritis (Noguchi et al., 1998), and Henoch-Schönlein purpura (Mrowka et al., 1999). Dysregulation of these cytokines and adhesion molecule cascades may occur in vasculitides, but have not yet been clearly documented. An imbalance between Th1 and Th2 lymphocyte immune pathways may be involved, as discussed below.

3.4. Other pathogenic factors

Other immunopathogenic factors and mechanisms may have roles to play in vasculitides. T cell-mediated immunity may contribute to the development of granulomatous vasculitides, i.e. WG and CSS. Infiltration by T lymphocytes secreting Th1 pro-inflammatory cytokines, essentially IFNγ, has been observed in granulomatous lesions of the nasal mucosa in WG patients. Thus, in WG, Th1 lymphocytes would play a major role in localized and granulomatous upper respiratory tract involvement, whereas a shift towards Th2 lymphocytes would tend to be more predominant in systemic forms (Balding et al., 2001; Csernok et al., 1999), which are thought to have a poorer prognosis (Bligny et al., 2003).

Antibody-mediated immunity is implied in some vasculitides, mainly through ANCA, but other autoantibodies may contribute to the vascular damage observed. Anti-endothelial cell antibodies (AECA) include a group of heterogeneous autoantibodies distinct from ANCA that have been detected in a wide variety of diseases, including systemic lupus erythematosus (Chan and Cheng, 1996), systemic sclerosis (Salojin et al., 1997) and WG, MPA, Kawasaki disease, Takayasu's arteritis, and small-vessel vasculitides (Falcini et al., 1997; Gobel et al., 1996; Praprotnik et al., 2000). AECA targets include a wide range of extracellular matrix antigens and phospholipids, but their precise identities in vasculitides remain to be determined and their pathogenicity are yet to be proven.

Viral etiologies for vasculitides have been clearly demonstrated in HBV-related PAN (Guillevin et al., 2001), mixed cryoglobulinemia related to HCV (Rieu et al., 2002), and in HIV-vasculitides (Gisselbrecht et al., 1997).

Genetic, hemodynamic, and environmental factors (Lane et al., 2003; Nuyts et al., 1995), and/or exposure to some drugs (Berbis et al., 1986; Guilpain et al., 2002; Holloway et al., 1998; Honsinger, 1998) may also be implicated in the development of various primary systemic vasculitides, but their respective roles remain to be elucidated.

4. Cardiovascular clinical manifestations in vasculitides

4.1. Main cardiovascular manifestations

Frequency, characteristics and severity of heart involvement vary according to the type of vasculitis. Each cardiac tissue may be affected, from myocardium

Table 2
Main cardiovascular manifestations and their reported frequencies in systemic necrotizing vasculitides

Cardiovascular manifestation	Frequency	References
Cardiomyopathy (specific and/or ischemia-related myocarditis)	Not mentioned, up to 78% (according to technique used for assessment)	Chumbley et al. (1977), Holsinger et al. (1962)
Coronary arteritis (with stenosis, thrombosis, aneurysm, or dissection)	9–50%	Schrader et al. (1985), Takahashi (1993)
Pericarditis	0–27%	Holsinger et al. (1962), Hu et al. (1997), Schrader et al. (1985)
Conduction tissue involvement (sinus or atrioventricular nodes) or arrhythmia (mostly supraventricular)	2–19%	Blétry et al. (1980), Holsinger et al. (1962)
Valve involvement (valvulitis, aseptic endocarditis)	Mostly anecdotal cases (up to 88% of patients may have valve involvement; but many have inorganic murmurs or non-specific valve involvement)	Greidinger et al. (1996), Morelli et al. (2000)
Aortic dissection (and dissection of proximal aortic arch branches)	Anecdotal in PAN and WG	Blockmans et al. (2000), Hautekeete et al. (1990)
Pulmonary hypertension	Anecdotal	Comparato and Toso, 1977; Marette et al. (1989)

to epicardium, endocardium, conductive nodal tissue and coronary arteries. Cardiovascular manifestations (Table 2) may thus be categorized as detailed below.

4.1.1. *Cardiomyopathy*

The reported frequencies of specific myocarditis vary widely from not-even-mentioned (Chumbley et al., 1977; Savage et al., 1985), up to 78% in an anatomical study (Holsinger et al., 1962), depending on the examinations used to diagnose small and medium-sized vessel vasculitides with a mean of 25–30% (Forstot et al., 1980; Lanham et al., 1985). In the context of vasculitis, specific cardiomyopathy mainly occurs in CSS, then WG, PAN, and MPA. However, cardiomyopathy leading to heart failure may reflect either specific myocardial involvement or myocardial ischemia in most patients or may be the consequence of associated conditions (e.g. hypertensive cardiomyopathy, steroid-induced coronary arteries atheromatosis). Specific cardiomyopathy could result from necrotizing vasculitis of the arterioles and venules supplying cardiac muscle (Fig. 1), with inflammatory infiltration and/or granulomas and/or fibrosis formation within cardiac tissue. It has been hypothesized that eosinophils play a direct pathogenic role in CSS, by infiltrating the myocardium, similar to what is seen in hypereosinophilic syndrome (Kendell et al., 1995; Kounis et al., 1989). Endoventricular biopsies are rarely obtained, even if the technique is now considered safe (Lanham et al., 1985; Leung et al., 1989) and may be helpful in understanding the causal process. However, vasculitis is rarely diagnosed based on the detection of granulomatous or necrotizing vasculitis in biopsy samples.

4.1.2. *Coronary arteritis*

Coronary arteritis may manifest as aneurysms, thromboses, dissections and/or stenoses, all of which can lead to myocardial infarction. Although coronary angiography may show some abnormalities, it is only occasionally performed, because angina is rare in vasculitides (Frohnert and Sheps, 1967; Holsinger et al., 1962). Nonetheless, an autopsy study has found coronary involvement in 50% of PAN patients (Schrader et al., 1985). In clinical practice, Kawasaki disease remains the vasculitis with the highest frequency of coronary arteritis, with up to 20% of the patients developing aneurysms (Kato et al., 1996).

4.1.3. Pericarditis

Pericardial effusion may be associated with cardiomyopathy, mainly in CSS (22% according to Hasley et al. (1990)), but also in WG (8% in Forstot et al. (1980)) and PAN (0–27% in Hu et al. (1997) and Schrader et al. (1985)). Tamponade may occur as can chronic constrictive pericarditis. Pertinently, an epicardial biopsy may provide the diagnosis of vasculitis, particularly of CSS (Sharma et al., 1993).

4.1.4. Endocarditis and valvular disease

Endocardium involvement is thought to be rare in vasculitides. Functional inorganic murmurs or valvular pathologies that are not related to vasculitis comprise most of the reported cases. Notably, myocardial vasculitis with subsequent thrombus formation or sterile valvulitis and immunosuppressive therapy for vasculitis may predispose to infectious endocarditis, which must be considered a highly likely diagnosis for a patient with an audible heart murmur. Nevertheless, specific valve damage may sometimes occur during the acute phase of the vasculitis, and progress to valve distortion during lesion repair and cicatrization, despite immunosuppressants (Davenport et al., 1994). Anecdotal cases with specific valve involvement have been reported over the past two decades at rapidly increasing frequency (Anthony et al., 1999; Bruno et al., 2000; Davenport et al., 1994; Fox and Robbins, 1994; Gerbracht et al., 1987; Greidinger et al., 1996; Morgan et al., 1989).

4.1.5. Conduction tissue involvement

Vasculitic or ischemic cardiomyopathy may involve nodal tissue, more frequently the sinus node than atrioventricular branches. Complete atrioventricular heart blocks and bundle-branch blocks have hence been mentioned, some requiring transient use of pacemaker in WG (Forstot et al., 1980; Handa et al., 1997; Schiavone et al., 1985), CSS (Rabusin et al., 1998), or PAN (Blétry et al., 1980).

4.1.6. Arrhythmia

Arrhythmias, mainly supraventricular, may occur and usually resolve within a few days of treatment for vasculitis (Balestrieri et al., 1992; Hu et al., 1997; Schiavone et al., 1985), as for conduction disorders.

4.1.7. Aortic dissections and aneurysms

The aorta and its proximal branches are the end-organs targeted in Takayasu's arteritis and Kawasaki disease and are frequently involved in GCA (Cormier et al., 2000; Kerr et al., 2000; Mohan and Kerr, 2000). Conversely, vasculitis of the small vessels in the vasa vasorum of the aorta may occasionally be involved in ANCA-associated vasculitides and progress to aortitis (Schildhaus et al., 2002).

4.1.8. Pulmonary hypertension

Pulmonary hypertension is rare, with only anecdotal episodes reported in PAN patients (Comparato and Toso, 1977; Marette et al., 1989). In some instances, it can be the consequence of constrictive pericarditis and/or restrictive cardiomyopathy (Grant et al., 1994; Schiavone et al., 1985) and/or lung involvement.

4.1.9. Thromboembolic and proximal vascular complications

In addition to heart and aortic involvement, thromboembolic events can complicate all these vasculitides (Somer, 1993), most commonly those with necrotizing vascular inflammation, i.e. Kawasaki disease, Behçet's disease, Buerger's disease, PAN and the vasculitis of rheumatoid arthritis. One of the characteristic features of Behçet's disease is aneurysms and thromboses of the pulmonary arteries, leading to caval syndrome and so-called Hughes–Stovin syndrome (Erkan et al., 2001, 2002). Granulomatous vasculitides are less frequently concerned. More peripheral vascular manifestations are beyond the scope of this chapter.

4.1.10. Secondary cardiovascular manifestations and differential diagnoses

All the cardiovascular manifestations that can occur in vasculitides must be distinguished from those which can occur as a consequence of other organ involvement or treatment side-effects. Infective endocarditis, hypertensive cardiomyopathy, uremic pericarditis (which is now a rare finding), traumatic perforation and dissection after endovascular investigations or biopsies, or long-term therapy with corticosteroid and immunosuppressants may be causative of, or at least may worsen, heart involvement in vasculitides.

4.2. Large vessel vasculitides

4.2.1. Giant cell arteritis

GCA is a chronic vasculitis of large and medium-sized vessels that occurs in persons over 50 years of age (Salvarani et al., 2002). The incidence increases with age and is higher in populations of northern European origin than in Mediterranean countries (Salvarani et al., 1991, 1995).

In approximately 10–15% of the cases, the branches of the aortic arch, particularly the subclavian and axillary arteries, become narrowed to produce upper extremity claudication (Klein et al., 1975; Salvarani et al., 2002). Bruits may be heard on auscultation over the carotid, subclavian, axillary, and brachial arteries. Absent or decreased pulses are present in the neck or arms. Such patients may have few of the usual symptoms of GCA, so the diagnosis may be initially overlooked.

Thoracic aortic aneurysms is 17 times more likely to develop in patients with GCA than in persons without this disease (Evans et al., 1995). This complication occurs as a late event, usually several years after the diagnosis and often after the patient's other symptoms have subsided. The aneurysm may rupture and cause the patient's death. However, the mortality rate in patients with GCA is similar to that expected in general populations of similar age and sex (Salvarani et al., 2002).

In the clinical suspicion of large-vessel GCA, arteriography, computerized tomography (CT) scanning and magnetic resonance (MR) angiography are the diagnostic modalities required (Stanson, 2000; Stanson et al., 1976). On arteriography, the typical pattern is represented by bilateral stenosis or occlusions with a smooth, tapered appearance in the subclavian, axillary and proximal brachial arteries. Femoral arteries and their branches are less commonly involved. Positron emission tomography (PET) using 18-fluoro-deoxyglucose (FDG) is a promising experimental technique for the diagnosis of large-vessel GCA (Blockmans et al., 1999) but is not routinely employed in clinical practice.

A chest X-ray at yearly intervals is adequate to screen for thoracic aortic aneurysm in patients with GCA. However, the best imaging modalities to evaluate aortic aneurysms or dissections are CT or MR scanning. A thickened aortic wall on CT or MRI is a direct finding of inflammation of the aortic wall, an indication that the disease is active (Stanson, 2000).

Pericardial effusion, coronary ischemia and occlusion are unusual manifestations of GCA (Guillaume et al., 1991; Paulley, 1980a,b).

4.2.2. Takayasu's arteritis

Takayasu's arteritis is an obliterative GCA, which is most frequently seen in young women, 15–25 years old, in Asian countries such as India, South America and Africa, rather than Europe and United States. It affects the aortic arch and its proximal branches. Distribution of the arteries involved also varies according to geography, since abdominal branch involvement is mostly seen in Europe, India and the United States. The disease characteristically evolves in three phases (Kerr, 1994). Systemic symptoms develop and then resolve over several weeks, while arteritis takes root. This arteritis also resolves, with an ensuing asymptomatic period (mean duration of 8 years) before vaso-occlusive signs and symptoms develop. During the initial phase, systemic symptoms are noted only in less than half of the cases, especially European patients, whereas they are rare in Japanese patients. The disease is monophasic and self-limited for 20% of the patients.

Severe cardiovascular complications of Takayasu's arteritis are caused by fibrotic thickening of the aortic arch and its branches and, more rarely, complicated by thromboembolic events. Aortic regurgitation and aneurysm formation, particularly in descending thoracic aorta have been described (Kumar et al., 1990). Histological findings are granulomatous inflammation and adventitial sclerosis, predominantly at the adventia-media junction. Necrosis is unusual. Occasionally, vascular inflammation spreads from the aorta to the proximal epicardial coronary arteries and may cause coronary insufficiency and myocardial infarctions (Rosen and Gaton, 1972).

4.3. Medium-sized vessel vasculitides

4.3.1. Polyarteritis nodosa

PAN is a systemic necrotizing vasculitis affecting medium-sized arteries of various organs, but which also often affects small vessels. Multiple organs or systems, most frequently kidneys, skin, muscle, gastrointestinal tract and the nervous system, may be involved. The diagnosis is made by biopsy of affected tissue(s) and/or by angiography revealing characteristic microaneurysms and/or stenoses.

Cardiac involvement in PAN, which was already mentioned in the first publication (Küssmaul and Maier, 1866) which described a case of 'nodular coronaritis', was subsequently reported with frequencies ranging from 10% in clinical studies of PAN patients (Frohnert and Sheps, 1967) to 78% in histopathological study (Holsinger et al., 1962). Main results of published clinical studies are listed in Table 3.

Congestive heart failure is the main manifestation, occurring in 6–57% in PAN (Frohnert and Sheps, 1967; Holsinger et al., 1962). It is specific and/or can result from other vasculitis-related organ involvement or disorders, mainly hypertension and/or renal involvement (Blétry et al., 1980). Specific cardiomyopathy could occur as early as the 3rd to 4th month after PAN onset. Interstitial myocarditis was seen in 14% of autopsied patients (Schrader et al., 1985).

Congestive heart failure may thus also be attributed to coronary artery or myocardial arteriolar infarcts, caused by immune complex deposition, resulting in disseminated necrotic foci, mostly in the left ventricle. The right ventricle may also be involved, as reported for 6/8 patients with heart involvement (Blétry et al., 1980). However, clinical angina is rare, reported in 2–18% of patients (Blétry et al., 1980; Frohnert and Sheps, 1967), as are myocardial infarctions diagnosed during patients' life in 1–12%, whereas the latter were a common finding at autopsy (Frohnert and Sheps, 1967). Among 66 autopsied patients, 41 had features of myocardial infarction, but only three of them had clinical symptoms and three had coronary atherosclerosis (Holsinger et al., 1962). Schrader et al. (1985) autopsied 36 PAN patients, 50% of whom had evidence of coronary arteritis, with severe lesions involving small subepicardial vessels just as they entered the myocardium and 8% had gross infarcts.

In 85% of the patients with clinical signs of infarction, angiography can prove coronary involvement (Fig. 2). In the remaining 15%, infarction may be due to arteritis in small coronary vessels or spasms (Rajani et al., 1991). Coronary aneurysms were found in 9% of children with PAN (Takahashi, 1993). To date, no guidelines regarding the indications and modes of exploration of the coronary arteries have been formulated for PAN patients without cardiac symptoms.

Murmurs are frequent, having been noted in 28% (Godeau et al., 1985) to 39% (Holsinger et al., 1962) of vasculitis patients. In most cases, they are innocuous, underlining the rarity of valve involvement in PAN. However, some patients with mitral and tricuspid regurgitation supposedly specifically related to PAN have been reported (Blétry et al., 1980; Gunal et al., 1997).

Pericardial involvement occurs in 0–5% of PAN patients (Hu et al., 1997), rising to 19% (Schrader et al., 1985) to one-third (Holsinger et al., 1962) in autopsy series. About half of the first reported cases of pericardial effusion were indeed secondary to uremia, which is much less frequent nowadays since diagnosis and therapeutic management of PAN patients have improved.

Sinus tachycardia is usual and non-specific. Arrhythmias and conduction disorders, mainly supraventricular, can occur in 2–19% of patients (Blétry et al., 1980; Holsinger et al., 1962) because of arteritis of the sinus node or neighboring nerve fibers.

Aortic dissection is a rare complication, resulting from diffuse vasculitis of the vasa vasorum, but was reported in one patient with HBV-related PAN which evolved to fatal tamponade (Iino et al., 1992). Dissections of proximal aortic branches have also been reported, but some were attributed to other causes, such as atherosclerotic aneurysms (Bookman et al., 1983; Hachulla et al., 1993; Hautekeete et al., 1990; Lomeo et al., 1989), syphilis, cystic media necrosis, trauma, sepsis, or hypertension.

4.3.2. Kawasaki disease

Kawasaki disease, or mucocutaneaous lymph-node syndrome (Kawasaki, 1967), affects children mostly those aged 8–24 months in North America and 6–11 months in Asia, and is associated with arterial vasculitis. Although inflammation is present in medium-sized and small arteries throughout the

Table 3
Frequencies of organ/system involvement in, or manifestation, of polyarteritis nodosa

Reference	No. of patients	Organ/system involved or manifestation (%)						
		Heart	HTA	Skin	CNS	PNS	Kidney	GI
Gunal et al. (1997)	15	67	20	20	0	0	13	47
Schrader et al. (1985)	36	61	72	–	–	–	76	–
Fortin et al. (1995)	45	18	–	44	24	51	44	53
Frohnert and Sheps (1967)	130	10	–	58	3	52	8	14
Guillevin et al. (1988)	165	23	31	46	17	67	29	31

CNS, central nervous system; HTA, hypertension; GI, gastrointestinal tract; PNS, peripheral nervous system.

body, coronary arteries are the main target. Kawasaki disease is now recognized as the leading cause of acquired heart disease in children in the developed world. Epidemiology (endemic clusters and epidemic flares) and clinical features of the disease strongly suggest an infectious triggering agent, consistent with superantigen activity. Many superantigen-producing organisms have already been isolated from patients with this entity, including *Propionibacterium acnes*, streptococci and staphylococci; and a murine model of coronary arteritis has been developed based on infection with *Lactobacillus casei* (Duong et al., 2003). However, the mechanisms leading to the localized coronary arteritis of Kawasaki disease remain to be elucidated.

Up to 20% of untreated children develop coronary artery aneurysms, with a peak 3–4 weeks into the illness. Because these lesions can be detected by echocardiography, it is recommended as early as the 7th day after first disease manifestations appear, since aneurysms can occur early. Fewer than 1–2% of the patients succumb to sudden death due to coronary artery thrombosis or aneurysm rupture with subsequent acute myocardial infarctions (responsible for 80% of the deaths), myopericarditis, congestive heart failure and/or arrhythmia. More than half of small and moderate-sized coronary artery aneurysms regress over several years (Kato et al., 1996). Patients with persistent large coronary artery aneurysms may, however, develop acute coronary syndromes in adulthood (Takahashi, 1993).

Half the patients may have electrocardiographic abnormalities (first degree atrioventricular block, or sinus tachycardia, but rarely ventricular arrhythmia). Myocarditis and pericarditis are rare, occurring in half and 25% of the patients with cardiac complications during the initial phase of the disease, respectively.

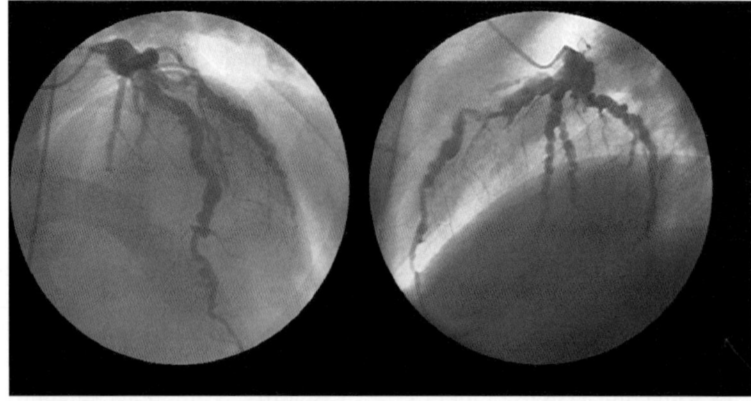

Figure 2. Multiple coronary artery aneurysms and irregular narrowing in a patient with polyarteritis nodosa.

Mitral insufficiency has been observed in less than 1% of the cases and aortic regurgitation even less frequently.

4.4. Small vessel vasculitides

4.4.1. Wegener's granulomatosis

WG is characterized by granulomatous-necrotizing vasculitis, which most commonly affects the upper and lower respiratory tracts and kidneys. Klinger (1931) was the first to describe the disorder, followed 5 years later by Wegener (1936). Evidence of C-ANCA, detected in the sera of more than 80% of WG patients with systemic forms (Kallenberg et al., 1992), is useful in making the diagnosis.

Cardiac involvement is traditionally thought to be rare in WG, even though it has been reported in 6% to almost 30% of autopsied cases (Pinching et al., 1983; Walton, 1958). In clinical studies, it varies from 0% (Anderson et al., 1992) to 12% (Fauci et al., 1983). Organ/system involvement in WG patients is summarized in Table 4. Pericarditis and coronary arteritis occur in half the patients with cardiac involvement and are the most common manifestations of it (Goodfield et al., 1995), but myocarditis (25%), valvulitis (21%), conduction system granulomata (17%), sinus node arteritis (13%), atrioventricular node arteritis (13%), myocardial infarction (11%), and epicarditis (8%) have also been reported (Forstot et al., 1980). An intracardiac mass was observed in one patient (Kosovsky et al., 1991).

Pericarditis is common, sometimes progressing to tamponade or to constrictive pericarditis (Grant et al., 1994; Schiavone et al., 1985).

Coronary arteritis, as in PAN, is clinically silent in most WG patients, but can nonetheless be responsible for foci of myocardial infarcts and eventually lead to congestive heart failure, with left ventricular systolic dysfunction detected echocardiographically in 22% of the patients (Morelli et al., 2000).

Valvular involvement, mostly affecting the aortic valve, has been more frequently reported during the past 10 years. This finding is extremely rare in our personal experience. Among 14 patients, eight had aortic regurgitation, and eight had mitral regurgitation (Greidinger et al., 1996). Systematic echocardiography of nine WG patients detected aortic valve

Table 4
Frequencies of organ/system involvement in, or manifestation, of Wegener's granulomatosis

Reference	No. of patients	Organ/system involved or manifestation (%)								
		Heart	Lung	Kidney	Skin	GI	ENT	CNS	PNS	NS
Morelli et al. (2000)[a]	9	88	55	44	44	44	78	–	–	44
Pinching et al. (1983)	18	44	100	100	67	–	94	44	67	–
Walton, 1958)[b]	56	–/11/28	48/81/78	25/67/78	46/–/17	–/–/24	89/52/26	–/7/–	–/29/7	–
Koldingsnes and Nossent (2003)	56	20	61	80	34	5	80	13	23	–
Fauci et al. (1983)	85	12	94	85	45	–	91	–	–	22
Reinhold-Keller et al. (2000)	155	12.9	55	53.5	23.2	–	93.5	–	20.6	–
Hoffman et al. (1992)	158	6	85	72	46	–	92	8	15	
Lie (1997)	216	2.8	69	48	12.4	6.5	87	8.3	–	–
Anderson et al. (1992)	265	<4	63	60	25	–	75	–	–	–

CNS, central nervous system; ENT, ear, nose and throat; GI, gastrointestinal tract; NS, nervous system; PNS, peripheral nervous system.

[a] Ultrasonographic study.

[b] Autopsy study (autopsy was performed in 54 out of the 56 patients). Percentages refer to clinical manifestations noted prior to death/presence of granulomas/arteritis observed at post-mortem histological examination.

abnormalities in 88% (ranging from mild non-specific thickening to more severe insufficiency requiring valve replacement in three), mitral involvement in 33%, tricuspid in 33%, and pulmonary in 11% (Morelli et al., 2000); only two of them had clinical symptoms. Valvular involvement was present at diagnosis in 40%, occurred during the first month of treatment in 40%, and later in 20%. Aortic valve insufficiency or regurgitation may be due to distortion and thickening of the aortic cusps and/or cusp perforation resulting from local vascular necrosis during the active phase of disease (Davenport et al., 1994), or to late dilatation of the aortic root (Grant et al., 1994). Rare aortic valve vegetations have been described, in which both vasculitis and bacteria-culture-negative endocarditis might have coexisted (Anthony et al., 1999; Wagner et al., 1991). Notably, histopathological examination of the valves usually revealed only non-specific abnormalities such as fibrinoid connective tissue damage with swelling and fragmentation of the collagen fibrils, and mononuclear cell and neutrophil infiltration.

The most common electrocardiographic manifestations are atrial arrhythmias (Forstot et al., 1980), which usually revert with treatment. Conduction tissue may be involved, affecting sinus rather than atrioventricular nodes or bundle branches. Complete heart blocks have been reported that also rapidly reverted under steroid and cyclophosphamide therapy, even though transient use of pacemaker was necessary in some cases (Forstot et al., 1980; Handa et al., 1997; Schiavone et al., 1985; Suleymenlar et al., 2002).

WG is a vasculitis of small and medium-sized and vessels and therefore involvement of the aorta and its proximal branches is not expected. However, they, as well as the more distal branches such as iliac or popliteal arteries (Allen et al., 1984) can sometimes be involved, causing proximal dilatation (Grant et al., 1994), dissection (Blockmans et al., 2000) or thickening (Fink et al., 1994; Goodfield et al., 1995). Associations of GCA and WG have been reported (Small and Brisson, 1991) and may explain some of these overlapping features.

4.4.2. Churg–Strauss Syndrome

The first description of CSS was published in 1951 (Churg and Strauss, 1951). This vasculitis usually occurs during the fourth decade of life and is characterized by a history of asthma and paranasal sinus disease, non-fixed pulmonary infiltrates on chest films, eosinophilia exceeding 10%, and may affect multiple organs or systems (Table 5).

Five-year survival of untreated CSS patients was 25%, compared to over 80% now with immunosuppressive therapy (Guillevin et al., 1996). Cardiac involvement is the major cause of mortality (Balestrieri et al., 1992), accounting for 48% of deaths (Lanham et al., 1985).

Heart involvement is frequent, 60% according to the princeps study (Churg and Strauss, 1951) and heart failure may affect up to 47% of CSS patients (Lanham et al., 1985). Cardiomyopathy may result from vasculitis-related ischemia affecting small myocardial vessels and coronary arteries (Hellemans et al., 1997), from myocardial eosinophilic infiltration sometimes followed by fibrotic scar tissue or, more rarely, from granulomatous infiltration of the myocardium (Cohen et al., 1995). We found heart involvement in 35% of 112 CSS patients enrolled in ongoing therapeutic trials (unpublished data). Preliminary analyses showed cardiac manifestations to be significantly more frequent in ANCA-negative patients, suggesting that different pathogenic mechanisms are at work in CSS affecting the heart rather than the kidney, e.g.

Many features of CSS cardiomyopathy are shared with eosinophilic endomyocardiopathy, which includes different pathologies: idiopathic hypereosinophilic syndrome, hypersensitivity myocarditis, Loeffler's disease and endomyocardial fibrosis, transplant rejection, giant cell myocarditis, toxic myocarditis, parasitic infections, eosinophilic leukemias, T-cell lymphomas and carcinomas (Pearce et al., 1999). During the first stage of these eosinophilic cardiomyopathies, eosinophils infiltrate the tissue and the proteins (major basic protein, cationic protein, eosinophil derived neurotoxin) they release induce local toxic reactions (Tai et al., 1984; Terasaki et al., 1997) that potentially evolve to scarring and fibrosis. However, CSS is distinguished from idiopathic hypersensitivity syndrome by its less intense eosinophilic infiltration, less frequent fibrosis, and the presence of myocardial foci of necrosis and angiitis.

Myocarditis can lead to restrictive (Kitschke et al., 1986; Lanham et al., 1985), congestive (Terasaki et al., 1997) or dilated cardiomyopathy (Morgan

Table 5
Frequencies of organ/system involvement in, or manifestation, of Churg–Strauss syndrome

Reference	No. of patients	Organ/system involved or manifestation (%)							
		Heart	Asthma	Kidney	Skin	GI	ENT	CNS	PNS
Lanham et al. (1984)	16	47	100	49	48	59	70	–	66
Haas et al. (2001)	20	50	100	35	75	50	45	–	65
Guillevin et al. (1999a)	96	Myocarditis 14 Pericarditis 23	100	26	51	33	61	8.3	78

CNS, central nervous system; ENT, ear, nose and throat; GI, gastrointestinal tract; PNS, peripheral nervous system.

et al., 1989; Terasaki et al., 1997) with heart failure, and myocardial infarction (Scolyer, 1999). By echocardiography, left ventricle dilatation was seen in 33% of CSS patients, the shortening fraction was reduced in 25%, and the amplitude of the overall wall echogenicity was increased in 100% (possibly related to a fibrotic process), and persisted even when disease has become inactive under therapy and other manifestations had subsided (Morgan et al., 1989). Endomyocardial biopsies from CSS patients may show acute inflammatory changes, with the presence of eosinophils or fibrosis, but rarely necrotizing vasculitis or extravascular granuloma (Alvarez-Sala et al., 1995; Hellemans et al., 1997; Leung et al., 1989). Cardiomyopathy can sometimes lead to the gradual build-up of large overlying intraventricular thrombi (Lanham et al., 1985) or masses (Yamashita et al., 1998), which usually decrease in size with therapy and could therefore be considered extra-vascular granulomas.

Acute and chronic constrictive pericarditides, valvular disease and sudden cardiac arrest are other known features of heart involvement in CSS (Azzopardi et al., 1999).

Pericardial effusion occurs in up to 22% of CSS patients. Tamponade has been reported and is usually easily controlled with corticosteroids, but may have a relapsing course (Hasley et al., 1990). Pericardial biopsy or pericardiectomy may show granulomatous nodules in the epicardium and can serve as the basis for a histological diagnosis of CSS (Sharma et al., 1993).

Among 12 CSS patients evaluated echocardiographically, half had mitral regurgitation, without cusp abnormalities, perhaps as a consequence of subendocardial fibrosis, and two of them required valve replacement (Morgan et al., 1989).

Conduction disorders and supraventricular arrhythmias may result from myocarditis, and usually respond to corticosteroids; however, some cases of ventricular fibrillation and fatal bradycardia have been reported (Fong et al., 1992; Rabusin et al., 1998).

Although steroids and immunosuppressants may be effective during the early stages of CSS myocarditis, fibrosis or residual cardiac insufficiency may thereafter progress on their own and require heart transplantation. The results of heart engraftments in CSS have been mitigated: one recipient had no CSS recurrence, but died of infectious complications 3 years post-transplant (Yeatman et al., 1996) and CSS reappeared either in the transplanted heart (Henderson et al., 1993) or at extracardiac sites (Thomson et al., 1989) despite potent immunosuppression in the other patients.

4.4.3. Microscopic polyangiitis

The rare reports on cardiovascular complications of MPA could, at least in part, be explained by the fact that some of the earlier patients diagnosed as having PAN probably had MPA. We described 85 MPA patients, in whom heart failure and pericarditis occurred at respective frequencies of 17.6 and 10% (Guillevin et al., 1999b). Severe acute congestive heart failure had been reported, but rarely with documented myocardial infarction due to small vessel arteritis (Wang et al., 2002). However, subclinical myocardial infarctions may be more frequent, as in PAN and other small vessel vasculitides. MPA with lung and kidney involvement appears to be associated with P-ANCA whereas heart involvement may be more frequent in ANCA-negative patients (Wang et al., 2002) as in CSS.

4.4.4. Henoch-Schönlein purpura

Henoch-Schönlein purpura affects people of all ages, but is mainly a disease of children under 10 years, and usually involves skin, gut, joints, and kidneys. Heart involvement is uncommon but can be severe, even if it generally responds to immunosuppressive therapy. IgA and C3 deposits have been detected in intramyocardial vessel walls in right ventricular endomyocardial biopsies from one patient; they resolved under immunosuppressive therapy (Kereiakes et al., 1984). Myocardial infarction (Agraharkar et al., 2000), conduction abnormalities and/or congestive heart failure (Imai and Matsumoto, 1970) have also been reported.

4.4.5. Cryoglobulinemic vasculitis

More than 80% of the cases of mixed cryoglobulinemia are now attributed to HCV infection (Ferri et al., 1991a; Rieu et al., 2002). The heart may be involved, as in other small vessel vasculitides. Congestive heart failure may be seen in up to 30% of the patients, even though myocardial infarction is often clinically silent, concerning less than 8.5% of the patients, and rarely diagnosed during the patients' lifetime (Rieu et al., 2002). Pericarditis, mitral and/or aortic insufficiencies have occasionally been reported (Brouet et al., 1974; Gorevic et al., 1980).

4.5. Other vasculitic diseases

4.5.1. Behçet's disease

Behçet's disease occurs in young patients, predominantly male (80%), with no other known cardiovascular risk factor. The underlying process is vasculitis of small vessels of the vasa vasorum, with subsequent damage, including thrombosis, occlusions and/or aneurysm formation, with a risk of rupture and hemorrhages (Somer, 1993). Cardiac and arterial manifestations have been reported, respectively, in 1–16% (Lakhanpal et al., 1985; Shimizu et al., 1979) and 2.2–34% (Hamza, 1987; Lakhanpal et al., 1985; Somer, 1993) of the patients with Behçet's disease. Cardiovascular manifestations occur within the first year after diagnosis in one-quarter of the cases, and can even reveal the disease. Venous lesions (30% of the patients) are more common than arterial disease. Most arterial involvement is clinically silent (Lakhanpal et al., 1985; Wechsler et al., 1999). The main localizations are the abdominal aorta and the pulmonary arteries. Pulmonary artery aneurysms and/or thrombosis, with subsequent caval syndrome (Hughes–Stovin syndrome), may occur in 1.1% of the patients and carries a poor prognosis (Durieux et al., 1981; Hamuryudan et al., 1994; Stricker and Malinverni, 1989). Cardiac involvement includes mainly pericarditis (40% of all cardiac manifestations), which usually responds to anti-inflammatory drugs or corticosteroids, and coronary artery disease (33% of the cardiac manifestations) (Blétry et al., 1988). Most of the coronary artery lesions are proximal and manifestations include occlusions, stenoses, aneurysms or spasms. Coronary thrombosing arteritis has been histologically documented in some cases (Lakhanpal et al., 1985; Schiff et al., 1982). Mortality of patients with coronary disease reaches 20% within the first months or years following diagnosis. Myocarditis is uncommon, representing only 7% of cardiac manifestations (Lakhanpal et al., 1985). However, echocardiographic diastolic dysfunction may occur in up to 37% of Behçet's disease patients (Calguneri et al., 1993). Fibrotic endomyocardiopathy has been reported infrequently (Huong et al., 1997), as were intraventricular thrombi, which usually regressed on anticoagulants (Islim et al., 1994). Valve involvement may occur (Chikamori et al., 1990), primarily aortic regurgitation (due to cusp perforation, prolapsus or aortic root dilatation), followed by mitral and/or tricuspid regurgitations.

4.5.2. Buerger's disease

Inflammation of the vessels of the hands and feet is commonly associated in Buerger's disease with thromboses and microabscesses, which are thought to be secondary to vasospastic arterial occlusions, responsible for chronic ischemia and tissue necroses. The coronary arteries and myocardium are rarely affected and may be seen only as another clinical consequence of tobacco toxicity, known to be the leading causative factor of this disease (Joyce, 1990; Shionoya, 1993; Somer, 1993).

4.5.3. Cogan's syndrome

Cogan's syndrome is a disease of young adults, with a median age at onset of 25 years, and of unknown etiology. It associates ocular manifestations, with interstitial keratitis being the hallmark of the disease, and audiovestibular symptoms like sensorineural hearing loss or vertigo. Half the patients may have systemic features (fever and/or weight loss) and up to 15% may have vasculitis involving small, medium-sized and/or large vessels (Vollertsen et al., 1986). In addition to a poor functional prognosis, patient outcome depends on the presence, or absence, of cardiovascular manifestations. The estimated 2-year overall mortality of patients with Cogan's syndrome is 9%. Aortic insufficiency may be seen in up to 14% of the patients, while inflammatory proximal aortitis, which involves all the aortic wall layers, may occur in 10%, and is usually associated with ostium coronary artery stenosis. Distal coronary artery stenoses and aneurysms, pericarditis, and conductive heart tissue involvement have also been reported (Cochrane and Tatoulis, 1991).

4.6. Restrictive myocardial idiopathic vasculitis

Rare cases of myocardial vasculitis have been published (Frustaci et al., 1997) that were characterized by idiopathic compromised diastolic function, mild increase of left ventricular wall thickness and pulmonary hypertension, with no ANCA, no extracardiac manifestations suggestive of vasculitis and a normal eosinophil count. Histology may reveal periarteriolar and perivenular inflammation with focal fibrinoid necrosis of the vascular wall and microaneurysm formation or only moderate interstitial fibrosis and cellular hypertrophy (Rapezzi et al., 1990). Although some cases evolved to restrictive cardiomyopathy requiring heart transplantation, most regressed under immunosuppression with cyclophosphamide and corticosteroids (Frustaci et al., 1997).

4.7. Hypersensitivity myocarditis

Hypersensitivity myocarditis is relatively rare. Its clinical signs are non-specific, occur in the setting of generalized drug reactions with eosinophilia, and can mimic vasculitis. Among many drugs that have been linked to the development of hypersensitivity myocarditis, the main ones include: sulfonamides, methyldopa, and penicillins, which are incriminated in 75% of cases (Kounis et al., 1989). Prior uneventful exposure to the suspected medication is one of the criteria for diagnosing hypersensitivity myocarditis. Reactive drugs metabolites would act as haptens, triggering a local antigenic response, when they bind to myocardial collagen fibrils, and an earlier systemic reaction, that finally activating macrophages and T lymphocytes (mainly CD45RO + memory T cells). In situ cytokine release would attract eosinophils to the interstitial and perivascular myocardium, where they in turn would release their toxic degranulation products. Diagnosis relies on endomyocardial biopsy (Kendell et al., 1995; Kounis et al., 1989). No vasculitis is seen and myocardial damage is usually less extensive than in CSS. Tachycardia, ST-segment or T-wave changes, mild cardiomegaly and slightly elevated cardiac enzymes can be observed. After withdrawal of the responsible medication, the majority of the patients recovers in a few days without sequelae. Immunosuppressive treatment may, however, be required when cardiac involvement is severe and/or because of late diagnosis.

5. Evolution and prognostic factors

The outcome of vasculitis differs from one disease to another and the relapse rate also varies, from 5% for HBV-related PAN (Guillevin et al., 1995b) to 23.4% for CSS (Guillevin et al., 1999b), 34.1% for MPA (Guillevin et al., 1999b) and more than 50% for WG (Guillevin et al., 1995c; Hoffman et al., 1992). Cardiac involvement may dramatically worsen the prognosis, particularly for CSS patients. Death due to acute heart failure, arrhythmia or massive myocardial infarction can occur during the initial acute phase, or later during the course of the disease, from refractory residual cardiac failure.

According to multivariate analysis of the characteristics of 342 patients with PAN or CSS, specific cardiac, renal, gastrointestinal and/or CNS involvements have been shown to be associated with poor outcome (Guillevin et al., 1996). A prognostic score,

Table 6a
The five factor score attributes, as established in 342 patients with polyarteritis nodosa or Churg–Strauss syndrome (Guillevin et al., 1996)

Proteinuria > 1 g/24 h
Creatininemia > 140 μmol/l
Specific gastrointestinal involvement
Specific cardiomyopathy
Specific CNS involvement

1 point for each of these five items when present.

the five-factor score (FFS, see Tables 6a and b), has thus been devised, which includes all these parameters. Five-year mortality is 12% when FFS is null, 26% when FFS is 1, and 46% when FFS is 2 or more ($p < 0.001$). Application of the FFS to MPA patients has also been validated (Gayraud et al., 2001).

Cardiac involvement has also been included in another scale aimed to assess the activity of systemic necrotizing vasculitis, the Birmingham vasculitis activity score (BVAS) (Luqmani et al., 1994; Stone et al., 2001). Cardiac manifestations included in the BVAS are new loss of pulse(s) with/without threatened loss of limb, aortic incompetence, myocardial infarction/angina, cardiomyopathy, bruits, and pericarditis. However, because this score was designed only to reflect the severity and current extent of active disease in patients, its use should be restricted to the evaluation of therapeutic efficacy, primarily in trials.

Cardiac involvement in vasculitides may leave sequelae, which can also hamper the overall outcome of the patients. A scoring system has been developed to assess organ damage in systemic necrotizing vasculitides, the vasculitis damage index (VDI) (Exley et al., 1997). It includes the following cardiovascular manifestations: angina/coronary bypass, myocardial infarction, second myocardial infarction, cardiomyopathy, valvular disease, pericarditis, and hypertension. Mortality was retrospectively shown to correlate with the VDI.

Table 6b

FFS	5-Year survival rate (%)	Relative risk
0	88.1	0.62
1	74.1*	1.35
≥2	54.1**	2.40

$*p < 0.005$ and $**p < 0.0001$ as compared to patients with FFS = 0.

6. Treatment

In combination with symptomatic therapies (e.g. angiotensin inhibitors, angiotensin II-receptor blockers, antiarrhythmic drugs, anticoagulants) or cardiac surgery (valve replacement, pericardiectomy) when needed, specific treatments for these vasculitides have to be used in patients with vasculitis and cardiovascular involvement. Before the introduction of corticosteroids (CS) in the 1970s, survival was 10% for untreated PAN patients (Frohnert and Sheps, 1967). Since then, it has increased to 55% with the use of CS alone, and to 82% at 5 years with combined CS and immunosuppressive therapy (Guillevin et al., 1988; Leib et al., 1979). Therapeutic decisions to treat and with which agents should rely on the presence or not of FFS factor(s) of poor prognosis. Evaluation of a patient's status under treatment and afterwards may be improved by using BVAS and VDI.

6.1. Large vessel vasculitides

6.1.1. Giant cell arteritis

CS are the drug of choice to treat GCA with or without large vessel disease. An initial daily dose of at least 40–60 mg of prednisone or equivalent in single or divided doses is adequate in most cases of GCA (Salvarani et al., 2002). Initial intravenous pulse methylprednisolone (1000 mg every day for 3 days) can be tried in patients with recent or impending visual loss. CS may prevent, but usually do not reverse fixed visual loss.

The response to CS is rapid, with resolution of many symptoms after a few days of therapy. The absence of improvement should alert physicians to question the diagnosis. The initial dose is usually maintained for 2–4 weeks, then it can be gradually reduced each week or every 2 weeks by a maximum of 10% of the total daily dose. If CS doses are reduced or withdrawn too quickly, a relapse or recurrence of symptoms usually occurs. However, in about 30–50%

of the patients spontaneous disease exacerbations occur, more frequently in the first 2 years, independent of the CS reduction schedule (Andersson et al., 1986a,b; Salvarani et al., 1987). Regular monitoring of clinical symptoms, erythrocyte sedimentation rate (ESR) or C-reactive protein (CRP) values is the most useful way of following the patients. A treatment course of 1–2 years is often required. However, some may have a more chronic, relapsing course and require low doses of CS for several years. No consistently reliable predictors of duration of CS therapy have been found. CS-related adverse events, in particular osteoporotic fractures, are frequently observed during treatment course. In a 15-year survey, 58% of GCA patients developed major CS-related complications, occurring more frequently in patients over 75 and in those with a prednisone starting dose more than 40 mg/day (Nesher et al., 1994).

Calcium and vitamin D supplementation should be added to CS therapy in all patients with GCA. In the case of reduced bone mineral density, bisphosphonates are indicated.

Among cytotoxic agents, methotrexate (MTX) has been proposed as a CS-sparing drug in GCA with conflicting results (Salvarani et al., 2002). However, this drug may be added in patients who need high CS doses to control active disease and have developed major side effects. A recent pilot study found that infliximab was efficacious in patients with CS-resistant GCA (Cantini et al., 2001).

6.1.2. Takayasu's arteritis

Treatment is mainly aimed at countering the ischemic manifestations and thus relies on interventional radiology and, when necessary, vascular surgery and bypass procedures. CS (1 mg/kg/day) may be prescribed to patients with general systemic symptoms or when arterial disease appears to be extensive, which in practice would represent up to 80% of the patients (Kerr, 1994). In these more severe forms, immunosuppression may also be required, and might include cyclophosphamide (CYC) or MTX (Hoffman et al., 1994). However, about half of the patients who achieve remission will have further relapse(s); thereby implying the need for long-term therapy in some patients.

6.2. Medium-sized and small vessel vasculitides

6.2.1. Kawasaki disease

At the initial stage, prompt administration of salicylate and intravenous immunoglobulins is necessary, as they prevent the development and progression of coronary aneurysms and their complications (Murphy and Huhta, 1987; Newburger et al., 1991). Immunoglobulins (2 g/kg) should be administered in a single perfusion, associated with high dose oral aspirin (80–100 mg/kg/day) for the first 10 days, then decreased to 3–5 mg/kg/day with long-term maintenance therapy in patients who have developed coronary aneurysms (Leung et al., 1998). Coronary angioplasty, endarterial procedures or coronary bypass surgery may be needed in severe progressing forms (Sugimura et al., 1997).

6.2.2. Primary systemic necrotizing vasculitides

The therapeutic strategy for systemic necrotizing vasculitides comprises CS and immunosuppressants, like CYC. However, the combination of CS and immunosuppressants should be prescribed only for patients with severe forms of PAN, MPA, and CSS. When factors of poor prognosis are absent, CS alone can be prescribed. For systemic WG, the combination of CS and CYC, oral or pulses, should always be prescribed. Maintenance therapy with azathioprine or MTX is recommended. Alternative treatments using other immunosuppressants or immunomodulating agents can be prescribed for relapses or patients who do not respond to conventional regimens. The different therapeutic modalities should also be adapted to the patient's age and general condition.

6.2.3. Corticosteroids

Initial therapy for all necrotizing vasculitides with cardiac manifestations, should first include 1–3 days of methylprednisolone pulse (15 mg/kg/day), followed by high-dose oral prednisone (at least 1 mg/kg/day). This full oral dose should be maintained until clinical and biological improvement is achieved, generally within 1 month, and then gradually tapered over 12–18 months.

6.2.4. Cyclophosphamide

Fauci et al. (1979) demonstrated the efficacy of adjunctive CYC in patients whose vasculitides were not controlled with CS alone. Pulse IV CYC should be combined with CS for patients with PAN, MPA, or CSS and a FFS ≥ 1, like those with cardiomyopathy and every patient with systemic WG. Pulse therapy acts more rapidly and engenders fewer side effects (hemorrhagic cystitis, leukopenia) than oral administration. However, oral CYC is also effective as first-line therapy for WG, and may nonetheless achieve remission in patients who did not respond to the pulse CYC regimen (Gayraud et al., 1997; Généreau et al., 1994; Reinhold-Keller et al., 1993). Doses, intervals between pulses, and duration of CYC treatment have to be adjusted for each patient. Briefly, each CYC pulse (0.5–0.7 mg/m^2) is administered every 15 days for the first three boluses, then every 3 weeks (for WG and MPA) or monthly (for PAN and CSS). When preferred (in WG) or needed (e.g. after failure of pulse CYC), oral CYC (2 mg/kg/day) should be prescribed. The duration of CYC therapy varies according to the patient's status and to local physicians' practice, between 3 (for pulse CYC) and 18 months (for oral CYC) and to the subsequent use or otherwise of a maintenance therapy (required for WG and MPA). Many trials have been and/or are still being conducted throughout the world to determine the most accurate, effective and safe therapy, for each of these vasculitides.

In patients with cardiac dysfunction, hydration during pulse CYC administration has to be carefully monitored. However, the potential but rarely reported cardiac side effects of CYC (Gharib and Burnett, 2002; Hochster et al., 1995) must definitely not prevent its use in patients with specific cardiomyopathy, because CYC is clearly the most effective drug used to date. It has been shown that delaying treatment can favor the progression to myocardial infarction, intractable cardiac failure and eventual myocardial fibrosis in CSS patients with heart involvement. Conversely, it has been reported that the rare cases of valvulitis occurring in the context of CSS or WG responded to therapy (Gerbracht et al., 1987), as did conductive heart blocks, even though a pacemaker might be needed temporarily (Forstot et al., 1980; Handa et al., 1997; Schiavone et al., 1985; Suleymenlar et al., 2002).

6.2.5. Intravenous immunoglobulins

Because they can prevent aneurysms formation in Kawasaki disease, it may be expected that parenteral immunoglobulins would also be effective in ANCA-associated vasculitides. First reports of their use in patients with refractory vasculitides have yielded encouraging but mixed results. Forty to 92% of the patients with the latter (Jayne et al., 1991, 2000) responded, at least partially, but rates of complete remission and their long-term maintenance, have to be more closely analyzed in ongoing trials.

6.2.6. Other therapies

Plasma exchanges may be useful as second-line therapy for refractory PAN or MPA with rapidly progressive glomerulonephritis (Guillevin and Bussel, 2000; Pusey et al., 1991), but are contraindicated for patients with unstable cardiac conditions. Other immunosuppressants (MTX, azathioprine, mycophenolate mofetil) should preferentially be kept for maintenance therapy, when indicated, i.e. for WG and MPA, or PAN and CSS with multiple relapses (De Groot et al., 1996; Nowack et al., 1999). Cotrimoxazole may be beneficial as an adjuvant therapy in patients with systemic WG (Israel, 1988) or limited nasal and/or oral forms of WG (Le Thi Huong et al., 1990; Reinhold-Keller et al., 1996; Sangle et al., 2002). Dapsone or colchicine can help control some relapsing cutaneous manifestations of vasculitides (Thomas-Golbanov and Sridharan, 2001). Treatment with anti-TNFα antibodies may be promising for patients with intractable vasculitides (Bartolucci et al., 2002), but they would have to be carefully monitored since these antibodies are theoretically contraindicated in patients with coronary artery disease and/or heart failure (Weisman, 2002). Other therapeutics are still experimental, in pilot studies or of anecdotal use in refractory cases (bone marrow auto- or allografts (Thomas-Golbanov and Sridharan, 2001), anti-CD20 which also appears to be a very promising drug for vasculitides (Specks et al., 2001) and anti-CD52 monoclonal antibodies (Lockwood, 1998; Lockwood et al., 1996)).

6.2.7. Virus-related vasculitides

When vasculitides are related to viral infection, a specific approach is needed, combining antiviral treatments and plasma exchanges.

6.2.7.1. HBV-related polyarteritis nodosa

Because classical treatment with CS and CYC may worsen hepatic disease and stimulate viral replication in HBV-related PAN, a specific therapy has been established and validated for these patients (Guillevin et al., 1994, 2001). The therapeutic sequence should be as follows: initial CS to rapidly control life-threatening manifestations of PAN, which are common during the first weeks of the disease, and their abrupt withdrawal to enhance immunological clearance of HBV-infected hepatocytes and favor HBe antigen to anti-HBe antibody seroconversion; plasma exchanges to control the course of PAN, in combination with antiviral agents (lamivudine or IFNα-2b) for several months (Guillevin et al., 2001; Gupta et al., 2001). Immunosuppressants should only be given to those patients whose PAN manifestations worsen despite well-conducted therapy, as recommended.

6.2.7.2. HCV-related mixed cryoglobulinemic vasculitis

As for HBV-related PAN, antiviral drugs (ribavirin, Pegylated-IFNα) are to be used in symptomatic patients with mixed cryoglobulinemia when HCV infection is proven. However, the probability of sustaining long-term disappearance of the virus and cryoglobulin remains low, despite good initial responses (Cohen et al., 1996; Ferri et al., 1991b). Plasma exchanges might prove beneficial in severe forms with visceral involvement, but a rebound phenomenon is common after their discontinuation (Durand et al., 1998; Guillevin and Lhote, 1997; Lunel and Cacoub, 2000; Naarendorp et al., 2001; Rieu et al., 2002). CS and immunosuppressants are indicated only for patients who do not respond to antiviral drugs and plasma exchanges (Guillevin et al., 2000).

6.2.8. Henoch-Schönlein purpura

Patients with Henoch-Schönlein purpura and cardiac involvement must receive at least CS. There are no clear-cut data for the need and benefit of combining immunosuppressive therapy in patients with severe visceral involvement(s). Ongoing, prospective therapeutic trials, comparing treatment with CS alone or combined with pulse CYC, will probably answer that question in the next few years.

6.3. Other vasculitides

6.3.1. Behçet's disease

One hallmark of the arterial and cardiac involvement in Behçet's disease is the high relapse rate, despite surgical or endovascular interventions. However, for patients with arterial and aneurysmal manifestations, the 2-year relapse rate fell from almost all cases to 67% since CS therapy has been used and to 20% since immunosuppressants have been prescribed in combination with CS (monthly parenteral CYC or azathioprine for 12–24 months, followed by colchicine) (Wechsler et al., 1999; Yazici and Barnes, 1991). Coronary artery aneurysms seem to carry a poorer prognosis than stenoses and may therefore warrant immunosuppression. Valve disease and myocardial dysfunction(s) may resolve with CS alone. Because of the high frequency of thromboses, anticoagulants are widely prescribed.

6.3.2. Buerger's disease

First of all, tobacco use must be stopped. Vasodilators may be used to treat peripheral disease, with anti-platelet-aggregating agents, such as aspirin, or anticoagulants. When cardiac ischemic manifestations occur, patients should be managed as for common coronary artery disease (Shionoya, 1993). There are no indications for CS or immunosuppressants use to treat this entity.

6.3.3. Cogan's syndrome

While ocular manifestations may sometimes be treated with topical CS alone, audiovestibular and systemic features of Cogan's syndrome require systemic therapy, with CS and often immunosuppressants. No trial data are available to guide the therapeutic decisions. MTX, azathioprine, cyclosporin A and CYC have been used. Surgical valve replacement, radiological or surgical treatment of coronary artery involvement may be necessary (Raza et al., 1998; Vollertsen et al., 1986).

Key points

- Heart involvement may occur in vasculitides, but its frequency and manifestations vary according to the type of vasculitis.
- Cardio-vascular manifestations include cardiomyopathy (specific or resulting from myocardial infarctions), coronary arteritis (with risk of aneurysms, stenoses and thrombosis formation or rupture), pericarditis, valvulitis, conduction tissue involvement (with heart blocks), arrhythmias (mainly supraventricular), dissection of the aorta (and/or its proximal branches).
- Many of these cardiac manifestations may be clinically silent, at least during their early stages. Therefore, heart function should be systematically assessed in these patients, at least with ECG, and echocardiography, then with more appropriate or invasive explorations when abnormal or when symptoms occur.
- Specific cardiomyopathy has been identified as a factor of poor outcome in small and medium-sized vessel vasculitides (FFS). In addition to symptomatic treatments, prescription of corticosteroids and immunosuppressants (mainly cyclophosphamide) is considered mandatory for these diseases. This therapy has dramatically improved the overall prognosis of the affected patients.

References

Agraharkar, M., Gokhale, S., Le, L., Rajaraman, S., Campbell, G.A. 2000. Cardiopulmonary manifestations of Henoch-Schönlein purpura. Am. J. Kidney Dis. 35, 319.

Allen, D.C., Doherty, C.C., O'Reilly, D.P. 1984. Pathology of the heart and the cardiac conduction system in Wegener's granulomatosis. Br. Heart J. 52, 674.

Alvarez-Sala, R., Prados, C., Armada, E., Del Arco, A., Villamor, J. 1995. Congestive cardiomyopathy and endobronchial granulomas as manifestations of Churg–Strauss syndrome. Postgrad. Med. J. 71, 365.

Andersson, R., Malmvall, B.E., Bengtsson, B.A. 1986a. Long-term corticosteroid treatment in giant cell arteritis. Acta Med. Scand. 220, 465.

Andersson, R., Malmvall, B.E., Bengtsson, B.A. 1986b. Long-term survival in giant cell arteritis including temporal arteritis and polymyalgia rheumatica. A follow-up study of 90 patients treated with corticosteroids. Acta Med. Scand. 220, 361.

Anderson, G., Coles, E.T., Crane, M., Douglas, A.C., Gibbs, A.R., Geddes, D.M., Gibbs, Peel, E.T., Wood, J.B. 1992. Wegener's granuloma. A series of 265 British cases seen between 1975 and 1985. A report by a sub-committee of the British Thoracic Society Research Committee. QJM 83, 427.

Anthony, D.D., Askari, A.D., Wolpaw, T., McComsey, G. 1999. Wegener granulomatosis simulating bacterial endocarditis. Arch. Intern. Med. 159, 1807.

Ara, J., Mirapeix, E., Arrizabalaga, P., Rodriguez, R., Ascaso, C., Abellana, R., Font, J., Darnell, A. 2001. Circulating soluble adhesion molecules in ANCA-associated vasculitis. Nephrol. Dial. Transpl. 16, 276.

Arend, W.P., Michel, B.A., Bloch, D.A., Hunder, G.G., Calabrese, L.H., Edworthy, S.M., Fauci, A.S., Leavitt, R.Y., Lie, J.T., Lightfoot, R.W. 1990. The American College of Rheumatology 1990 criteria for the classification of Takayasu arteritis. Arthritis Rheum. 33, 1129.

Azzopardi, C., Montefort, S., Mallia, C. 1999. Cardiac involvement and left ventricular failure in a patient with the Churg–Strauss syndrome. Adv. Exp. Med. Biol. 455, 547.

Balding, C.E., Howie, A.J., Drake-Lee, A.B., Savage, C.O. 2001. Th2 dominance in nasal mucosa in patients with Wegener's granulomatosis. Clin. Exp. Immunol. 125, 332.

Balestrieri, G.P., Valentini, U., Cerudelli, B., Spandrio, S., Renaldini, E. 1992. Reversible myocardial impairment in the Churg–Strauss syndrome: report of a case. Clin. Exp. Rheumatol. 10, 75.

Bartolucci, P., Ramanoelina, J., Cohen, P., Mahr, A., Godmer, P., Le Hello, C., Guillevin, L. 2002. Efficacy of the anti-TNF-alpha antibody infliximab against refractory systemic vasculitides: an open pilot study on 10 patients. Rheumatology (Oxford) 41, 1126.

Becvar, R., Paleckova, A., Tesar, V., Rychlik, I., Masek, Z. 1997. Von Willebrand factor antigen and adhesive molecules in Wegener's granulomatosis and microscopic polyangiitis. Clin. Rheumatol. 16, 324.

Bely, M., Apathy, A. 1996. Vasculitis in rheumatoid arthritis. Orv. Hetil. 137, 1571 (in Czech).

Berbis, P., Carena, M.C., Auffranc, J.C., Privat, Y. 1986. Cutaneo-systemic necrotizing vasculitis occurring during desensitization. Ann. Dermatol. Venereol. 113, 805.

Blétry, O., Godeau, P., Charpentier, G., Guillevin, L., Herreman, G. 1980. Manifestations cardiaques de la périartérite noueuse. Fréquence de la cardiomyopathie non hypertensive. Arch. Mal. Cœur. Vaiss. 73, 1027.

Blétry, O., Mohattane, A., Wechsler, B., Beaufils, P., Valere, P., Petit, J., Gourgon, R., Grosgogeat, Y., Godeau, P. 1988. Cardiac involvement in Behçet's disease. 12 cases. Presse Méd 17, 2388 (in French).

Bligny, D., Mahr, A., Le Toumelin, P., Mouthon, L., Guillevin, L. 2003. Is the prognosis of Wegener's granulomatosis determined by the balance between granulomatosis and vasculitis? An analysis of survival in 93 patients with systemic Wegener's granulomatosis. Arthritis care and Research. 93 in press.

Bloch, D.A., Michel, B.A., Hunder, G.G., McShane, D.J., Arend, W.P., Calabrese, L.H. 1990. The American College of Rheumatology 1990 criteria for the classification of vasculitis. Patients and methods. Arthritis Rheum. 33, 1068.

Blockmans, D., Maes, A., Stroobants, S., Nuyts, J., Bormans, G., Knockaert, D., Bobbaers, H., Mortelmans, L. 1999. New arguments for a vasculitic nature of polymyalgia rheumatica using positron emission tomography. Rheumatology (Oxford) 38, 444.

Blockmans, D., Baeyens, H., Van Loon, R., Lauwers, G., Bobbaers, H. 2000. Periaortitis and aortic dissection due to Wegener's granulomatosis. Clin. Rheumatol. 19, 161.

Bookman, A.A., Goode, E., McLoughlin, M.J., Cohen, Z. 1983. Polyarteritis nodosa complicated by a ruptured intrahepatic aneurysm. Arthritis Rheum. 26, 106.

Brouet, J.C., Clauvel, J.P., Danon, F., Klein, M., Seligmann, M. 1974. Biologic and clinical significance of cryoglobulins. A report of 86 cases. Am. J. Med. 57, 775.

Bruno, P., Le Hello, C., Massetti, M., Babatasi, G., Saloux, E., Galateau, F., Khayat, A. 2000. Necrotizing granulomata of the aortic valve in Wegener's disease. J. Heart Valve Dis. 9, 633.

Calabrese, L.H., Michel, B.A., Bloch, D.A., Arend, W.P., Edworthy, S.M., Fauci, A.S., Fries, J.F., Hunder, G.G., Leavitt, R.Y., Lie, J.T. 1990. The American College of Rheumatology 1990 criteria for the classification of hypersensitivity vasculitis. Arthritis Rheum. 33, 1108.

Calguneri, M., Erbas, B., Kes, S., Karaaslan, Y. 1993. Alterations in left ventricular function in patients with Behçet's disease using radionuclide ventriculography and Doppler echocardiography. Cardiology 82, 309.

Cantini, F., Niccoli, L., Salvarani, C., Padula, A., Olivieri, I. 2001. Treatment of longstanding active giant cell arteritis with infliximab: report of four cases. Arthritis Rheum. 44, 2933.

Chan, T.M., Cheng, I.K. 1996. A prospective study on anti-endothelial cell antibodies in patients with systemic lupus erythematosus. Clin. Immunol. Immunopathol. 78, 41.

Chikamori, T., Doi, Y.L., Yonezawa, Y., Takata, J., Kawamura, M., Ozawa, T. 1990. Aortic regurgitation secondary to Behçet's disease. A case report and review of the literature. Eur. Heart J. 11, 572.

Chomette, G., Auriol, M., Tranbaloc, P. 1983. Anatomopathology of inflammatory arteriopathies. Peculiar aspects of giant cell arteritis. Ann. Méd. Interne (Paris) 134, 421 (in French).

Chumbley, L.C., Harrison, E.G. Jr., DeRemee, R.A. 1977. Allergic granulomatosis and angiitis (Churg–Strauss syndrome). Report and analysis of 30 cases. Mayo Clin. Proc. 52, 477.

Churg, J., Strauss, L. 1951. Allergic granulomatosis, allergic angiitis and periarteritis nodosa. Am. J. Pathol. 27, 277.

Cochrane, A.D., Tatoulis, J. 1991. Cogan's syndrome with aortitis, aortic regurgitation, and aortic arch vessel stenoses. Ann. Thorac. Surg. 52, 1166.

Cohen, A., Johnson, N., Prier, A., Zerbib, E., Chauvel, C., Kaplan, G., Valty, J. 1995. Segmental myocarditis in Churg–Strauss syndrome. Review of the literature apropos of a case. Rev. Méd. Interne 16, 58 (in French).

Cohen, P., Nguyen, Q.T., Dény, P., Ferriere, F., Roulot, D., Lortholary, O., Jarrousse, B., Danon, F., Barrier, J.H., Ceccaldi, J., Constans, J., Crickx, B., Fiessinger, J.N., Hachulla, E., Jaccard, A., Seligmann, M., Kazatchkine, M., Laroche, L., Subra, J.F., Turlure, P., Guillevin, L. 1996. Treatment of mixed cryoglobulinemia with recombinant interferon alpha and adjuvant therapies. A prospective study on 20 patients. Ann. Méd. Interne (Paris) 147, 81.

Comparato, E., Toso, M. 1977. A case of polyarteritis nodosa associated with pulmonary hypertension. Minerva Med. 68, 2963 (in Italian).

Cormier, J.M., Cormier, F., Laridon, D., Vuong, P.N. 2000. Horton's disease and aortic aneurysm: coincidence or causality? 5 cases. J. Mal. Vasc. 25, 92 (in French).

Csernok, E., Trabandt, A., Muller, A., Wang, G.C., Moosig, F., Paulsen, J., Schnabel, A., Gross, W.L. 1999. Cytokine profiles in Wegener's granulomatosis: predominance of type 1 (Th1) in the granulomatous inflammation. Arthritis Rheum. 42, 742.

Davenport, A., Goodfellow, J., Goel, S., Maciver, A.G., Walker, P. 1994. Aortic valve disease in patients with Wegener's granulomatosis. Am. J. Kidney Dis. 24, 205.

Davies, D.J., Moran, J.E., Niall, J.F., Ryan, G.B. 1982. Segmental necrotising glomerulonephritis with antineutrophil antibody: possible arbovirus aetiology? Br. Med. J. (Clin. Res. Ed.) 285, 606.

D'Cruz, D. 1998. Vasculitis in systemic lupus erythematosus. Lupus 7, 270.

De Groot, K., Reinhold-Keller, E., Tatsis, E., Paulsen, J., Heller, M., Nolle, B., Gross, W.L. 1996. Therapy for the maintenance of remission in sixty-five patients with generalized Wegener's granulomatosis. Methotrexate versus trimethoprim/sulfamethoxazole. Arthritis Rheum. 39, 2052.

D'Izarn, J.J., Boulet, C.P., Convard, J.P., Bonnin, A., Ledoux-Lebard, G. 1976. Arteriography in polyarteritis nodosa. 15 cases. J. Radiol. Electrol. Med. Nucl. 57, 505 (in French).

Drenkard, C., Villa, A.R., Reyes, E., Abello, M., Alarcon-Segovia, D. 1997. Vasculitis in systemic lupus erythematosus. Lupus 6, 235.

Duong, T.T., Silverman, E.D., Bissessar, M.V., Yeung, R.S. 2003. Superantigenic activity is responsible for induction of coronary arteritis in mice: an animal model of Kawasaki disease. Int. Immunol. 15, 79.

Durand, J.M., Cacoub, P., Lunel-Fabiani, F., Cosserat, J., Cretel, E., Kaplanski, G., Frances, C., Bletry, O., Soubeyrand, J., Godeau, P. 1998. Ribavirin in hepatitis C related cryoglobulinemia. J. Rheumatol. 25, 1115.

Durieux, P., Blétry, O., Huchon, G., Wechsler, B., Chrétien, J., Godeau, P. 1981. Multiple pulmonary arterial aneurysms in Behçet's disease and Hughes–Stovin syndrome. Am. J. Med. 71, 736.

Erkan, F., Gul, A., Tasali, E. 2001. Pulmonary manifestations of Behçet's disease. Thorax 56, 572.

Erkan, F., Kiyan, E., Tunaci, A. 2002. Pulmonary complications of Behçet's disease. Clin. Chest Med. 23, 493.

Evans, J.M., O'Fallon, W.M., Hunder, G.G. 1995. Increased incidence of aortic aneurysm and dissection in giant cell (temporal) arteritis. A population-based study. Ann. Intern. Med. 122, 502.

Ewert, B.H., Jennette, J.C., Falk, R.J. 1991. The pathogenic role of antineutrophil cytoplasmic autoantibodies. Am. J. Kidney Dis. 18, 188.

Exley, A.R., Bacon, P.A., Luqmani, R.A., Kitas, G.D., Gordon, C., Savage, C.O., Adu, D. 1997. Development and initial validation of the vasculitis damage index for the standardized clinical assessment of damage in the systemic vasculitides. Arthritis Rheum. 40, 371.

Falcini, F., Trapani, S., Turchini, S., Farsi, A., Ermini, M., Keser, G., Khamashta, M.A., Hughes, G.R. 1997. Immunological findings in Kawasaki disease: an evaluation in a cohort of Italian children. Clin. Exp. Rheumatol. 15, 685.

Falk, R.J., Jennette, J.C. 1988. Anti-neutrophil cytoplasmic autoantibodies with specificity for myeloperoxidase in patients with systemic vasculitis and idiopathic necrotizing and crescentic glomerulonephritis. N. Engl. J. Med. 318, 1651.

Fauci, A., Katz, P., Haynes, B., Wolff, S. 1979. Cyclophosphamide therapy of severe necrotizing vasculitis. N. Engl. J. Med. 301, 235–238.

Fauci, A.S., Haynes, B.F., Katz, P., Wolff, S.M. 1983. Wegener's granulomatosis: prospective clinical and therapeutic experience with 85 patients for 21 years. Ann. Intern. Med. 98, 76.

Ferri, C., Greco, F., Longombardo, G., Palla, P., Moretti, A., Marzo, E., Mazzoni, A., Pasero, G., Bombardieri, S., Highfield, P. 1991a. Association between hepatitis C virus and mixed cryoglobulinemia. Clin. Exp. Rheumatol. 9, 621.

Ferri, C., Marzo, E., Longombardo, G., Lombardini, F., Greco, F., Bombardieri, S. 1991b. Alpha interferon in the treatment of mixed cryoglobulinaemia patients. Eur. J. Cancer 27, S81.

Fink, A.M., Miles, K.A., Wraight, E.P. 1994. Indium-111 labelled leucocyte uptake in aortitis. Clin. Radiol. 49, 863.

Flores-Suarez, L.F., Cabiedes, J., Villa, A.R., van der Woude, F.J., Alcocer-Varela, J. 2003. Prevalence of antineutrophil cytoplasmic autoantibodies in patients with tuberculosis. Rheumatology (Oxford) 42, 223.

Fong, C., Schmidt, G., Cain, N., Cranswick, P., Tonkin, A.M. 1992. Churg–Strauss syndrome, cardiac involvement and life threatening ventricular arrhythmias. Aust. NZ J. Med. 22, 167.

Forstot, J.Z., Overlie, P.A., Neufeld, G.K., Harmon, C.E., Forstot, S.L. 1980. Cardiac complications of Wegener granulomatosis: a case report of complete heart block and review of the literature. Semin. Arthritis Rheum. 10, 148. Echocardiographic study in nine patients with WG revealing cardiac valve disease in eight of them.

Fortin, P.R., Larson, M.G., Watters, A.K., Yeadon, C.A., Choquette, D., Esdaile, J.M. 1995. Prognostic factors in systemic necrotizing vasculitis of the polyarteritis nodosa group—a review of 45 cases. J. Rheumatol. 22, 78–84.

Fox, A.D., Robbins, S.E. 1994. Aortic valvulitis complicating Wegener's granulomatosis. Thorax 49, 1176.

Fries, J.F., Hunder, G.G., Bloch, D.A., Michel, B.A., Arend, W.P., Calabrese, L.H. 1990. The American College of Rheumatology 1990 criteria for the classification of vasculitis. Arthritis Rheum. 33, 1135 (Summary).

Frohnert, P., Sheps, S. 1967. Long term follow-up study of periarteritis nodosa. Am. J. Med. 43, 8.

Frustaci, A., Chimenti, C., Pieroni, M. 1997. Idiopathic myocardial vasculitis presenting as restrictive cardiomyopathy. Chest 111, 1462.

Garcia-Porrua, C., Llorca, J., Gonzalez-Louzao, C., Gonzalez-Gay, M.A. 2001. Hypersensitivity vasculitis in adults: a benign disease usually limited to skin. Clin. Exp. Rheumatol. 19, 85.

Gayraud, M., Guillevin, L., Cohen, P., Lhote, F., Cacoub, P., Deblois, P., Godeau, B., Ruel, M., Vidal, E., Piontud, M., Ducroix, J.P., Lassoued, S., Christoforov, B., Babinet, P. 1997. Treatment of good-prognosis polyarteritis nodosa and Churg–Strauss syndrome: comparison of steroids and oral or pulse cyclophosphamide in 25 patients. French Cooperative Study Group for Vasculitides. Br. J. Rheumatol. 36, 1290.

Gayraud, M., Guillevin, L., Le Toumelin, P., Cohen, P., Lhote, F., Casassus, P., Jarousse, B. 2001. Long-term followup of polyarteritis nodosa, microscopic polyangiitis, and Churg–Strauss syndrome: analysis of four prospective trials including 278 patients. Arthritis Rheum. 44, 666.

Généreau, T., Lortholary, O., Leclerq, P., Grenet, D., Tubery, M., Sicard, D., Caubarrére, I., Guillevin, L. 1994. Treatment of systemic vasculitis with cyclophosphamide and steroids: daily oral low-dose cyclophosphamide administration after failure of a pulse intravenous high-dose regimen in four patients. Br. J. Rheumatol. 33, 959.

Généreau, T., Lortholary, O., Pottier, M.A., Michon-Pasturel, U., Ponge, T., de Wazières, B., Liozon, E., Pinède, L., Hachulla, E., Roblot, P., Barrier, J.H., Herson, S., Guillevin, L. 1999. Temporal artery biopsy: a diagnostic tool for systemic necrotizing vasculitis. French Vasculitis Study Group. Arthritis Rheum. 42, 2674.

Gerbracht, D.D., Savage, R.W., Scharff, N. 1987. Reversible valvulitis in Wegener's granulomatosis. Chest 92, 182.

Gharib, M.I., Burnett, A.K. 2002. Chemotherapy-induced cardiotoxicity: current practice and prospects of prophylaxis. Eur. J. Heart Fail. 4, 235.

Girard, T., Mahr, A., Noël, L.H., Cordier, J.F., Lesavre, P., André, M.H., Guillevin, L. 2001. Are antineutrophil cytoplasmic antibodies a marker predictive of relapse in Wegener's granulomatosis? A prospective study. Rheumatology (Oxford) 40, 147.

Gisselbrecht, M., Cohen, P., Lortholary, O., Jarrousse, B., Gayraud, M., Gherardi, R., Baudrimont, M., Guillevin, L. 1997. HIV-related vasculitis: clinical presentation and therapeutic approach on six patients. AIDS 11, 121.

Gobel, U., Eichhorn, J., Kettritz, R., Briedigkeit, L., Sima, D., Lindschau, C., Haller, H., Luft, F.C. 1996. Disease activity and autoantibodies to endothelial cells in patients with Wegener's granulomatosis. Am. J. Kidney Dis. 28, 186.

Godeau, P., Blétry, O., Guillevin, L., Herson, S., Piette, J.C. 1985. Le coeur des collagénoses. Ann. Méd. Interne (Paris) 136, 496.

Golan, T.D. 2002. Lupus vasculitis: differential diagnosis with antiphospholipid syndrome. Curr. Rheumatol. Rep. 4, 18.

Goodfield, N.E., Bhandari, S., Plant, W.D., Morley-Davies, A., Sutherland, G.R. 1995. Cardiac involvement in Wegener's granulomatosis. Br. Heart J. 73, 110.

Gorevic, P.D., Kassab, H.J., Levo, Y., Kohn, R., Meltzer, M., Prose, P. 1980. Mixed cryoglobulinemia: clinical aspects and long-term follow-up of 40 patients. Am. J. Med. 69, 287.

Goronzy, J.J., Weyand, C.M. 1994. Vasculitis in rheumatoid arthritis. Curr. Opin. Rheumatol. 6, 290.

Gower, R.G., Sausker, W.F., Kohler, P.F., Thorne, G.E., McIntosh, R.M. 1978. Small vessel vasculitis caused by hepatitis B virus immune complexes. Small vessel vasculitis and HBsAG. J. Allergy Clin. Immunol. 62, 222.

Grant, S.C., Levy, R.D., Venning, M.C., Ward, C., Brooks, N.H. 1994. Wegener's granulomatosis and the heart. Br. Heart J. 71, 82.

Greidinger, E.L., Lemes, V., Hellmann, D.B. 1996. Cardiac valve disease in Wegener's granulomatosis. J. Rheumatol. 23, 1485.

Guillaume, M., Vachiery, F., Cogan, E. 1991. Pericarditis: an unusual manifestation of giant cell arteritis. Am. J. Med. 91, 662.

Guillevin, L., Bussel, A. 2000. Indications of plasma exchanges in 2000. Ann. Méd. Interne (Paris) 151, 123.

Guillevin, L., Lhote, F. 1997. Classification and management of necrotising vasculitides. Drugs 53, 805.

Guillevin, L., Le Thi Huong, D., Godeau, P., Jais, P., Wechsler, B. 1988. Clinical findings and prognosis of polyarteritis nodosa and Churg–Strauss angiitis: a study in 165 patients. Br. J. Rheumatol. 27, 258.

Guillevin, L., Lhote, F., Léon, A., Fauvelle, F., Vivitski, L., Trepo, C. 1993. Treatment of polyarteritis nodosa related to hepatitis B virus with short term steroid therapy associated with antiviral agents and plasma exchanges. A prospective trial in 33 patients. J. Rheumatol. 20, 289.

Guillevin, L., Lhote, F., Sauvaget, F., Deblois, P., Rossi, F., Levallois, D., Pourrat, J., Christoforov, B., Trepo, C. 1994. Treatment of polyarteritis nodosa related to hepatitis B virus with interferon-alpha and plasma exchanges. Ann. Rheum. Dis. 53, 334.

Guillevin, L., Lhote, F., Brauner, M., Casassus, P. 1995a. Antineutrophil cytoplasmic antibodies (ANCA) and abnormal angiograms in polyarteritis nodosa and Churg–Strauss syndrome: indications for the diagnosis of microscopic polyangiitis. Ann. Méd. Interne (Paris) 146, 548.

Guillevin, L., Lhote, F., Cohen, P., Sauvaget, F., Jarrousse, B., Lortholary, O., Noel, L.H., Trep, C. 1995b. Polyarteritis nodosa related to hepatitis B virus. A prospective study with long-term observation of 41 patients. Medicine (Baltimore) 74, 238.

Guillevin, L., Lhote, F., Jarrousse, B., Cohen, P., Jacquot, C., Lesavre, P. 1995c. Treatment of Wegener's granulomatosis: a prospective trial in 50 patients comparing prednisone, pulse cyclophosphamide versus prednisone and oral cyclophosphamide. Clin. Exp. Rheumatol. 101, 43 (Abstract).

Guillevin, L., Lhote, F., Gayraud, M., Cohen, P., Jarrousse, B., Lortholary, O., Thibult, N., Casassus, P. 1996. Prognostic factors in polyarteritis nodosa and Churg–Strauss syndrome. A prospective study in 342 patients. Medicine (Baltimore) 75, 17.

Five clinical and biological parameters, defining the five factor score, have marked prognostic value in CSS and PAN.

Guillevin, L., Lhote, F., Gherardi, R. 1997. The spectrum and treatment of virus-associated vasculitides. Curr. Opin. Rheumatol. 9, 31.

Guillevin, L., Cohen, P., Gayraud, M., Lhote, F., Jarrousse, B., Casassus, P. 1999a. Churg–Strauss syndrome. Clinical study and long-term follow-up of 96 patients. Medicine (Baltimore) 78, 26.

Guillevin, L., Durand Gasselin, B., Cevallos, R., Gayraud, M., Lhote, F., Callard, P., Amouroux, J., Casassus, P., Jarrousse, B. 1999b. Microscopic polyangiitis: clinical and laboratory findings in eighty-five patients. Arthritis Rheum. 42, 421.

Guillevin, L., Lhote, F., Mouthon, L., Cohen, P. 2000. How to optimize the treatment of systemic vasculitides. Ann. Méd. Interne (Paris) 151, 199.

Guillevin, L., Cohen, P., Larroche, C., Queyrel, V., Loustaud-Ratti, V., Imbert, B., Hausfater, P., Ramanoealina, J., Lacombe, F., Roudier, J., Bielefeld, P., Petitjean, P., Smadja, D. 2001. Treatment of HBV-related polyarteritis nodosa (PAN) with lamivudine and plasma exchanges: a prospective, multicenter, pilot trial in 10 patients. Arthritis Rheum. 44, S271.

Guilpain, P., Viallard, J.F., Lagarde, P., Cohen, P., Kambouchner, M., Pellegrin, J.L., Guillevin, L. 2002. Churg–Strauss syndrome in two patients receiving montelukast. Rheumatology (Oxford) 41, 535.

Gunal, N., Kara, N., Cakar, N., Kocak, H., Kahramanyol, O., Cetinkaya, E. 1997. Cardiac involvement in childhood polyarteritis nodosa. Int. J. Cardiol. 60, 257.

Gupta, S., Piraka, C., Jaffe, M. 2001. Lamivudine in the treatment of polyarteritis nodosa associated with acute hepatitis B. N. Engl. J. Med. 344, 1645 (letter).

Ha, H.K., Lee, S.H., Rha, S.E., Kim, J.H., Byun, J.Y., Lim, H.K., Chung, J.W., Kim, J.G., Kim, P.N., Lee, M.G., Auh, Y.H. 2000. Radiologic features of vasculitis involving the gastrointestinal tract. Radiographics 20, 779.

Haas, C., Le Jeunne, C., Choubrac, P., Durand, H., Hugues, F.C. 2001. Churg–Strauss syndrome. Retrospective study of 20 cases. Bull. Acad. Natl Med. 185, 1113 (in French).

Hachulla, E., Bourdon, F., Taieb, S., Robert, Y., Amrouni, N., Steckolorom, T., Jabinet, J.L., Hatron, P.Y., Devulder, B. 1993. Embolization of two bleeding aneurysms with platinum coils in a patient with polyarteritis nodosa. J. Rheumatol. 20, 158.

Hagen, E.C., Daha, M.R., Hermans, J., Andrassy, K., Csernok, E., Gaskin, G., Lesavre, P., Ludemann, J., Rasmussen, N., Sinico, R.A., Wiik, A., van der Woude, F.J. 1998. Diagnostic value of standardized assays for anti-neutrophil cytoplasmic antibodies in idiopathic systemic vasculitis. EC/BCR Project for ANCA assay standardization. Kidney Int. 53, 743.

Halbwachs-Mecarelli, L., Nusbaum, P., Noël, L.H., Reumaux, D., Erlinger, S., Grunfeld, J.P., Lesavre, P. 1992. Antineutrophil cytoplasmic antibodies (ANCA) directed against cathepsin G in ulcerative colitis. Crohn's disease and primary sclerosing cholangitis. Clin. Exp. Immunol. 90, 79.

Hamuryudan, V., Yurdakul, S., Moral, F., Numan, F., Tuzun, H., Tuzuner, N., Mat, C., Tuzun, Y., Ozyazgan, Y., Yazici, H. 1994. Pulmonary arterial aneurysms in Behçet's syndrome: a report of 24 cases. Br. J. Rheumatol. 33, 48.

Hamza, M. 1987. Large artery involvement in Behçet's disease. J. Rheumatol. 14, 554.

Handa, R., Wali, J.P., Aggarwal, P., Wig, N., Biswas, A., Kumar, A.K. 1997. Wegener's granulomatosis with complete heart block. Clin. Exp. Rheumatol. 15, 97.

Hasley, P.B., Follansbee, W.P., Coulehan, J.L. 1990. Cardiac manifestations of Churg–Strauss syndrome: report of a case and review of the literature. Am. Heart J. 120, 996.

Hautekeete, M.L., Babany, G., Marcellin, P., Gayno, S., Palazzo, E., Erlinger, S., Benhamou, J.P. 1990. Retroperitoneal fibrosis after surgery for aortic aneurysm in a patient with periarteritis nodosa: successful treatment with corticosteroids. J. Intern. Med. 228, 533.

Heeringa, P., Brouwer, E., Tervaert, J.W., Weening, J.J., Kallenberg, C.G. 1998. Animal models of anti-neutrophil cytoplasmic antibody associated vasculitis. Kidney Int. 53, 253.

Hellemans, S., Dens, J., Knockaert, D. 1997. Coronary involvement in the Churg–Strauss syndrome. Heart 77, 576.

Henderson, R.A., Hasleton, P., Hamid, B.N. 1993. Recurrence of Churg Strauss vasculitis in a transplanted heart. Br. Heart J. 70, 553.

Hochster, H., Wasserheit, C., Speyer, J. 1995. Cardiotoxicity and cardioprotection during chemotherapy. Curr. Opin. Oncol. 7, 304.

Hoffman, G.S., Kerr, G.S., Leavitt, R.Y., Hallahan, C.W., Lebovics, R.S., Travis, W.D., Rottem, M., Fauci, A.S. 1992. Wegener granulomatosis: an analysis of 158 patients. Ann. Intern. Med. 116, 488.

Hoffman, G.S., Leavitt, R.Y., Kerr, G.S., Rottem, M., Sneller, M.C., Fauci, A.S. 1994. Treatment of glucocorticoid-resistant or relapsing Takayasu arteritis with methotrexate. Arthritis Rheum. 37, 578.

Holloway, J., Ferriss, J., Groff, J., Craig, T.J., Klinek, M., Klinik, M. 1998. Churg–Strauss syndrome associated with zafirlukast. J. Am. Osteopath. Assoc. 98, 275.

Holsinger, D., Osmundson, P., Edward, J. 1962. The heart in periarteritis nodosa. Circulation 25, 610.

Honsinger, R.W. 1998. Zafirlukast and Churg–Strauss syndrome. JAMA 279, 1949 (author reply 1950).

Hu, P.J., Shih, I.M., Hutchins, G.M., Hellmann, D.B. 1997. Polyarteritis nodosa of the pericardium: antemortem diagnosis in a pericardiectomy specimen. J. Rheumatol. 24, 2042.

Hunder, G.G., Arend, W.P., Bloch, D.A., Calabrese, L.H., Fauci, A.S., Fries, J.F., Leavitt, R.Y., Lie, J.T., Lightfoot, R.W., Masi, A.T. 1990a. The American College of Rheumatology 1990 criteria for the classification of vasculitis. Introduction. Arthritis Rheum. 33, 1065.

Hunder, G.G., Bloch, D.A., Michel, B.A., Stevens, M.B., Arend, W.P., Calabrese, L.H., Leavitt, R.Y., Lie, J.T., Lightfoot, R.W., Masi, A.T. 1990b. The American College of Rheumatology 1990 criteria for the classification of giant cell arteritis. Arthritis Rheum. 33, 1122.

Huong, D.L., Wechsler, B., Papo, T., de Zuttere, D., Blétry, O., Hernigou, A., Delcourt , A., Godeau, P., Piette, J.C. 1997. Endomyocardial fibrosis in Behçet's disease. Ann. Rheum. Dis. 56, 205.

Iino, T., Eguchi, K., Sakai, M., Nagataki, S., Ishijima, M., Toriyama, K. 1992. Polyarteritis nodosa with aortic dissection: necrotizing vasculitis of the vasa vasorum. J. Rheumatol. 19, 1632.

Imai, T., Matsumoto, S. 1970. Anaphylactoid purpura with cardiac involvement. Arch. Dis. Child. 45, 727.

Islim, I.F., Gill, M.D., Situnayake, D., Watson, R.D. 1994. Successful treatment of right atrial thrombus in a patient with Behçet's disease. Ann. Rheum. Dis. 53, 550.

Israel, H.L. 1988. Sulfamethoxazole-trimethoprim therapy for Wegener's granulomatosis. Arch. Intern. Med. 148, 2293.

Jayne, D.R., Davies, M.J., Fox, C.J., Black, C.M., Lockwood, C.M. 1991. Treatment of systemic vasculitis with pooled intravenous immunoglobulin. Lancet 337, 1137.

Jayne, D.R., Chapel, H., Adu, D., Misbah, S., O'Donoghue, D., Scott, D. 2000. Intravenous immunoglobulin for ANCA-associated systemic vasculitis with persistent disease activity. QJM 93, 433.

Jee, K.N., Ha, H.K., Lee, I.J., Klim, J.K., Sung, K.B., Cho, K.S., Kim, P.N., Lee, M.G., Lim, H.K., Choi, C.S., Auh, Y.H. 2000. Radiologic findings of abdominal polyarteritis nodosa. Am. J. Roentgenol. 174, 1675.

Jennette, J.C., Falk, R.J., Andrassy, K., Bacan, P.A., Churg, J., Gross, W.L., Hagen, E.C., Hoffman, G.S., Hunder, G.G., Kallenberg, C.G. 1994. Nomenclature of systemic vasculitides. Proposal of an international consensus conference. Arthritis Rheum. 37, 187.

Joyce, J.W. 1990. Buerger's disease (thromboangiitis obliterans). Rheum. Dis. Clin. North Am. 16, 463.

Kallenberg, C.G., Mulder, A.H., Tervaert, J.W. 1992. Antineutrophil cytoplasmic antibodies: a still-growing class of autoantibodies in inflammatory disorders. Am. J. Med. 93, 675.

Kato, H., Sugimura, T., Akagi, T., Sato, N., Hashino, K., Maeno, Y., Kazue, T., Eto, G., Yamakawa, R. 1996. Long-term consequences of Kawasaki disease. A 10- to 21-year follow-up study of 594 patients. Circulation 94, 1379.

Kawasaki, T. 1967. Acute febrile mucocutaneous syndrome with lymphoid involvement with specific desquamation of the fingers and toes in children. Arerugi 16, 178 (in Japanese).

Kendell, K.R., Day, J.D., Hruban, R.H., Olson, J.L., Rosenblum, W.D., Kasper, E.K., Baughman, K.L., Hutchins, G.M. 1995. Intimate association of eosinophils to collagen bundles in eosinophilic myocarditis and ranitidine-induced hypersensitivity myocarditis. Arch. Pathol. Lab. Med. 119, 1154.

Kereiakes, D.J., Ports, T.A., Finkbeiner, W. 1984. Endomyocardial biopsy in Henoch-Schönlein purpura. Am. Heart J. 107, 382.

Kerr, G. 1994. Takayasu's arteritis. Curr. Opin. Rheumatol. 6, 32.

Kerr, L.D., Chang, Y.J., Spiera, H., Fallon, J.T. 2000. Occult active giant cell aortitis necessitating surgical repair. J. Thorac. Cardiovasc. Surg. 120, 813.

Kitschke, B., Ferrière, M., Vaucher, E., Duhamel, O., Monnin, E., Blanc, F. 1986. Allergic granulomatosis (Churg–Strauss syndrome). Apropos of a case diagnosed by endomyocardial biopsy. Ann. Méd. Interne (Paris) 137, 170 (in French).

Klein, R.G., Hunder, G.G., Stanson, A.W., Sheps, S.G. 1975. Large artery involvement in giant cell (temporal) arteritis. Ann. Intern. Med. 83, 806.

Klinger, H. 1931. Grenzformen der Periarteritis Nodosa. Frankfurter Zeitschrife für Pathologie 42, 455.

Koldingsnes, W., Nossent, J.C. 2003. Baseline features and initial treatment as predictors of remission and relapse in Wegener's granulomatosis. J. Rheumatol 30, 80.

Kosovsky, P.A., Ehlers, K.H., Rafal, R.B., Williams, W.M., O'Loughlin, J.E., Markisz, J.A. 1991. MR imaging of cardiac mass in Wegener granulomatosis. J. Comput. Assist. Tomogr. 15, 1028.

Kounis, N.G., Zavras, G.M., Soufras, G.D., Kitrou, M.P. 1989. Hypersensitivity myocarditis. Ann. Allergy 62, 71.

Kumar, S., Subramanyan, R., Mandalam, K.R., Rao, V.R., Gupta, A.K., Joseph, S., Unni, N.M., Rao, A.S. 1990. Aneurysmal form of aortoarteritis (Takayasu's disease): analysis of thirty cases. Clin. Radiol. 42, 342.

Küssmaul, A., Maier, K. 1866. Uber eine bischer nicht beschreibene eigenthumliche Arterienerkrankung (Periarteritis Nodosa), die mit Morbus Brightii und rapid fortschreitender allgemeiner Muskellähmung einhergeht. Dtsch. Arch. Klein. Med. 1, 484.

Lakhanpal, S., Tani, K., Lie, J.T., Katoh, K., Ishigatsubo, Y., Ohokubo, T. 1985. Pathologic features of Behçet's syndrome: a review of Japanese autopsy registry data. Hum. Pathol. 16, 790.

Lane, S.E., Watts, R.A., Bentham, G., Innes, N.J., Scott, D.G. 2003. Are environmental factors important in primary systemic vasculitis? A case-control study. Arthritis Rheum. 48, 814.

Lanham, J.G., Elkon, K.B., Pusey, C.D., Hughes, G.R. 1984. Systemic vasculitis with asthma and eosinophilia: a clinical approach to the Churg–Strauss syndrome. Medicine (Baltimore) 63, 65.

Lanham, J.G., Cooke, S., Davies, J., Hughes, G.R. 1985. Endomyocardial complications of the Churg–Strauss syndrome. Postgrad. Med. J. 61, 341.

Le Thi Huong, D., Wechsler, B., De Gennes, C., Raguin, G., Piette, J.C., Blétry, O., Godeau, P. 1990. Treatment of Wegener's granulomatosis with cotrimoxazole (7 cases). Rev. Méd. Interne 11, 87 (in French).

Leavitt, R.Y., Fauci, A.S., Bloch, D.A., Michel, B.A., Hunder, G.G., Arend, W.P., Calabrese, L.H., Fries, J.F., Lie, J.T., Lightfoot, R.W. 1990. The American College of Rheumatology 1990 criteria for the classification of Wegener's granulomatosis. Arthritis Rheum. 33, 1101.

Ledford, D.K. 1997. Immunologic aspects of vasculitis and cardiovascular disease. JAMA 278, 1962.

Leib, E.S., Restivo, C., Paulus, H.E. 1979. Immunosuppressive and corticosteroid therapy of polyarteritis nodosa. Am. J. Med. 67, 941.

Leung, W.H., Wong, K.K., Lau, C.P., Wong, C.K., Cheng, C.H., So, K.F. 1989. Myocardial involvement in Churg–Strauss syndrome: the role of endomyocardial biopsy. J. Rheumatol. 16, 828.

Leung, D.Y., Schlievert, P.M., Meissner, H.C. 1998. The immunopathogenesis and management of Kawasaki syndrome. Arthritis Rheum. 41, 1538.

Lie, J.T. 1997. Wegener's granulomatosis: histological documentation of common and uncommon manifestations in 216 patients. Vasa 26, 261.

Lightfoot, R.W. Jr., Michel, B.A., Bloch, D.A., Hunder, G.G., Zvaifler, N.J., McShane, D.J. 1990. The American College of Rheumatology 1990 criteria for the classification of polyarteritis nodosa. Arthritis Rheum. 33, 1088.

Lockwood, C.M. 1998. Refractory Wegener's granulomatosis: a model for shorter immunotherapy of autoimmune diseases. J. R. Coll. Phys. Lond. 32, 473–478.

Lockwood, C.M., Thiru, S., Stewart, S., Hale, G., Isaacs, J., Wraight, P., Elliott, J., Waldmann, H. 1996. Treatment of refractory Wegener's granulomatosis with humanized monoclonal antibodies. QJM 89, 903.

Lomeo, R.M., Silver, R.M., Brothers, M. 1989. Spontaneous dissection of the internal carotid artery in a patient with polyarteritis nodosa. Arthritis Rheum. 32, 1625.

Lortholary, O., Généreau, T., Guillevin, I. 1999. Viral vasculitis not related to HBV, HCV and HIV. Pathol. Biol. (Paris) 47, 248 (in French).

Lunel, F., Cacoub, P. 2000. Treatment of autoimmune and extrahepatic manifestations of HCV infection. Ann. Méd. Interne (Paris) 151, 58.

Luqmani, R.A., Bacon, P.A., Moots, R.J., Janssen, B.A., Pall, A., Emery, P., Savage, C., Adu, D. 1994. Birmingham vasculitis activity score (BVAS) in systemic necrotizing vasculitis. QJM 87, 671.

Marette, P., Molle, B., Mas, J.L., Kahan, A., Devaux, J.Y., Toussaint, M., Volkringer, P., Fouchard, J. 1989. Angina without involvement of large coronary trunks and precapillary pulmonary hypertension in a patient with periarteritis nodosa. Ann. Cardiol. Angeiol. (Paris) 38, 305 (in French).

Masi, A.T., Hunder, G.G., Lie, J.T., Michel, B.A., Bloch, D.A., Arend, W.P., Calabrese, L.H., Edworthy, S.M., Fauci, A.S., Leavitt, R.Y. 1990. The American College of Rheumatology 1990 criteria for the classification of Churg–Strauss syndrome (allergic granulomatosis and angiitis). Arthritis Rheum. 33, 1094.

McLaren, J.S., McRorie, E.R., Luqmani, R.A. 2002. Diagnosis and assessment of systemic vasculitis. Clin. Exp. Rheumatol. 20, 854.

Miller, D.L. 2000. Angiography in polyarteritis nodosa. Am. J. Roentgenol. 175, 1747.

Mills, J.A., Michel, B.A., Bloch, D.A., Calabrese, L.H., Hunder, G.G., Arend, W.P. 1990. The American College of Rheumatology 1990 criteria for the classification of Henoch-Schönlein purpura. Arthritis Rheum. 33, 1114.

Mohan, N., Kerr, G. 2000. Spectrum of giant cell vasculitis. Curr. Rheumatol. Rep. 2, 390.

Morelli, S., Gurgo Di Castelmenardo, A.M., Conti, F., Sgreccia, A., Alessandri, C., Bernardo, M.L. 2000. Cardiac involvement in patients with Wegener's granulomatosis. Rheumatol. Int. 19, 209.

Morgan, J.M., Raposo, L., Gibson, D.G. 1989. Cardiac involvement in Churg–Strauss syndrome shown by echocardiography. Br. Heart J. 62, 462.

Mrowka, C., Sieberth, H.G. 1994. Circulating adhesion molecules ICAM-1, VCAM-1 and E-selectin in systemic vasculitis: marked differences between Wegener's granulomatosis and systemic lupus erythematosus. Clin. Investig. 72, 762.

Mrowka, C., Sieberth, H.G. 1995. Detection of circulating adhesion molecules ICAM-1, VCAM-1 and E-selectin in Wegener's granulomatosis, systemic lupus erythematosus and chronic renal failure. Clin. Nephrol. 43, 288.

Mrowka, C., Heintz, B., Sieberth, H.G. 1999. VCAM-1, ICAM-1, and E-selectin in IgA nephropathy and Schonlein-Henoch syndrome: differences between tissue expression and serum concentration. Nephrology 81, 256.

Murphy, D.J., Huhta, J.C. 1987. Treatment of Kawasaki syndrome with intravenous gamma globulin. N. Engl. J. Med. 316, 881 (Letter).

Naarendorp, M., Kallemuchikkal, U., Nuovo, G.J., Gorevic, P.D. 2001. Longterm efficacy of interferon-alpha for extrahepatic disease associated with hepatitis C virus infection. J. Rheumatol. 28, 2466.

Nesher, G., Sonnenblick, M., Friedlander, Y. 1994. Analysis of steroid related complications and mortality in temporal arteritis: a 15-year survey of 43 patients. J. Rheumatol. 21, 1283.

Newburger, J.W., Takahashi, M., Beiser, A.S., Burns, J.C., Bastian, J., Chung, K.J., Colan, S.D., Duffy, C.E., Fulton, D.R., Glode, M.P. 1991. A single intravenous infusion of gamma globulin as compared with four infusions in the treatment of acute Kawasaki syndrome. N. Engl. J. Med. 324, 1633.

Noguchi, S., Numano, F., Gravanis, M.B., Wilcox, J.N. 1998. Increased levels of soluble forms of adhesion molecules in Takayasu arteritis. Int. J. Cardiol. 66, S23.

Nowack, R., Gobel, U., Klooker, P., Hergesell, O., Andrassy, K., van der Woude, F.J. 1999. Mycophenolate mofetil for maintenance therapy of Wegener's granulomatosis and microscopic polyangiitis: a pilot study in 11 patients with renal involvement. J. Am. Soc. Nephrol. 10, 1965.

Nuyts, G.D., Van Vlem, E., De Vos, A., Daelemans, R.A., Rorive, G., Elseviers, M.M., Schurgers, M., Segaert, M., D'Haese, P.C., De Broe, M.E. 1995. Wegener granulomatosis is associated to exposure to silicon compounds: a case-control study. Nephrol. Dial. Transplant. 10, 1162.

Ohta, N., Fukase, S., Aoyagi, M. 2001. Serum levels of soluble adhesion molecules ICAM-1, VCAM-1 and E-selectin in patients with Wegener's granulomatosis. Auris Nasus Larynx 28, 311.

Pall, A.A., Adu, D., Drayson, M., Taylor, C.M., Richards, N.T., Michael, J. 1994. Circulating soluble adhesion molecules in systemic vasculitis. Nephrol. Dial. Transpl. 9, 770.

Paulley, J.W. 1980a. Ischaemic heart disease in giant cell arteritis. Lancet 1, 421.

Paulley, J.W. 1980b. Coronary ischaemia and occlusion in giant cell (temporal) arteritis. Acta Med. Scand. 208, 257.

Pearce, C.B., McMeekin, J.D., Moyana, T.N., Sibley, J. 1999. A case of peripartum eosinophilic myocarditis. Can. J. Cardiol. 15, 465.

Pinching, A.J., Lockwood, C.M., Pussell, B.A., Rees, A.J., Sweny, P., Evans, D.J., Bowley, N., Peters, D.K. 1983. Wegener's granulomatosis: observations on 18 patients with severe renal disease. QJM 52, 435.

Praprotnik, S., Rozman, B., Blank, M., Shoenfeld, Y. 2000. Pathogenic role of anti-endothelial cell antibodies in systemic vasculitis. Wien Klin. Wochenschr. 112, 660.

Pusey, C.D., Rees, A.J., Evans, D.J., Peters, D.K., Lockwood, C.M. 1991. Plasma exchange in focal necrotizing glomerulonephritis without anti-GBM antibodies. Kidney Int. 40, 757.

Rabusin, M., Lepore, L., Costantinides, F., Bussani, R. 1998. A child with severe asthma. Lancet 351, 32.

Rajani, R.M., Dalvi, B.V., D'Silva, S.A., Lokhandwala, Y.Y., Kale, P.A. 1991. Acute myocardial infarction with normal coronary arteries in a case of polyarteritis nodosa: possible role of coronary artery spasm. Postgrad. Med. J. 67, 78.

Rapezzi, C., Ortolani, P., Binetti, G., Picchio, F.M., Magnani, B. 1990. Idiopathic restrictive cardiomyopathy in the young: report of two cases. Int. J. Cardiol. 29, 121.

Raza, K., Karokis, D., Kitas, G.D. 1998. Cogan's syndrome with Takayasu's arteritis. Br. J. Rheumatol. 37, 369.

Reinhold-Keller, E., Kekow, J., Schnabel, A., Schwarz-Eywill, M., Schmitt, W.H., Gross, W.L. 1993. Effectiveness of cyclophosphamide pulse treatment in Wegener's granulomatosis. Adv. Exp. Med. Biol. 336, 483.

Reinhold-Keller, E., de Groot, K., Rudert, H., Nolle, B., Heller, M., Gross, W.L. 1996. Response to trimethoprim/sulfamethoxazole in Wegener's granulomatosis depends on the phase of disease. QJM 89, 15.

Reinhold-Keller, E., Beuge, N., Latza, U., de Groot, K., Rudert, H., Nolle, B., Heller, M., Gross, W.L. 2000. An interdisciplinary approach to the care of patients with Wegener's granulomatosis: long-term outcome in 155 patients. Arthritis Rheum. 43, 1021.

Rieu, V., Cohen, P., Andre, M.H., Mouthon, L., Godmer, P., Jarrousse, B., Lhote, F., Ferriere, F., Démy, P., Buchet, P., Guillevin, L. 2002. Characteristics and outcome of 49 patients with symptomatic cryoglobulinaemia. Rheumatology (Oxford) 41, 290.

Rosen, N., Gaton, E. 1972. Takayasu's arteritis of coronary arteries. Arch. Pathol. 94, 225.

Salojin, K.V., Le Tonqueze, M., Saraux, A., Nassonov, E.L., Dueymes, M., Piette, J.C., Youinou, P.Y. 1997. Antiendothelial cell antibodies: useful markers of systemic sclerosis. Am. J. Med. 102, 178.

Salvarani, C., Macchioni, P.L., Tartoni, P.L., Rossi, F., Baricchi, R., Castri, C., Chiaravalloti, F., Portioli, I. 1987. Polymyalgia rheumatica and giant cell arteritis: a 5-year epidemiologic and clinical study in Reggio Emilia, Italy. Clin. Exp. Rheumatol. 5, 205.

Salvarani, C., Macchioni, P., Zizzi, F., Mantovani, W., Rossi, F., Castri, C., Chiravalloti, F., Portioli, I. 1991. Epidemiologic and immunogenetic aspects of polymyalgia rheumatica and giant cell arteritis in northern Italy. Arthritis Rheum. 34, 351.

Salvarani, C., Gabriel, S.E., O'Fallon, W.M., Hunder, G.G. 1995. The incidence of giant cell arteritis in Olmsted County, Minnesota: apparent fluctuations in a cyclic pattern. Ann. Intern. Med. 123, 192.

Salvarani, C., Cantini, F., Boiardi, L., Hunder, G.G. 2002. Polymyalgia rheumatica and giant-cell arteritis. N. Engl. J. Med. 347, 261.

Sangle, S., Karim, M.Y., Hughes, G.R., D'Cruz, D.P. 2002. Sulphamethoxazole-trimethoprim in the treatment of limited paranasal Wegener's granulomatosis. Rheumatology (Oxford) 41, 589.

Savage, C.O., Winearls, C.G., Evans, D.J., Rees, A.J., Lockwood, C.M. 1985. Microscopic polyarteritis: presentation, pathology and prognosis. QJM 56, 467.

Saveuse, H., Dorra, M., Dechy, H., Baglin, C., Rouveix, E., Betourne, C. 1988. Temporal arteritis: a syndrome. From Horton's disease to periarteritis nodosa. Presse Méd. 17, 517 (in French).

Schiavone, W.A., Ahmad, M., Ockner, S.A. 1985. Unusual cardiac complications of Wegener's granulomatosis. Chest 88, 745.

Schiff, S., Moffatt, R., Mandel, W.J., Rubin, S.A. 1982. Acute myocardial infarction and recurrent ventricular arrhythmias in Behcet's syndrome. Am. Heart J. 103, 438.

Schildhaus, H.U., Von Netzer, B., Dombrowski, F., Pfeifer, U. 2002. Atypical manifestation of a cytoplasmic antineutrophil cytoplasmic antibody (PR3-ANCA)-associated vasculitis with involvement of aortic intima and parietal endocardium. Hum. Pathol. 33, 441.

Schrader, M.L., Hochman, J.S., Bulkley, B.H. 1985. The heart in polyarteritis nodosa: a clinicopathologic study. Am. Heart J. 109, 1353.

Scolyer, R.A. 1999. Test and teach. Number ninety-four: Part 1. Churg–Strauss syndrome. Pathology 31, 217.

Sharma, A., De Varennes, B., Sniderman, A.D. 1993. Churg–Strauss syndrome presenting with marked eosinophilia and pericardial effusion. Can. J. Cardiol. 9, 329.

Shimizu, T., Ehrlich, G.E., Inaba, G., Hayashi, K. 1979. Behçet disease (Behçet syndrome). Semin. Arthritis Rheum. 8, 223.

Shionoya, S. 1993. Buerger's disease: diagnosis and management. Cardiovasc. Surg. 1, 207.

Small, P., Brisson, M.L. 1991. Wegener's granulomatosis presenting as temporal arteritis. Arthritis Rheum. 34, 220.

Somer, T. 1993. Thrombo-embolic and vascular complications in vasculitis syndromes. Eur. Heart J. 14, 24.

Specks, U., Homburger, H.A., DeRemee, R.A. 1993. Implications of c-ANCA testing for the classification of Wegener's granulomatosis: performance of different detection systems. Adv. Exp. Med. Biol. 336, 65.

Specks, U., Fervenza, F.C., McDonald, T.J., Hogan, M.C. 2001. Response of Wegener's granulomatosis to anti-CD20 chimeric monoclonal antibody therapy. Arthritis Rheum. 44, 2836.

Stanson, A.W. 2000. Imaging findings in extracranial (giant cell) temporal arteritis. Clin. Exp. Rheumatol. 18, S43.

Stanson, A.W., Klein, R.G., Hunder, G.G. 1976. Extracranial angiographic findings in giant cell (temporal) arteritis. Am. J. Roentgenol. 127, 957.

Stegeman, C.A., Tervaert, J.W., Huitema, M.G., de Jong, P.E., Kallenberg, C.G. 1994. Serum levels of soluble adhesion molecules intercellular adhesion molecule 1, vascular cell adhesion molecule 1, and E-selectin in patients with Wegener's granulomatosis. Relationship to disease activity and relevance during followup. Arthritis Rheum. 37, 1228.

Stone, J.H., Hoffman, G.S., Merkel, P.A., Min, Y.I., Uhlfelder, M.L., Hellmann, D.B., Allen, N.B., Davis, J.C., Spiera, R.R., Calabrese, L.H., Wigley, F.M., Maiden, N., Valente, R.M., Niles, J.L., Fye, K.H., McCune, J.W., St Clair, E.W., Luqmani, R.A. 2001. A disease-specific activity index for Wegener's granulomatosis: modification of the Birmingham Vasculitis Activity Score. International Network for the Study of the Systemic Vasculitides (INSSYS). Arthritis Rheum. 44, 912.

Stricker, H., Malinverni, R. 1989. Multiple, large aneurysms of pulmonary arteries in Behçet's disease. Clinical remission and radiologic resolution after corticosteroid therapy. Arch. Intern. Med. 149, 925.

Sugimura, T., Yokoi, H., Sato, N., Akagi, T., Kimura, T., Iemura, M. 1997. Interventional treatment for children with severe coronary artery stenosis with calcification after long-term Kawasaki disease. Circulation 96, 3928.

Suleymenlar, G., Sarikaya, M., Sari, R., Tuncer, M., Sevinc, A. 2002. Complete heart block in a patient with Wegener's granulomatosis in remission—a case report. Angiology 53, 337.

Sundy, J.S., Haynes, B.F. 2000. Cytokines and adhesion molecules in the pathogenesis of vasculitis. Curr. Rheumatol. Rep. 2, 402.

Tai, P.C., Holt, M.E., Denny, P., Gibbs, A.R., Williams, B.D., Spry, C.J. 1984. Deposition of eosinophil cationic protein in granulomas in allergic granulomatosis and vasculitis: the Churg–Strauss syndrome. Br. Med J. (Clin. Res. Ed.) 289, 400.

Takahashi, M. 1993. Inflammatory diseases of the coronary artery in children. Coron. Artery Dis. 4, 133–138.

Terasaki, F., Hayashi, T., Hirota, Y., Okabe, M., Suwa, M., Deguchi, H., Kitaura, Y., Kawamura, K. 1997. Evolution to dilated cardiomyopathy from acute eosinophilic pancarditis in Churg–Strauss syndrome. Heart Vessels 12, 43 (Physiopathogenesis of cardiac involvement in CSS).

Tervaert, J.W., Huitema, M.G., Hene, R.J., Sluiter, W.J., The, T.H., van der Hem, G.K., Kallenberg, C.G. 1990. Prevention of relapses in Wegener's granulomatosis by treatment based on antineutrophil cytoplasmic antibody titre. Lancet 336, 709.

Tesar, V., Jelinkova, E., Masek, Z., Jirsa, M., Jr., Zabka, J., Bartunkova, J., Stejskalova, A., Janatkova, I., Zima, T. 1998. Influence of plasma exchange on serum levels of cytokines and adhesion molecules in ANCA-positive renal vasculitis. Blood Purif. 16, 72.

Thomas-Golbanov, C., Sridharan, S. 2001. Novel therapies in vasculitis. Exp. Opin. Investig. Drugs 10, 1279.

Thomson, D., Chamsi-Pasha, H., Hasleton, P. 1989. Heart transplantation for Churg–Strauss syndrome. Br. Heart J. 62, 409.

Van der Woude, F.J., Rasmussen, N., Lobatto, S., Wiik, A., Permin, H., van Es, L.A van der Giessen, M., van der Hem, G.K., The, T.H. 1985. Autoantibodies against neutrophils and monocytes: tool for diagnosis and marker of disease activity in Wegener's granulomatosis. Lancet 1, 425.

Vollertsen, R.S., Conn, D.L. 1990. Vasculitis associated with rheumatoid arthritis. Rheum. Dis. Clin. North Am. 16, 445.

Vollertsen, R.S., McDonald, T.J., Younge, B.R., Banks, P.M., Stanson, A.W., Ilstrup, D.M. 1986. Cogan's syndrome: 18 cases and a review of the literature. Mayo Clin. Proc. 61, 344.

Wagner, J., Andrassy, K., Ritz, E. 1991. Is vasculitis in subacute bacterial endocarditis associated with ANCA? Lancet 337, 799.

Walton, E.W. 1958. Giant-cell granuloma of the respiratory tract (Wegener's granulomatosis). Br. Med. J. 2, 265–270.

Wang, L., Thelmo, W.L., Axiotis, C.A. 2002. Microscopic polyangiitis with massive myocardial necrosis and diffuse pulmonary hemorrhage. Virchows Arch. 441, 202.

Wechsler, B., Du, L.T., Kieffer, E. 1999. Cardiovascular manifestations of Behcet's disease. Ann. Méd. Interne (Paris) 150, 542 (in French).

Wegener, F. 1936. Uber generalisierte, septische Gefasserkrankungen. Verh. Dtsch. Ges. Pathol. 29, 202.

Weisman, M.H. 2002. What are the risks of biologic therapy in rheumatoid arthritis? An update on safety. J. Rheumatol. Suppl. 65, 33.

Woywodt, A., Streiber, F., de Groot, K., Regelsberger, H., Haller, H., Haubitz, M. 2003. Circulating endothelial cells as markers for ANCA-associated small-vessel vasculitis. Lancet 361, 206.

Xiao, H., Heeringa, P., Hu, P., Liu, Z., Zhao, M., Aratani, Y., Maeda, N., Falk, R.J., Jennette, J.C. 2002. Antineutrophil cytoplasmic autoantibodies specific for myeloperoxidase cause glomerulonephritis and vasculitis in mice. J. Clin. Invest. 110, 955.

Yamashita, Y., Yorioka, N., Taniguchi, Y., Yamakido, M., Watanabe, C., Kitamura, T., Nakamura, S. 1998. Nonasthmatic case of Churg–Strauss syndrome with rapidly progressive glomerulonephritis. Intern. Med. 37, 561.

Yazici, H., Barnes, C.G. 1991. Practical treatment recommendations for pharmacotherapy of Behcet's syndrome. Drugs 42, 796.

Yeatman, M., McNeil, K., Smith, J.A., Stewart, S., Sharples, L.D., Higenbottam, T., Wells, F.C., Wallwork, J. 1996. Lung transplantation in patients with systemic diseases: an eleven-year experience at Papworth Hospital. J. Heart Lung Transpl. 15, 144.

Index

2D and Doppler echocardiography 111
5-HT_4 receptor 63

A

aCL antibodies 99
Hughes–Stovin syndrome 240
MTXazathioprinemycophenolate mofetil 244
actin 28
activation/damage 43
active rheumatic fever 25
acute rheumatic fever 25
adenine nucleotide translocator (ANT) 29, 30
aetiology 124
ambulatory ECG monitoring 133
angina questionnaires 127
angiogenesis 117
angiotensin converting enzyme (ACE) inhibitors 137
animal models 43
ANT 29, 30
anti-52 kDa Ro/SSA 171
anti-60 kDa Ro/SSA 172
anti-ANT antibodies 29, 30
anti-β-receptor antibodies 30
anti-β_1-adrenoceptor antibodies 30
anti-β_1-receptor antibodies 31, 32
anti-β_1-receptor 31
anti-endothelial cell antibodies (AECA) 45, 231
anti-fibrillary 28
anti-heart antibodies 20, 23, 25
anti-heart autoantibodies 20, 23, 24, 25, 26, 28, 33
anti-heart autoantibodies by s-I IFL 34
anti-intercalated disks 28
anti-Jo-1 antibody 206
anti-La/SSB 171
anti-M2 antibodies 30
anti-Mi-2 206
anti-mitochondrial antibodies 28
anti-myosin antibodies 28, 32
anti-Na-K-ATPase autoantibodies 29
anti-Na-K-ATPase 29
anti-oxidized LDL 44
anti-receptor antibodies 32
anti-receptor 32
anti-ribonucleoprotein 198
anti-RNP 206
anti-Ro/SSA 164
anti-SSA/Ro-SSB/La antibodies 60
anti-streptococcal antibodies 24
anti-TNFα antibodies 244
antibodies against α_1-adrenergic receptor 34
antibodies against the β_1-adrenoceptor 30
antibodies against the heat shock protein 44
antibodies 19, 20, 23, 26
antibody repertoires 99
antibody-specific murine model 67
anticardiolipin antibodies 113, 213
antinuclear antibodies 206
antiphospholipid antibodies 148, 213
antiphospholipid syndrome 102, 109, 213
aortic dissections and aneurysms 233
aortic valve nodulosis 126
aPL 42, 47
apoptosis 54, 59
arrhythmias 200, 233
arthritis 102
asymptomatic cardiac abnormalities 112
AT1 receptor antibody 34
atherogenesis 132
atherosclerosis 44, 77, 131, 217
atherosclerotic plaque 132
atorvastatin 103
atrial and ventricular arrhythmias 111, 127
atypical verrucous endocarditis 147
autoantibodies 25, 29, 34
autoantibodies against laminin 29
autoantibodies to M_2-muscarinic receptors 30
autoantibodies to mitochondrial 29
autoantibody-associated congenital heart block 53
autoimmune disease 4, 19
autoimmune encephalomyelitis 103
autoimmune polyendocrinopathy 27, 34
autoimmunity 30
autonomic nervous system 127
autopsy studies 123
AV groove, 58
azathioprine 147

B

β MHC 28
β-adrenoceptors 30
β_1- and β_2-adrenergic receptors 30
β_1-receptor antibodies 30, 32
B_6B_{12} and folate 130
BCKD-E2 antibodies 30
Behçet's disease 240
betamethasone 177
biologic agents 136
Birmingham vasculitis activity score (BVAS) 242

blocking and stimulating autoantibodies to β-adrenergic receptors 30
blood pressure 136
brady or tachyarrhythmiassystemic arterial hypertension 20
branched chain α-ketoacid dehydrogenase dihydrolipoyl transacylase (BCKD-E2) 29
Buerger's disease 240

C

C reactive protein 79, 112, 131
CAMs 133
cancer 102
cardiac 146
cardiac antibodies 27
cardiac autoantibodies 26, 31
cardiac failure (see heart failure)
cardiac imaging techniques 110
cardiac involvement 198
cardiac MRI 219
cardiac murmurs 112
cardiac myosin 26
cardiac performance 201
cardiac tamponade 125
cardiac troponin-T 134
cardiac valve replacements 221
cardiac-specific antibodies 30, 31
cardiac-specific antigens 31
cardiac-specific autoantibodies 31
cardiomyopathy 167, 232
cardiovascular 121
cardiovascular disease 77, 122, 204
cardiovascular surgery 220
carotid intima-media thickness 134, 215
causes of death 122, 203
CB3-induced myocarditis 7
CD4 + T-cells 200
CD8 + T-cells 200
cerebrovascular accidents 127
Churg–Strauss Syndrome 46, 238
classification of vasculitides 227
cogan's syndrome 241
colchicine 126
comorbid CHD 127
comorbid CVD burden 133
complete heart block 53, 155, 163, 165, 207
computer tomography 147
conducting system 126
conduction abnormalities 154, 200, 207
conduction tissue involvement 233
congestive heart failure 126, 136, 151, 202, 207, 215, 232
constrictive pericarditis 125, 146
contraction band necrosis 190
contrast echocardiography 114
coronary arteritis 127, 232
coronary artery disease 109, 111, 122, 123, 127, 152, 200, 203, 207
corticosteroid treatment 206
corticosteroids 135, 147, 243
cotrimoxazole 244
counseling 175, 179
coxsackievirus B3 (CB3) 3
creatine kinase 205
criteria 197
cross-reactive 26, 27
cross-reactive 1 or partially organ-specific 27
cross-reactive 1 type 27, 28
cross-reactive 2 type 27, 28
CRP 102, 134
cryoglobulinemic vasculitis 240
CT scanning 134
cyclophosphamide 244
cytokines 82
cytokines and adhesion molecules 231
cytomegalovirus (CMV) 3

D

DCM 25, 26, 28, 29, 30, 31, 32
DCM/myocarditis 26, 27
dexamethasone 176
diabetes 129
diastolic function 111, 115, 192
diffuse 28
diffuse/striatednonmyasthenic 28
dilated cardiomyopathy (DCM) 3, 25, 150
dilated cardiomyopathy and myocarditis 25
dipyridamole thallium 114
disease modifying anti-rheumatic drugs 124
DMARD 126, 136
dobutamine 114
Doppler 189
Doppler echocardiography 218
Doppler velocimetry 170
Dressler's and post-pericardiotomy syndromes 20, 23, 25, 26, 27

E

E-selectin 102
echocardiography 113, 123, 125, 146, 151, 190, 205
embolism 149
endocardial and valve involvement 126
endocardial fibroelastosis 47, 167
endocarditis 233
endomyocardial biopsy 26, 151
endomysial 28
endothelial cells 42, 43
endothelial dysfunction 102, 131, 134
enzyme-linked immunosorbent assay (ELISA) 28, 29, 31
erythema marginatum 23
ESR 132
exercise SPECT 113

extra-articular manifestations 124
extracellular matrix antigens 29

F

family history 129
family members 26, 27
Fcγ receptors 56
FcR neonatal/β_2m (FcRn/β_2m) 57
fetal echocardiography 170
fetal/neonatal autoimmune diseases in pregnancy 53
fibrinogen 217
fibrinous pericarditis 191
five-factor score 242
fluorinated glucocorticoids 177
fluvastatin 97
folate 130

G

Gadolinium diethylenetriaminepentaacetic enhanced magnetic resonance imaging 204
GAS 24
genetic factors 199
giant cell arteritis 234
granulomatous disease 126
group A streptococcal 23

H

HBV-related polyarteritis nodosa 245
HCV-related mixed cryoglobulinemic vasculitis 245
HDL-cholesterol 100, 131
heart and skeletal muscle 27
heart failure 126, 136, 151, 202, 207, 215, 232
heart valve lesion 109
heart-specific (organ-specific) 27, 28
heat shock protein-60 (HSP-60) 28
Henoch-Schönlein purpura 240, 245
HLA-DRBI 64
HMG-CoA reductase 97
homocysteine 129, 130, 153, 217
hydrops 177
hydroxychloroquine 129, 136, 153, 220
hyperdynamic left ventricular contraction 202
hypersensitivity myocarditis 241
hypertension 33, 34, 128
hypertrophic cardiomyopathy 29

I

IBM 198
Ibuprofen 135
idiopathic hypereosinophilic syndrome 238
IFL 31
IL-1 and TNFα 82
IL-12 10
IL-18 11
IL-1beta 200
IL-6 82
ILD 206
imaging techniques 109
immune-mediated mechanisms 199
immunoadsorption 32
immunoblotting 28, 31
immunofluorescent 193
inception studies 121
incidence 198
incomplete AV block 177
infection 23
infectious agents 99
infectious endocarditis 149
infective causes of pericardial effusion 126
infiltration of T-lymphocytes 197
inflammation 77, 127, 130
innate immunity 77
interleukin (IL)-1β 6
interleukin—(IL) 1 alpha 200
intracardiac thrombosis 112, 216
intracellular signaling 102
intrauterine growth restriction 177
intravenous immunoglobulins 147, 244
ischaemic heart disease (see coronary artery disease)
iso-volumetic relaxation time 216
isolated CHB 164

J

juvenile dermatomyositis 203

K

Kawasaki disease 235, 243, 244
KD 45
kidney transplant 102

L

lamin B1 60
LDL receptor 98
learning disabilities 170
Libman–Sacks endocarditis 41, 147, 218
lifestyle advice 136
lipids 128
lipopolysaccharide (LPS) 6
lipoprotein (a) 130
long QT syndrome 164
lovastatin, simvastatin and atorvastatin 97, 103
low-dose aspirin 219
L-type calcium channel 63
lung involvement 206

lupus-anticoagulant test 213
lyme disease 69

M

M protein 24
M7 antibodies 29, 30
macrophage proliferation 100
macrophages 54
macrophages in skeletal muscle 197
magnetic resonance imaging 147
MCTD 198
membrane cofactor protein 65
meta-analyses 98
metalloproteinases 100
methotrexate 130, 136
microbubble contrast 115
microscopic polyangiitis 239
mitochondrial antigens 29
mitochondrial antigensthe M7 29
mitral regurgitation 218
mitral valve 126, 214
mitral valve prolapse 199, 202
mixed connective tissue disease 198
MMP-9 100
molecular mimicry 24
mortality 121
MSAs 206
mucocutaneaous lymph-node syndrome 235
multiple sclerosis 103
muscle-specific 23, 32
myasthenia gravis 27
mycophenolate mofetil 147
myocardial 47
myocardial contrast echocardiography 115
myocardial dysfunction 150
myocardial infarction 111, 215
myocardial perfusion 133
myocardial stunning 115
myocarditis 3, 26, 28, 29, 30, 31, 32, 47, 150, 177, 200, 208
myocarditis and dilated cardiomyopathy 26
myocarditis/DCM 26, 27, 28, 29, 30, 31, 32
myofibroblasts 60
myosin 24, 28, 30, 31, 32
myosin antibodies 31
myosin-induced EAM 7
myosin heavy chain 28
myositis 197
myositis specific autoantibodies 206

N

Na-K-ATPase 29
naproxen 135
neonatal cholestasis 166
neonatal 'hemochromatosis' 166
neonatal lupus Syndrome 46, 163, 180
NK 8
nodules on mitral or aortic 113
non-infective vegetations 113
non-traditional risk factors 153
nonorgan-specific mitochondrial or smooth muscle antibodies 27
not macrovascular 192
'novel' CVD risk factors 128
NSAIDs 128, 135

O

oligohydramnios 177
organ 26, 30
organ-specific 27, 28, 32
organ-specific antibodies 27
organ-specific autoimmunity 19, 20, 26, 31
organ-specific cardiac 23
organ-specific cardiac autoantibodies 27, 28, 34
organ-specific cardiac autoantigens 29, 30
outcome of vasculitis 241
oxidised LDL 99, 131, 154
oxidized low-density lipoproteins 217

P

pacemaker 181, 207
paraoxonase 1 131
partial organ-specificity 27
pathobiology 190
Pathogenesis 216
pathogenesis of vasculitides 230
percutaneous coronary intervention or coronary artery bypass graft surgery 117
pericardectomy 126
pericardial chest pain 125
pericardial disease 123
pericardial effusion 48, 124
pericardiocentesis 126
pericarditis 48, 109, 123, 145, 199, 201, 202, 233
phagocyte receptors 54
pharmacological stress test 114
phonocardiography 205
plaque rupture 100
plasma exchanges 244
polyarteritis nodosa 46, 234
positive troponin assay results 135
PR interval 171
pravastatin 101, 97
prednisone 219
preeclampsia 34, 180
premature atherosclerosis 153
premature rupture of membranes 180
prenatal counseling 175, 179

primary APS 215
pro-inflammatory cytokines 200
prophylactic therapy 175
protein isoprenylation 98
pseudoinfective endocarditis 218
PTX3 80
pulmonary arteries, 233
pulmonary hypertension 189, 199, 202, 233

Q

q waves 190
QT prolongation 168

R

radionuclide perfusion studies 116
reactive autoantibodies 32
recurrence rate 179
restrictive myocardial idiopathic vasculitis 241
rheumatic fever 24, 25
rheumatic heart disease, 23, 24, 25, 27, 218
rheumatoid arthritis 109, 121
rheumatoid factor 135
rheumatoid nodules 124
rheumatoid pericarditis 123
rhythm abnormality 154
ribonucleoproteins 165
rosuvastatin and pravastatin 97

S

s-I IFLELISA 31
s-I IFL 20, 25, 26, 27
salbutamol 178
sarcolemmal Na-K-ATPase 29
scavenger receptors 81
selective COX-2 inhibitors 135
seropositive disease 124
silent IHD 133
simvastatin 101, 102
sinus bradycardia 169
skeletal muscle 27
skeletal muscle cross-reactive 27
SLE 214
small dense LDL particles 131
small vessel vasculitides 237
smoking 128
SPECT 116
spontaneous echocontrast 113
standard indirect immunofluorescence (s-I IFL) 20
standardised mortality rates 121
statins 97, 101, 103, 137, 220
steroids 126
stimulating anti-α_1-antibodies 34
stimulating anti-β_1-receptor antibodies 30
stimulating autoantibodies to α_1-adrenergic receptors 34
stimulating autoantibodies to the angiotensin receptor (AT1) 34
streptococcal 24
streptococci 24
stress MUGA 191
striatedmyasthenic 28
striatednonmyasthenic 28
subacute cutaneous lupus 166
sustained inflammation 132
sympathomimetics 178
systemic arterial hypertension (see hypertension)
systemic autoimmune diseases 109
systemic lupus erythematosus 99, 109, 145, 163
systemic sclerosis 111
systemic vasculitides 227 (see vasculitis)

T

T cell-mediated immunity 231
T cells 100
Takayasu's arteritis 234, 243
Technetium 99m-pyrophosphate scintigraphy 204
TEE 113
Tei index 171
terbutaline 179
Th1 101
Th1 and Th2 response 12
Th2 101
thallium scintigraphy 191
thromboembolism 218
thrombotic markers 130
thrombotic/atherosclerotic coronary occlusion 215, 220
thyroid autoimmunity 98, 99
tissue Doppler imaging 115
TLR4 11
TNF-α 200
TNF-receptors 200
TNF2 polymorphism 65
Toll-like receptors 81
total cholesterol 129
traditional CVD risk factors 127, 129, 153
traditional rheumatoid heart 123
translocation of intracellular antigens 59
trans-thoracic 2D Doppler echocardiography 125 (see also echocardiography)
transdifferentiation of cardiac fibroblasts 60
transforming growth factor 65
transmyocardial laser revascularization 117
treat GCA 242
treatment 219, 242, 243
triglycerides 131
tropomyosin 28
troponin T 192
troponins 205
tumor necrosis factor (TNF)-α 6, 133

U

ultrasonic videodensitometric analysis 115
upregulation of CTGF 191

V

valve abnormalities 42, 112, 149, 214, 219
valve repair 150
valve replacement 150
vasculitis damage index (VDI) 242
vasculitis 201, 227, 230, 242
vasospastic angina 190, 201
ventricular diastolic dysfunction 202, 216
ventricular hypertrophy and dysfunction 216

W

warfarin 219
Wegener's granulomatosis 237